Manual of Pediatric Nursing Procedures

LIST OF VIDEOS

www.jaypeelearningsolutions.com
Online Learning Resource

1. Preparation for neonatal resuscitation.
2. Initial steps and bag and mask ventilation of neonatal resuscitation.
3. Discontinuation of bag and mask ventilation.
4. Weight recording of infant using digital weight machine.
5. Use of radiant warmer.
6. Phototherapy for the treatment of unconjugated hyperbilirubinemia.
7. Capillary blood glucose estimation of neonate.
8. Assessment of neonate's body temperature by human touch and capillary refill time (CRT).
9. IV cannulation.
10. Intramuscular injection to infant.
11. Gavage feeding of a baby.
12. Paladai feeding of a neonate.

Manual of Pediatric Nursing Procedures

As per Revised INC Syllabus

Parul Datta MSc (Nsg)
Retired Principal Nursing Officer
Formerly Senior Sister Tutor at IPGMER and SSKM MCH
Kolkata, West Bengal, India

JAYPEE
JAYPEE BROTHERS MEDICAL PUBLISHERS
The Health Sciences Publisher
New Delhi | London

JAYPEE **Jaypee Brothers Medical Publishers (P) Ltd**

Headquarters
Jaypee Brothers Medical Publishers (P) Ltd
EMCA House, 23/23-B
Ansari Road, Daryaganj
New Delhi 110 002, India
Landline: +91-11-23272143, +91-11-23272703
+91-11-23282021, +91-11-23245672
Email: jaypee@jaypeebrothers.com

Corporate Office
Jaypee Brothers Medical Publishers (P) Ltd
4838/24, Ansari Road, Daryaganj
New Delhi 110 002, India
Phone: +91-11-43574357
Fax: +91-11-43574314
Email: jaypee@jaypeebrothers.com

Overseas Office
J.P. Medical Ltd
83 Victoria Street, London
SW1H 0HW (UK)
Phone: +44 20 3170 8910
Fax: +44 (0)20 3008 6180
Email: info@jpmedpub.com

Website: www.jaypeebrothers.com
Website: www.jaypeedigital.com

Inquiries for bulk sales may be solicited at: jaypee@jaypeebrothers.com

Manual of Pediatric Nursing Procedures

First Edition: 2022

Reprint **2023**

ISBN: 978-93-5465-520-3

Printed at: Sterling Graphics Pvt. Ltd.

Preface

Children require comprehensive special care to survive and thrive. Improvement of child health status is possible with quality improvement in both curative management and preventive care. Health promotion and rehabilitation of disabled children also require special attention in all stages of growth and development towards optimal health outcome of all children. Changing trends in child health care strategies and advanced technology in health sciences make the child health care management a challenging task.

Nursing professionals require knowledge and understanding of the nature of childhood illnesses in respect to developmental variations and individual difference of the children within their environmental influence. In pediatric and neonatal care units curative and diagnostic interventions are performed for the treatment of hospitalized children. Healthcare professionals including nursing personnel require competent clinical skills and practice to perform these curative and diagnostic procedures.

This book is prepared to present important pediatric and neonatal nursing procedures to guide nursing professionals and other child healthcare providers to perform need-based priority interventions following scientific principles and rationale with recommended evidence-based clinical guidelines.

The overall objective of *Manual of Pediatric Nursing Procedures* is to enrich the undergraduate and postgraduate nursing students and also to support clinical nursing professionals to provide evidence-based competent skilled care to the children confidently.

In this title, clinical procedures are arranged considering the priority needs of the sick and hospitalized children from the time of admission in healthcare facility to transitional care at discharge or transfer-out from healthcare institutions. For newborn infants, procedures are organized from delivery room care to advice on discharge from postnatal units or neonatal units for continued care at home.

All procedures in this manual are presented with the following highlighted points—(a) Clinical guidelines, (b) Equipments required to perform the procedure, (c) Assessment of the child before performing procedure and preparation of procedure (for performer, environment, supplies, equipments, parents/family and the child), (d) Performance of steps of procedure with rationale and point of emphasis, (e) Evaluation and documentation, and (f) Communication and related teaching to parents/family and child.

For preparation of the content I consulted International and Indian reference books, journals, articles and websites. Personal working experience in neonatal and pediatric clinical units/areas along with discussion and experience sharing with child health care team members help me in the preparation of the book.

Constructive suggestions will be heartily received for further enrichment of the content of this book. Comments are always welcomed. I believe that this book will be a definite guide to perform pediatric nursing procedures to all child healthcare providers, especially for hospitalized children.

Parul Datta

Preface

Acknowledgments

I would like to acknowledge all neonates, infants and children along with their parents and family members who really help me to learn every aspects of child health.

It is a great pleasure to acknowledge all eminent authors and renowned publishers of different nursing and medical books, journals, manuals, periodicals and websites which I have taken as reference during preparation of this book.

I would like to convey my sincere thanks to all members of Jaypee Brothers Medical Publishers (P) Ltd, New Delhi for their excellent expertise in publication and promotion of book. I wish to convey special thanks to all members of Kolkata branch of Jaypee Brothers Medical Publishers for their continuous motivation and support for preparation of this book.

I would also like to express my sincere gratitude to all my teachers, seniors, colleagues, friends, students and well wishers for their constructive suggestions to make me confident to prepare this book.

It is immense pleasure to convey indebtedness to my parents, teachers and family members who inspired me to accept this challenging work of writing this book.

Above all, I am really grateful to Almighty God and Goddess for their grace.

Acknowledgments

Contents

Child Health Nursing - I and II Clinical (3 Credits – 240 Hours)

Placement: V and VI Semester

Practicum: Skill Lab: 1 Credit (40 hours)

Clinical: V Semester – 2 Credits (160 hours)
VI Semester – 1 Credit (80 hours)

Practice Competencies: On completion of the course, the students will be able to:

1. Perform assessment of children: Health, developmental and anthropometric.
2. Provide nursing care to children with various medical disorders.
3. Provide pre- and postoperative care to children with common pediatric surgical conditions/ malformation.
4. Perform immunization as per National Immunization Schedule (NIS).
5. Provide nursing care to critically ill children.
6. Give health education/nutritional education to parents.
7. Counsel parents according to identified counseling needs.

Skill Lab

Use of Manikins and Simulators
PLS, CPAP, Endotracheal Suction

Pediatric Nursing Procedures:

- Administration of medication – Oral, IM and IV
- Oxygen administration
- Application of restraints
- Specimen collection
- Urinary catheterization and drainage
- Ostomy care
- Feeding – NG, gastrostomy, Jejunostomy
- Wound dressing
- Suture removal

Clinical Postings

8 weeks × 30 hours per week (5 weeks + 3 weeks)

Clinical Area/Unit	*Duration (Weeks)*	*Learning Outcomes*	*Procedural Competencies/ Clinical Skills*	*Clinical Requirements*	*Assessment Methods*
Pediatric Medical Ward	V Sem – 2 weeks VI Sem – 1 week	➢ Provide nursing care to children with various medical disorders	➢ Taking pediatric history ➢ Physical examination and assessment of children ➢ Administration of oral, I/M and I/V medicine/fluids ➢ Calculation of fluid replacement ➢ Preparation of different strengths of I/V fluids	➢ Nursing care plan – 1 ➢ Case study presentation – 1 ➢ Health talk – 1	➢ Assess performance with rating scale ➢ Assess each skill with checklist OSCE/ OSPE
			➢ Application of restraints ➢ Administration of O_2 inhalation by different methods ➢ Baby bath/sponge bath ➢ Feeding children by Katori-spoon, Paladai cup ➢ Collection of specimens for common investigations ➢ Assisting with common diagnostic procedures ➢ Teaching mothers/ parents – Malnutrition – Oral rehydration therapy – Feeding and Weaning – Immunization schedule ➢ Play therapy		➢ Evaluation of case study/ presentation and health education session ➢ Completion of activity record
Pediatric Surgical Ward	V Sem – 2 weeks VI Sem – 1 week	➢ Recognize different pediatric surgical conditions/ malformations ➢ Provide pre- and postoperative care to children with common pediatric surgical conditions/ malformation ➢ Counsel and educate parents	➢ Calculation, preparation and administration of I/V fluids ➢ Bowel wash, insertion of suppositories ➢ Care for ostomies: – Colostomy Irrigation – Ureterostomy – Gastrostomy – Enterostomy ➢ Urinary catheterization and drainage ➢ Feeding – Nasogastric – Gastrostomy – Jejunostomy ➢ Care of surgical wounds – Dressing – Suture removal	➢ Nursing care plan – 1 ➢ Case study/ presentation – 1	➢ Assess performance with rating scale ➢ Assess each skill with checklist OSCE/ OSPE ➢ Evaluation of case study/ presentation ➢ Completion of activity record

Clinical Area/Unit	*Duration (Weeks)*	*Learning Outcomes*	*Procedural Competencies/ Clinical Skills*	*Clinical Requirements*	*Assessment Methods*
Pediatric OPD/ Immunization room	V Sem – 1 week	➢ Perform assessment of children: Health, developmental and anthropometric ➢ Perform immunization ➢ Give health education/ nutritional education	➢ Assessment of children – Health assessment – Developmental assessment – Anthropometric assessment – Nutritional assessment ➢ Immunization ➢ Health/Nutritional education	➢ Growth and developmental study: Infant – 1 Toddler – 1 Preschooler – 1 Schooler – 1 Adolescent – 1	➢ Assess performance with rating scale ➢ Completion of activity record.
NICU and PICU	VI Sem – 1 week	➢ Provide nursing care to critically ill children	➢ Care of a baby in incubator/warmer ➢ Care of a child on ventilator, CPAP ➢ Endotracheal suction ➢ Chest physiotherapy ➢ Administration of fluids with infusion pumps ➢ Total parenteral nutrition ➢ Phototherapy ➢ Monitoring of babies ➢ Recording and reporting ➢ Cardiopulmonary resuscitation (PLS)	➢ Newborn assessment – 1 ➢ Nursing Care Plan – 1	➢ Assess performance with rating scale ➢ Evaluation of observation report ➢ Completion of activity record

PLATE 1

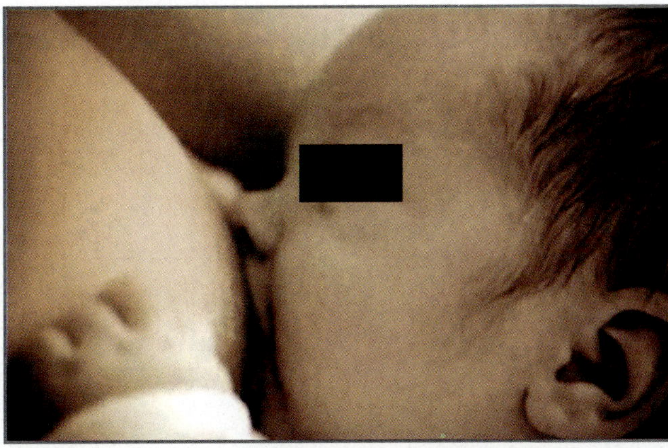

Fig. 2.1: Good attachment in breastfeeding.

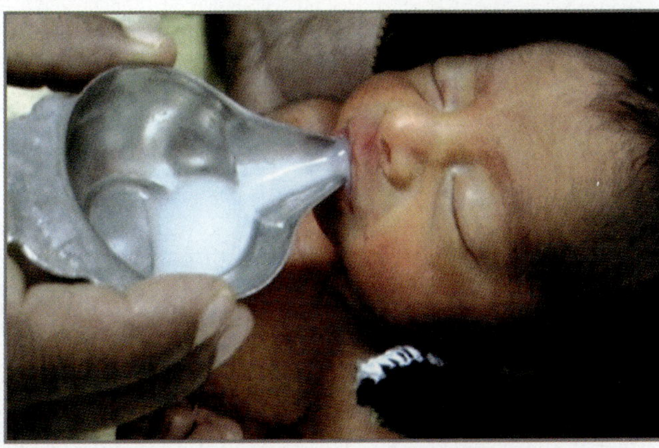

Fig. 2.3: Paladai feeding of a neonate.

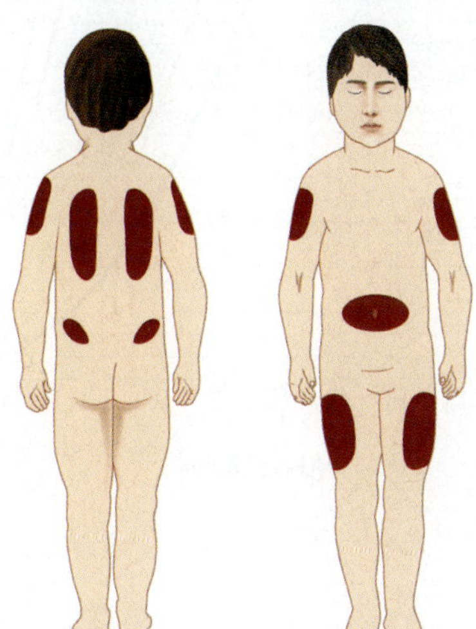

Fig. 3.5: Sites for subcutaneous injections.

PLATE 2

WHO Growth Chart for Boys

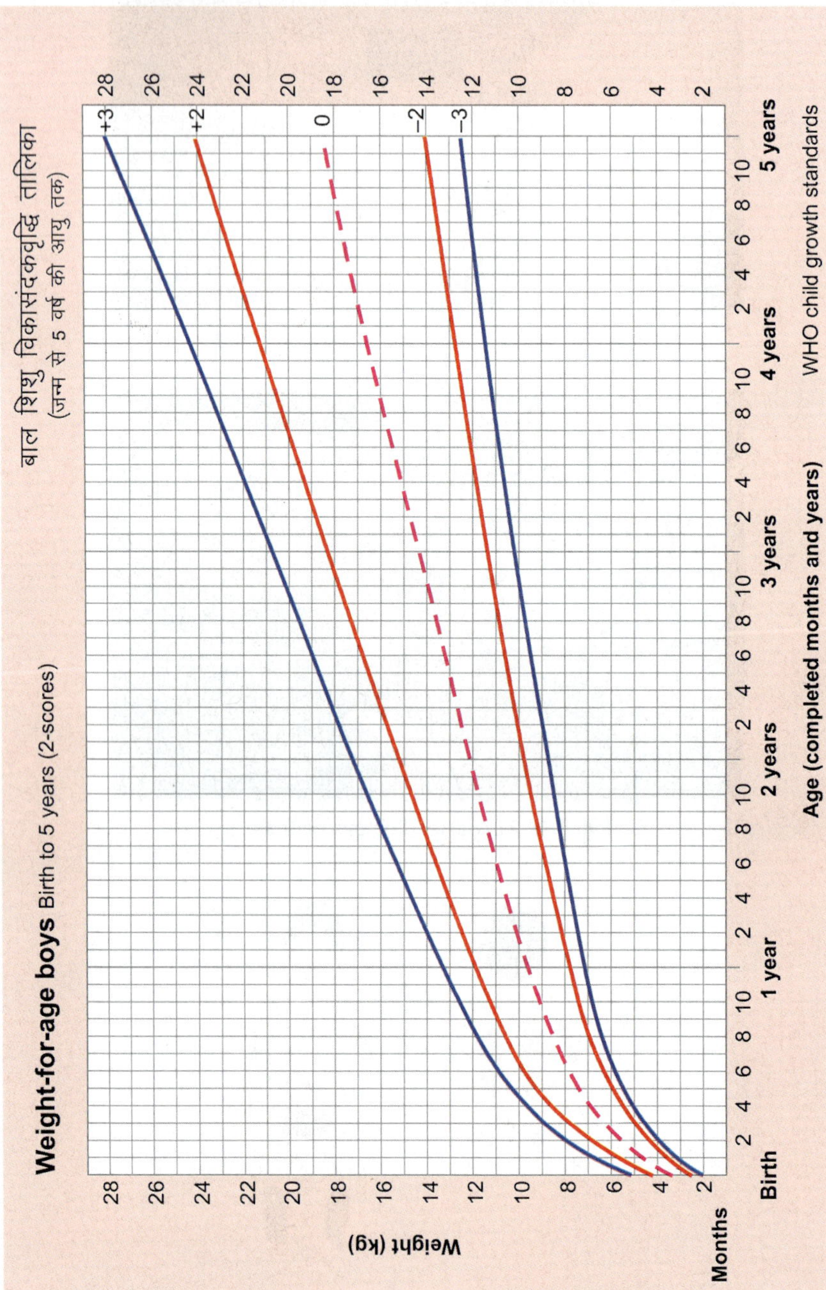

PLATE 3

WHO Growth Chart for Girls

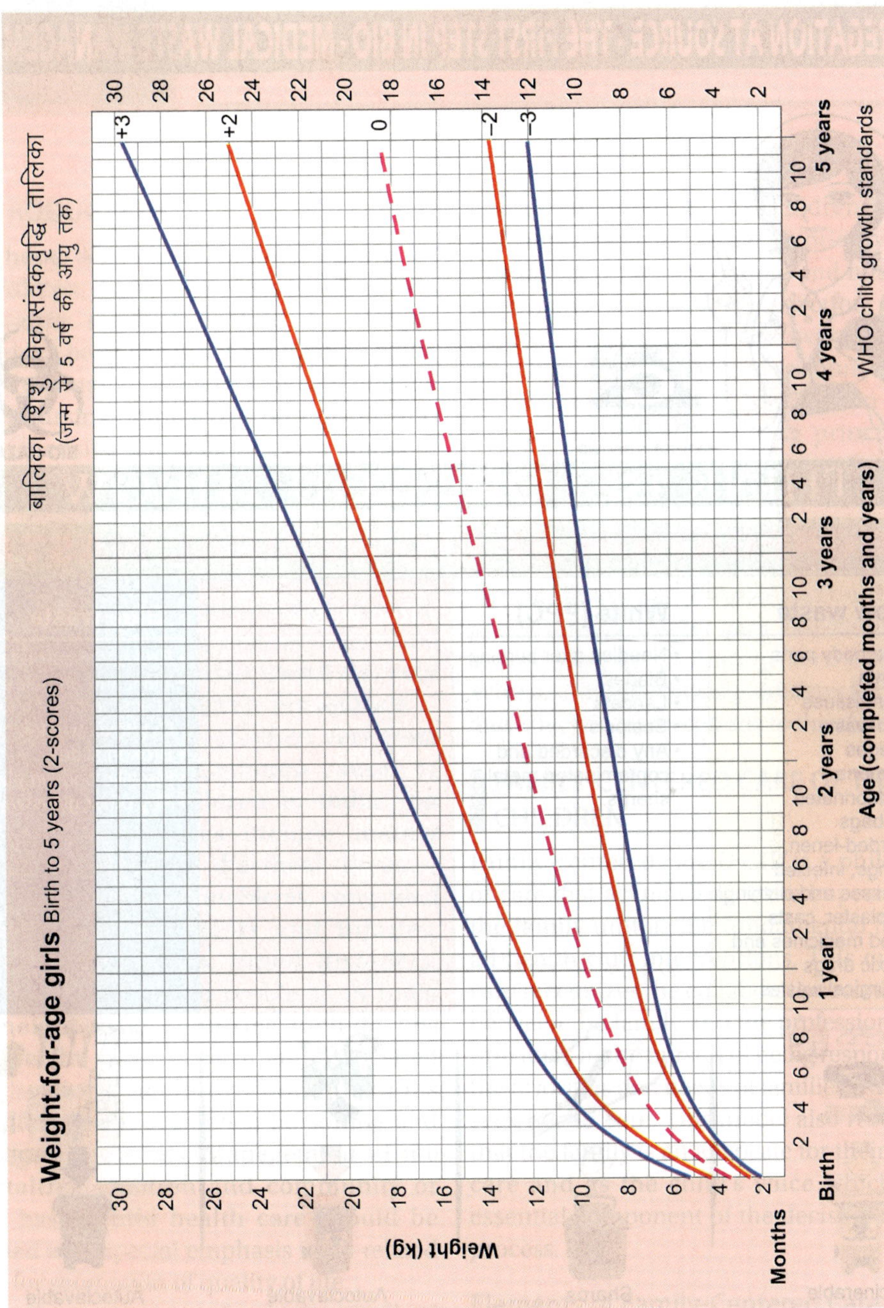

move an individual or an institution toward providing a family-centered approach. Each of these eight elements serves to reinforce, facilitate, and complement the implementation of the other elements. In child health care services, these elements of family - centered care give emphasis on each family's uniqueness, acknowledge the influence of the family as a constant in the child's life and emphasize the importance of providing services that demonstrate the value of collaboration between the health care providers, the child and the family. Family-centered care is based on the premise that a positive adjustment to the child's level of health and well-being requires the involvement of the whole family. These elements must be incorporated in health care policy and practices (Refer "Key Elements of Family-Centered Care" below).

Key Elements of Family-Centered Care

1. *The family at the center:* Family is the constant in the child's life and family members are at the center in child care. The service systems and the supportive health care providers within those systems can fluctuate.
2. *Family-professional collaboration:* Family-professional collaboration must be facilitated at all levels of hospital, home and community care of the individual child. It should also be included in program development, implementation, and evaluation and also for policy formation.
3. *Family-professional communication:* Effective communication for exchanging complete and unbiased information between families and professionals is essential in a supportive manner at all times.
4. *Cultural diversity of the families:* Recognition and honoring the cultural diversity, strengths and individuality within and across all families including ethnic, racial, spiritual, social, economic, educational and geographic diversity.
5. *Coping difference and support:* Respecting different methods of coping and implementing comprehensive policies and programs that provide developmental, educational, emotional, environmental, and financial supports to meet the diverse needs of the families.
6. *Family-centered peer support:* Encouraging and facilitating family to family support and networking.
7. *Specialized service and support systems:* Ensuring that hospital, home and community services and support systems for children needing special health care and developmental care and their families are flexible, accessible and comprehensive in responding to diverse family identified needs.
8. *Holistic perspective of FCC:* Appreciating families as families and children as children and recognizing that they possess a wide range of strengths, concerns, emotions, and aspirations beyond their need for specialized health and developmental services and support.

Strategies to Enhance Family-Centered Care

Family-centered care must be translated into action. The relevance to the child and family goes unnoticed unless active measures are taken to ensure that FCC practices are integrated into every aspect of the health care areas. The following strategies should be emphasized:

- Allow the presence of the parents or other family members at the bedside
- Establish family support groups and arrange meeting or discussion sessions
- Plan for the activities to support the family during transition from one unit to another such as from pediatric intensive care unit to the pediatric general ward
- Be sure that there is space for rest and sleep for the parents
- Establish the visiting policy for the sibling in the hospital
- Encourage family visiting in the intensive care units and in the post-anesthesia room
- Identify and understand the family needs using parents questions

- Create a parents information and orientation program to familiarize the parents with the hospital and necessary health care interventions
- Plan and implement the preoperative training program to minimize the fear of the child and the family about preoperative and postoperative interventions
- Encourage the parents to note the child's progress and to report to the care providers
- Recognize and integrate ethnic, racial and cultural activities as appropriate into the clinical setting, e.g., food, play items, pictures on the wall, etc.
- Teach the parents to provide routine care during day time as per their level of understanding and capabilities
- Involve parents in playroom and other recreational activities
- Establish discharge plan from the hospital to home and teach the parents about home care and follow-up activities
- Encourage all family members to participate in home care activities.

Family-centered care strategies need to be continued in hospital practices to identify their effectiveness in meeting family needs. Health care providers also need to continue to assess family needs, documents the implementation of the FCC, identify the factors that facilitate or hinder the process and establish its cost-effectiveness.

The implementation of *FCC interventions:*

- Facilitates growth and development of the children with special health care needs
- Optimizes the family's ability to interact, intervene and nurture the child during both physical and psychological stress
- Empowered the parents to make informed decision about their child's care within their available resources
- Elicited positive feelings among health care providers
- Increased parent and child satisfaction and reduce family anxiety.

Implementation of FCC is essential for the health well-being of the children and their family at all health care setting. It must be incorporated into policy and program for optimum child health care.

PROMOTING COPING OF CHILDREN DURING HOSPITALIZATION

Sick children tend to respond to hospitalization with emotional upset. Usually hospitalized children react negatively to the stress of hospitalization due to development of separation anxiety, unrealistic fears and feeling of loss of control. During illness the children also experience discomfort, pain, fatigue, frustration, mistrust, and anger. These responses often manifested as withdrawal or aggressive behaviors including crying, screaming, hitting, kicking, biting or physically resisting for procedures or simply ignoring the request for cooperation during any interventions.

Common Response of the Hospitalized Children

a. ***Separation Anxiety***

Separation anxiety in hospitalized children is common in the age group of 6 months to 4 years. Older children are still at risk of separation anxiety, but increasing the cognitive abilities and concept of time and place help them to cope with the situation. Due to separation from the parents, the hospitalized children respond with the phases of protest, despair and denial or detachment.

In the phase of protest, the children search for the lost parent and protest with anger, crying and rejecting the hospital staff. When parent returns, the child readily goes to him or her. In the phase of despair, the child becomes more sad and apathetic, mourning the lost parent but crying less and searching the environment less. They make few demands from the environment. When the parent returns, the child may not readily approach him or her or may cling to the parent. In the phase of denial, the children become cheerful, interested to the environment and new persons around them and become seemingly unaware of the lost parents. In detachment phase, the child is friendly with the hospital staff and begins to develop superficial relationship. The hospitalized children who progress to denial and detachment phase may suffer with long-term impaired parental relationship and impaired trust. They can have problems in establishment of close relationships, attention deficits, self-centeredness, and decreased intellectual functioning. Therefore the pediatric nurse must promote and practice interventions that reduce the separation anxiety of the children.

b. ***Loss of Control***

Hospitalized children commonly experience loss of control. Toddlers and preschoolers are at highest risk for loss of control. Toddlers are just gaining the ability to explore their environment and learning potty training and self-feeding as their developmental task. Hospitalization may interfere with the toddlers search for autonomy. For example, a toddler who has broken leg and immobilized, may experience limitations of the ability to ambulate or feed own self or to control the bowel movement. This loss of control can be very stressful for the parents also.

Nursing personnel can help to alleviate this stress by allowing choices, whenever possible. If the toddler is potty trained at home, continue with the routine when hospitalized. Allow the children to feed and dress themselves as much as possible. Try to maintain the home schedule and positive reinforcement for the children when in hospital.

c. ***Unrealistic Fears***

General fears of the children are found as the followings:

- Infants fear loud noises, sudden movements and loss of physical and emotional support
- Older infants fear separation from parents, strangers and heights
- Toddlers fear the dark, being alone, animals, machines and draining tubes
- Preschoolers fear the mutilation, the unknown person or events, the supernatural ideas or story and separation from family members
- School-aged children fear bodily injury, death, unsafe situation, loss of control of body functions, parental death and school related concerns
- Adolescents fear loss of peer relationships, body disfigurement, loss of physical abilities and death in the family

Sick and hospitalized children can have more fear such as procedural discomfort, needle injury, other painful events, and body distortion. So, health care providers must pay attention to the child's fear during all interventions.

Enhancing Strategies for Coping in the Hospitalized Children

Development of effective coping behaviors is mostly considered as nursing responsibility to support the children while in hospital. Children use many different strategies to cope with the stress of illness by information seeking, limiting and avoiding information, social support, emotional behaviors, and physical exercise. These responses emphasize on the need for the individualized interventions. It is believed that well prepared children cope better in the hospital having necessary information and need-based teaching to them.

To promote better coping, children should be supported with the following strategies:

i. Reduction of stress by relaxation, distraction, imagery and positive talk.
ii. Involvement of the parents to help the children to cope with the situation.
iii. Allow the children to reveal their fears and concerns by drawings that can help in better communication and correction of misconceptions which support coping skill.
iv. Music can also be used to promote coping as distraction from the stressful conditions and for promoting relaxation and reducing tension

v. Using therapeutic play to promote coping behaviors with hospital experience. The child feels sense of control and mastery over the situation when able to manipulate the equipment as play materials. Play room must be available for the hospitalized children with age appropriate play items.
vi. Organizing "Child Life Programs" to cope successfully and to minimize stress of the children and families during hospitalization. This can be done by the interventions such as preparation for hospitalization, diversional activities, continuation of school activities, emotional support, and promotion of FCC.
vii. Promoting effective coping skills of the family members helps them to adjust better during the child's hospitalization. Parent's coping is just as important as the child's coping, especially during acute illness. By providing appropriate information, establishing rapport, involving parents in planning of care, assessing the parent's needs and preferences for participation in care, parents' visits, and need-based teaching to the parents promote parental coping and satisfaction.

Minimizing Separation Anxiety

The stress due to separation anxiety can be reduced:

- *For infant:* By promoting rooming-in, minimizing the numbers of care takers, supporting by holding during parent's absence, providing stimulations with toys and comfort measures as talking in soothing voice, cuddling, holding, rocking, etc.
- *For toddlers and preschoolers:* By encouraging rooming-in, using doll-play, hide-and-seek play, allowing favorite toys and clothes from home, providing comfort measures by the parents, etc.
- *For school-aged children:* By promoting communication with siblings and friends, allowing homework of school, parents visit and play room activities.
- *For adolescent:* By promoting peer interactions and parent visits, allowing recreational and diversional activities, etc.

Reducing Loss of Control

The stress due to loss of control can be minimized:

- For infant: By allowing freedom of movements (as permissible), providing toys and altering environment as much as possible.
- *For toddlers:* By promoting dietary practices of home and home rituals, encouraging autonomy with child's choice for toys and game, providing opportunity for medical or therapeutic play and teaching the parents about the regressive behaviors which usually resolves when the child returns home.
- *For preschoolers:* By encouraging autonomy with the choices and participation in self-care, allowing playroom activities and therapeutic play and being truthful with the child.
- *For school-aged children:* By providing opportunities to discuss the medical situation with the children, encouraging to express their understanding, providing explanations for child's condition, helping to perform developmental tasks and promoting choices.
- *For adolescent:* By discussing plan of care and medical situation, respecting the need for independence and allowing for privacy.

Preventing Fears

Provide developmental appropriate explanations according to the level of understanding to counter the unrealistic fears and to intervene to minimize trauma caused by the real fear. These can be done as parental presence during procedures, allow expressing child's choice and concerns, use non-pharmacological measures for pain reduction, use of topical anesthetics and/or oral medications to reduce pain from needle sticks.

Therefore, interventions and strategies for effective coping by the children and the family members during the period of hospitalization are significant for optimum growth and development of the children and toward a positive beneficial experience of the family at the hospitals or at any healthcare settings

CHILDHOOD GROWTH AND DEVELOPMENTAL MILESTONES

Growth and development of the children are closely interrelated. Each child has individualized pattern of growth and development. Understanding the age-specific growth and development is very important for the nursing professionals to provide age-appropriate care to the children.

Growth is the process of physical maturation resulting in an increase in size of the body and various organs. It occurs by multiplication of cells and by increase in intracellular substance. It is quantitative changes of the body which is progressive and measurable phenomenon.

Development is the process of functional and physiological maturation of the individual. It is progressive increase in skill and capacity to do function and also includes psychological, emotional and social changes. It is related to maturation and myelination of the nervous system and considered as qualitative aspect of maturation.

Maturation is the increase in competence and change in behavior and ability to do function at higher level, depending upon the genetic inheritance.

Stages of Growth and Development

Prenatal period, i.e., intrauterine life:

- Ovum: 0–14 days after conception
- Embryo: 14 days to 8 weeks of gestation
- Fetus: 8 weeks of gestation to birth

Postnatal period, i.e., extrauterine life:

- Neonates: from birth to 4 weeks of life
- Infancy: Up to 12 months age
- Toddler: 1-3 years of age
- Preschooler: 3-6 years of age
- School-going children: 6–12 years of age
- Adolescence: From puberty to adulthood
- Prepubescent (early adolescent/late childhood): 10–12 years of age in girls and 12–14 years of age in boys
- Pubescent (middle adolescent): 12–14 years of age in girls and 14–16 years of age in boys
- Post-pubescent (late adolescent): 14–18 years of age in girls and 16–20 years of age in boys.

Factors Influencing Growth and Development

Growth and development depends upon multiple factors or determinants. These factors influence growth and development directly or indirectly by promoting and hindering the process. The factors are grouped as hereditary factors and environmental factors. Hereditary factors determine the extent of growth and development that is possible for the individual but environment determines the degree to which the potential of the individual is achieved.

- ***Genetic factors:*** Each child has a different genetic potential inherited from parents. Genetic predisposition is the important factor which influence the growth and development of the children. Different characteristics such as height, body structure, intelligence, color of skin, eyes and hair, etc., depend upon inherited gene from parents.
  Abnormal gene from ancestors may produce different familial diseases which usually hinders the growth and development of the children. The inherited diseases are thalassemia, hemophilia, galactosemia, sickle cell anemia, etc.
  The process of growth and development of the children is also affected by the chromosomal abnormalities such as Down's syndrome, Turner's syndrome, etc.
  Sex, race, and nationality are also found as influencing genetic factors for growth and development on an individual. Sex of the children influences their physical attributes and patterns of growth. Growth potential of different racial group is distinct in varying extent. Physical characteristics

of the individual of different country also vary due to difference in nationality.

- ***Prenatal factors:*** Intrauterine environment is an important predominant factor for optimal growth and development of the children. This factor includes different maternal health problems which have adverse effects on fetal growth that ultimately affect growth and development in extrauterine life.
  Several maternal health problems influence the fetal growth in intrauterine life, such as maternal malnutrition and anemia, maternal infections (STORCH, HIV, HBV), maternal illness (PIH, heart disease, chronic renal disease, hyperpyrexia, iodine deficiency), maternal substance abuse (tobacco chewing, smoking), exposure to drugs and toxins, uterine malformations, malpresentation, oligohydramnios, polyhydramnios, influence of maternal hormonal deficiency (hypothyroidism, diabetes mellitus), maternal emotional problems, and inadequate prenatal care.
- ***Postnatal factors***: Important postnatal factors which influence growth and development of the children include growth potential at birth (low birth weight, preterm birth, perinatal asphyxia, neonatal sepsis, neonatal complications, congenital anomalies), poor nutritional status (iron deficiency, iodine deficiency), accidental injury and childhood illnesses [e.g., acute respiratory infection (ARI), diarrhea, infections and parasitic infestations, tuberculosis, nephrotic syndrome, blood disorders, malabsorption syndrome, endocrinal abnormalities, etc.].
  Other factors which influence growth and development of the children include physical environment, psychological environment, birth order of the child, intelligence of the child, hormonal effects, mental health, play and exercise, culture and customs, socioeconomic status, climate and season.

Thus, the growth and development is a complex process with influence of various factors and determinants. Favorable conditions promote growth and development of the children, whereas unfavorable conditions inhibit the process leading to developmental delay, growth retardation, growth failure or failure to thrive.

Systemic changes occur with favorable situations during growth and development of the children. All body systems gradually developed as age increases toward maturity.

Responsibility of the child health nursing professionals includes early detection of deviations from expected growth and development of the individual child with prompt initiation of required interventions to overcome the problems related to growth and development.

Assessment of Growth

Measurement of various growth parameters is the important nursing responsibility in child health care both in facility and in community. The criteria for assessment of physical growth are mainly anthropometric measurements [body weight, length or height, head circumference (HC), chest circumference (CC), and mid-upper arm circumference (MUAC)], fontanel closure, dentition, and assessment of body mass index (BMI), body ratio, skinfold thickness, and bone age.

Body Weight of the Children

- Body weight is one of the best criteria for assessment of growth. It is a good indicator of health and nutritional status of the child. Measurement of body weight of the children should be done using weighing scale accurately. Electronic weighing scale, beam balance or spring balance and adult weighing machine can be used for measurement of body weight of the children according to the child's age, ability, health status and availability of the equipment. Precautions must be followed during weighing the child to prevent transmission of microorganisms, loss of body heat and accidental fall.

- Growth chart should be maintained by recording body weight to detect any deviations and to manage the abnormal conditions as early as feasible.
- In Indian children, normal birth weight in full-term neonate is about 2,500–4,000 g. There is about 5–10% loss of body weight in first week of life which regains by 10 days of age. After that in normal infant, the weight gain follows an average pattern. The healthy infants doubled their birth weight by 5 months of age and trebled by 1 year of age. Birth weight increases by 4 times 2 years, 5 times by 3 years, 6 times by 5 years, 7 times by 7 years and 10 times by 10 years. Then weight increases rapidly during puberty followed by gradual increase to adult size according to the height *(Refer WHO Child Growth Standard Chart as Weight-for-age for boys and girls up to 5 years of age, in Appendix – I and II).*

Length and Height

- Length or height of the children is measured for detection of skeletal growth. Yearly increase in height gradually diminished from birth to maturity. Recumbent length is measured up to 2 years of age. Infantometer or simple tape measure is used to assess the crown-heel length by placing the child on hard surface in supine position with extended legs. For older children, standing height is measured using vertical height scale or stadiometer or with simple tape-measure. The older child should stand on the floor in bare feet against the scale. Child's arms should hang by the side and occiput, upper back, buttocks and heels should touch the scale or wall with straight head in parallel vision. A flat object is placed top of the head and the height is then marked.
- Recording of length or height should be done in child's health card and must be compared with weight to assess weight-for-height and BMI.
- Average length of a healthy Indian infant at birth is 50 cm. It increases to 60 cm at 3 months, 70 cm at 9 months and 75 cm at 1 year of age. In second year of age, there is 12 cm increase, in third year of age the increment is 9 cm, in fourth year it is 7 cm and in fifth year it is 6 cm. The child doubles the birth length by 4–4.5 years of age. Afterwards, there is about 5 cm increase in height in every year till onset of puberty and then there is slow increase in height in adolescence period *(Refer Appendix – III for average height and weight of Indian boys and girls up to 18 years of age).*

Assessment of Body Mass Index

- BMI is an important criterion to assess normal growth of the children and its deviations as malnutrition, underweight, overweight and obesity. BMI is calculated as the body weight divided by the square of the body height.
- BMI remains constant up to 5 years of age. Normal BMI is 18.5 to < 25 kg/m^2. If BMI is less than 15 kg/m^2, then it indicates malnutrition. BMI less than 18.5 kg/m^2 is underweight and 25–29.9 kg/m^2 indicate overweight. When BMI is more than 30 kg/m^2, then it indicates obesity.
- BMI is calculated with the formula using measured weight and height of the child, as given here:

$$\text{BMI} = \frac{\text{Weight in Kg}}{(\text{Height in meter})^2}$$

Head Circumference

- Measurement of HC is done to assess brain growth and development of intracranial volume. HC is measured using ordinary tape-measure placing over the occipital protuberance at the back, above the ears on the sides and just over the supraorbital ridges in front and measuring the point of highest circumference
- Average HC of the infant at birth is 35 cm. At 3 months of age HC is about 40 cm, at 6 months of age it is 43 cm and at 1 year of age it is 45 cm. HC increases to about 48 cm at 2 years age, 50 cm at 7 years of age and about 52 cm at 12 years of age, which is almost same as adult's HC

- If head circumference increases more than 1 cm in 2 weeks period, during the first 3 months of life, then hydrocephalus should be suspected. Abnormal HC may be found as large size of head (macrocephaly or hydrocephaly) or small size of head (microcephaly) indicating different disease conditions and cranial abnormalities. Abnormal growth of head in children may be found as abnormal shape such as tomb-shaped (oxycephaly), boat-shaped (scaphocephaly) and asymmetrical (plagiocephaly).

Fontanel Closure

- Fontanel closure indicates bony development of the skull. Posterior fontanel closes early within a few weeks (6–8 weeks) of age in infants. Anterior fontanel normally closes by 12–18 months of age of the children. Early closure of fontanels indicates craniostenosis due to immature closure of skull sutures. Delayed closure of fontanels may be found in rickets, malnutrition, hydrocephalus, cretinism and congenital cyanotic heart disease.

Chest Circumference

- Chest circumference or thoracic diameter is an important growth parameter which indicates nutritional status of the children and their growth status. At birth, chest is about round in shape with equal transverse and anteroposterior diameters. Thereafter, width of chest becomes larger than depth, due to rapid increase of transverse diameter. Abnormal shape of chest is found in rickets, malnutrition and congenital heart diseases.
- Chest circumference is measured by placing the ordinary tape-measure around the chest at the level of the nipples, in between inspiration and expiration.
- Normal chest circumference at birth is 2–3 cm less than the head circumference of the neonate. At 6–12 months of age of the infant both become equal. After first year of age, the chest circumference is greater than the head circumference by 2.5 cm and by the age of 5 years of the child, CC is about 5 cm larger than HC.

Mid-Upper Arm Circumference

- Measurement of MUAC helps to assess the nutritional and growth status of the children. If there is any growth retardation due to inadequate nutrition, that can be detected by this simple useful measurement. If MUAC measurement is < 11.5 cm in children of 6 months to 59 months age group (under-5 age group) along with bilateral pedal edema, it indicates severe acute malnutrition (SAM).
- To assess MUAC, the left upper arm is measured firmly and gently without compressing the arm. The simple tape-measure or MUAC measuring special tape can be used. The arm is measured while the hand is allowed to hang freely. The MUAC measurement is taken at mid-point between the tip of acromion process of scapula and olecranon process of ulna. There should be no cloths on the arm.
- The average MUAC of normal healthy infants at birth is 11–12 cm and at 1 year of age it is 12–16 cm. Normally MUAC at 5 years of age becomes 16–17 cm, at 12 years of age, it is 17–18 cm and at 15 years of age of the children, it is 20–21 cm.

Dentition

- Dentition is not a dependable parameter for assessment of growth, as there is a variation for the time of eruption of teeth. There are two sets of teeth, i.e., temporary teeth and permanent teeth. There is a phase of mixed dentition with two sets of teeth.
- First teeth may erupt commonly at 6–7 months of age of the infant. By the age of 2.5–3 years, the children have full set of temporary teeth with total number 20. The first permanent teeth usually appear at the age of 6 years. Total permanent teeth numbering 32 usually erupt within 12 years of age of the children, except third molars which may appear at 18 years of age or later.

- Delayed dentition may be found in children due to familial tendency, poor nutritional status, bottle feeding, rickets and osteogenesis imperfecta. No teething may occur as congenital anomalies. No dentition beyond 1.5 years of age requires special attention.

Body Proportion

Body proportion is the ratio between the upper and lower segment of the body, which is measured from symphysis pubis. At birth, the body ratio is 1.7:1.0 due to less growth of legs and more development of head and upper segment of the body in intrauterine life. This ratio becomes 1.3:1.0 at 3 years of age and 1.0:1.0 at the age of 10–12 years of age of the children.

Skin-fold Thickness

Measurement of skin-fold thickness is used in evaluating nutritional status of the children by estimating the amount of subcutaneous fat. Calibrated calipers are used to measure the thickness of a fold of skin at defined body sites that include upper arm or triceps, subscapular region and upper abdomen. The triceps site is the most commonly used single-site skinfold measurement as it is easy to measure and reference data are available for comparison (e.g., WHO triceps skin-fold thickness for age).

Bone Age or Osseous Growth

Bone age is the degree of maturation of the bones. The bone age is estimated to assess the maturity of the child's skeletal system. Skeletal maturation or bone growth is an indicator of physiological development. As an individual grows from fetal life through childhood, puberty and completes as a young adult, there is skeletal changes in size and shape. These skeletal changes or bone growth is calculated by appearance of ossification center and can be seen by X-ray study. It is usually done by a single X-ray of the left wrist, hand and fingers. It is safe and painless procedure that uses a small amount of radiation only.

Advanced bone age may be found in precocious puberty, thyrotoxicosis and adrenal hyperplasia. Retardation of bony growth is found in cretinism.

Domains/Aspects of Childhood Development

Childhood development has various aspects which includes physical development, gross motor development, fine motor development, language and speech development, vision development, hearing development, sensory development (taste, smell, touch), sexual development, personal and social development, interpersonal development, play development, cognitive development, intellectual development, emotional development, personality development, development of body image, moral development and spiritual development.

Study of childhood development and understanding of its different aspects helps the nursing professionals to provide holistic and comprehensive care to the children in health and illness. It assures early detection of developmental delays for prompt initiation of individualized priority-based management of the affected children.

Important Expected Developmental Milestones of Children

Development is the functional maturation of organs and body systems. It depends upon neuromuscular maturity, genetic determinants, and environmental influences. Developmental milestones are accomplished by the children at an anticipated age. There may be great variations in time of achievement of different levels of development with extreme ranges. The average achievement levels in different age group of children are found as follows:

At 3 months of age:

- The infant is able to lift head and front part of chest by supporting weight on extended arms. Infant can follow moving object with steady eye movements and able to focus eyes. Produces "cooing" sound and enjoy people taking with him/her. Able to recognize mother and turn head to sound. Infant will have social smile and steady head holding.

At 6 months of age:

- The infant will be able to sit with support. Infant can hold a cube and transfer from one hand to other. Reach out with arms and grasp a toy. Turn head to follow an object. Try to imitate sound and enjoy own mirror image. Recognize strangers and show stranger anxiety.

At 9 months of age:

- The infants are able to crawl on abdomen. Sit without support. Can stand with support. Can hold small object between index finger and thumb. Speak "Da-Da" and "Ma-Ma" combing syllables without meaning. Waves "bye-bye".

At 12 months of age:

- The infant can stand without support, creeps well and walk holding furniture. Able to feed himself/herself with spilling. Can pick up small bits of food and take to mouth. Able to push toy car alone and play simple ball game. Can speak 3-5 meaningful words and understand meaning of several words. Respond for affection by kiss.

At 2 years of age:

- The toddlers are able run and try to climb upstairs by resting on each step and then climbing up on next. Walk backward. Able to put shoes and socks on and can remove pants. Build tower of six to seven blocks. Point to parts of doll. Pull people to show toys. Able to copy and draw horizontal and vertical lines. Able to control bladder at day time. Can ask for food, drink and toilet. Speak simple sentences without use of verbs.

At 3 years of age:

- The toddlers can walk on tip-toes and stand on one leg for seconds. Able to jump with both feet. Climb upstairs by coordinated manner. Ride tricycle. Can dress and undress. Brush teeth with help. Can draw a circle. Build tower of nine blocks. Has vocabulary of about 250 words. Able to repeat three numbers. Know own name and sex. Achieve bladder control by night. Fear dark. Interact and play simple games with peers.

At 6 years of age:

- The preschoolers can jump and hop. Able to draw a cross (+) and tilted cross (X). Can draw rectangle and triangle. Able to copy letters. Can tell stories and describe recent experience. Become independent, impatient and aggressive both physically and verbally. Jealous of sibling but gradually improve in behavior and manners.

At 12 years of age:

- The children of the age develop coordinated, skillful manipulative activities and games. Able to use "parts of speech" correctly. Accepts suggestions and instructions obediently. May show short burst of anger. Participate in family discussion. Able to do peer group involvement and have increased awareness about sex role.

Puberty

Puberty is the stage of life at which members of both sexes become functionally capable of reproduction. It is the sequence of events by which an individual is transformed into a young adult by a series of biological changes. Adolescence begins with the onset of puberty. The age of onset of puberty and sexual maturation vary widely in different individual depending upon the genetic and environmental factors.

Common order of puberty changes in girls are found as follows:

- Accelerated growth in weight and height gain
- Breast changes such as pigmentation of areola and enlargement of breast tissue and nipples
- Increase in pelvic girth mainly in the transverse diameter
- Appearance of pubic hair and change in vaginal secretions

- Activation of axillary sweat glands and appearance of axillary hair
- Onset of menstruation (menarche). First menstrual bleeding occurs usually 2 years after the onset of first manifestation of puberty
- Abrupt slowing of height gain.

Common order of puberty changes in boys are found as follows:

- Accelerated increase in weight and height gain
- Increase in the size of external genitalia
- Appearance of pubic hair followed by hair in axillae, upper lip, groin, thigh, and between symphysis pubis and umbilicus
- Appearance of facial hair, 2 years after the pubic hair
- Changes in voice as cracking and then deepening
- Nocturnal discharge of semen during sleep
- Abrupt slowing in height gain.

Assessment of childhood development must be performed at regular interval to detect developmental delays or any other abnormalities. The mostly used screening test for detection of developmental delays in infancy and preschool children is Denver Developmental Screening Test (DDST). At present Denver-II scale is used. Other developmental screening tests used for the children are Bayley's Scale, DASII (Developmental Assessment Scale of Indian Infant), Trivandrum Scale, Baroda DST, Early language milestones scale, cognitive adaptive test, Stanford-Binet Intelligence Scale, etc.

Nursing personnel should support the children and their family members to promote optimal childhood growth and development. Assessment of growth and development, early identification of deviations and abnormalities, prompt management of health problems, keeping health record, counseling, and guidance to parents for child care are considered as important nursing responsibilities for promotion of child health status.

PRINCIPLES OF FLUID AND NUTRITIONAL MANAGEMENT OF CHILDREN

Requirements of Fluid in Children

Stable internal environment is maintained by the balance of body water and electrolytes. Water balance represents the difference between water intake (including that generated from endogenous metabolism) and water losses. Water output involves losses in urine, stool, sweating and by evaporation from moist surfaces of the skin and respiratory tract (i.e., insensible losses). Kidneys are major regulators of water output.

Growing children are more susceptible to disturbances of fluid and electrolyte balance during their illness. Correction of fluid and electrolyte imbalance and maintenance of appropriate fluid and electrolyte balance are the significant approach in the management of any childhood disease conditions.

The normal maintenance water requirement is equal to the insensible and urinary water losses. Fluid requirements change considerably in different clinical conditions. Conditions that lead to increased fluid requirement are fever, use of radiant warmer, phototherapy, very low birth weight baby, diarrhea, vomiting, polyuria, hyperventilation, etc. Decreased fluid requirement is indicated in oliguria, anuria, caring in incubator, hypothyroidism, etc.

Distribution of Total Body Water

Water is the largest component of human body. Total body water (TBW) in full-term neonates at birth is about 75–80% of body weight which gradually reduces to 60% by 1–2 years of age and remains so till puberty. TBW consists of two major compartments, i.e., intracellular fluid (ICF) and extracellular fluid (ECF) and two minor compartments, i.e., transcellular fluid (TCF) and slowly exchangeable fluid (SEF). Distribution of TBW as percent of body weight is shown in **Table 1.1.**

TABLE 1.1: Distribution of total body water.

Fluid Compartments	*Infants*	*Older Children*
Intracellular fluid (ICF)	40%	35–40%
Extracellular fluid (ECF) Interstitial Transvascular (Plasma) Transcellular	35–40% - - -	20–25% 15% 5% 1–3%
Total body water	75–80%	60%

Fluid Requirements of Neonates

- Fluid requirements in neonates depend upon birth weight, gestational age, postnatal age and presence of disease conditions. Fluid requirement in preterm neonates is more as compared to term neonates due to higher insensible losses.
- Use birth weight for fluid calculations as long as the infant's postnatal weight remains below birth weight. Once the birth weight is regained then use actual body weight for all weight-based calculations. Daily requirement of water/fluid in different age groups are given in the **Table 1.2.**
- When the infant is treated with both intravenous (IV) fluid therapy and enteral feeding, then calculate fluid requirements by adjusting IV fluid amount with enteral feeding. Subtract the daily volume of feed intake from total calculated fluid requirement and administer the remaining fluid requirement as IV fluid.

TABLE 1.2: Daily requirements of water and calories in infants and children.

Age range	*Water requirement (mL/kg)*	*Calorie requirement (cal/kg)*
Day 7 to 3 months	150	120
3–12 months	150	110
1–3 years	125	100
4–6 years	100	90
7–9 years	75	80
10–12 years	50	70
13–15 years	50	60
16–19 years	50	50

- Monitor the neonates for daily body weight and urine output (normal urine output in neonate is 1–4 mL/kg body weight/hour). If the neonate is receiving IV fluid therapy then we should monitor IV site, total intake and total output, signs of dehydration and overhydration, electrolytes, biochemical parameters, and blood glucose level at regular interval, as per standard protocol or institutional policy.
- Discontinue the infusion of IV fluid when the neonate is receiving 100 mL/kg body weight/day or about two-thirds of the daily calculated fluid volume as oral feeds and has no abdominal distension or vomiting.

Fluid requirements of neonates can be calculated as follows:

- On day 1, if neonates are having birth weight 1,500 g or more, fluid requirement of those neonates is 60 mL/kg body weight/day. If neonates are having birth weight less than 1,500 g, fluid requirement of those neonates is 80 mL/kg body weight/day
- Daily increment of fluid requirements in all groups is about 15 mL/kg/day till it reached 150 mL/kg/day
- On day 7, neonates should have calculated total fluid requirement as 150 mL/kg of body weight per day.

Overhydration

Overhydration or excess of fluids in the body may occur especially during fluid therapy in sick children. Signs of overhydration should be monitor for detection of the problems and for prompt initiation of management **(Table 1.3)**. Overhydration is detected in children having puffiness of eyes, edema on dependent parts, excessive weight gain and respiratory distress due to pulmonary edema.

Nutritional Requirements in Children

Nutritional requirements may vary from one child to another child and depends upon metabolic and genetic difference. No single food provides all essential nutrients for children, except mother's milk which provides all nutritional requirements to the

TABLE 1.3: Clinical assessment of dehydration.

	No dehydration	*Some dehydration*	*Severe dehydration*
Decrease in body weight	< 5% in infants, < 3% in older children	5–10% in infants, 3–6% in older children	>10% in infants, > 6% in older children
Mental status	Normal	Irritable	Lethargic to comatosed
Thirst	Normal	Increased	Unable to drink
Skin color and elasticity (turgor)	Normal	Cool, pale, mild delay in turgor	Cold, mottled, tenting
Sunken eyes	Normal	Sunken	Very sunken
Mucous membrane	Normal	Dry	Very dry
Pulse rate	Normal	Slightly increased	Tachycardia
Capillary refill time	2–3 seconds	3–4 seconds	>4 seconds
Blood pressure	Normal	Normal	Normal or low
Urine output	Slightly decreased	Decreased	Oliguria, anuria

infants up to 6 months of age. Complementary feeding should be started after 6 months of age of the children and afterward balanced diet should be provided for optimal growth and development and to prevent nutritional deficiency and developmental delay.

Children's diet should be planned and arranged by the parents or family members with sufficient amount of fluids, calories, proteins, carbohydrates, fats, vitamins, minerals and salts to meet their daily nutritional requirements. Food items should be digestible, palatable, attractive, choiceable and easily available. Healthy dietary habit depends upon cultural, social, and economic influence. Nutritional requirements should be maintained with safety and with appropriate balance. A deficit or excess intake of nutrients could be harmful and should be avoided. "Recommended daily intake of nutrients" should be provided to the children to maintain needs of the body and to promote good and optimal health.

Dietary Recommendations for Children

Effective Breastfeeding Practices

- Breastfeeding is the best feeding for the infant up to 6 months of age. It should be continued up to 2 years of age or beyond along with complementary feeding.
- Feeding with mother's own milk is natural and appropriate for her own infant
- Breastfeeding must be initiated within one hour of birth or as soon as possible as breast crawl techniques, irrespective of mode of delivery, when both mother and neonate are not sick. *Early initiation of breastfeeding (EIBF)* prevents hypothermia, hypoglycemia, infections, and other neonatal problems.
- Breastfeeding is beneficial for infants, mother, family and society
- *Benefits of breastfeeding to the infants:* (a) Provides optimum nutrition for growth and development, (b) protects from infections such as diarrhea, respiratory infections and other infections, (c) protects from allergies, including eczema and asthma, (d) enhances emotional bonding between mother and baby, (e) easily digested and available at appropriate temperature, (f) promotes development of higher IQ and feeling of security, and (g) breastfed babies have less chance of developing hypertension, diabetes mellitus, coronary heart disease and cancer in later life
- *Benefits of breastfeeding to the mothers:* (a) Accelerates the process of involution of uterus reducing chances of postpartum hemorrhage (PPH), (b) lowers the risk

of breast and ovarian cancer in mother, (c) reduces workload of mother and (d) delays next pregnancy, if the baby is getting exclusive breastfeeding

- *Benefits to family and society:* It is more economical and promotes family planning. It helps to reduce infant mortality and morbidity and hospitalization of the children.
- *Colostrum feeding* in first few days of life protects the neonate with anti-infective proteins and considered as "first immunization" to the newborn baby. Colostrum has mild purgative effect which helps to clear meconium from the neonate's gut and helps to prevent neonatal hyperbilirubinemia.
- No prelacteal feeding should be given to the neonates such as honey, sweet drinks, gripe water, animal milk, formula milk, etc.
- *Exclusive breastfeeding* should be provided to the infant up to 6 months of life with only breast milk feeding. Only medications can be given if required. Any food or drinks, even water in hot summer season, should not be given to the infant up to 6 months of age
- *Correct positioning* during breastfeeding is important to ensure correct attachment and effective suckling. This helps to prevent sore nipples and breast engorgement. Correct positioning of the infant is done by ensuring: (i) Baby's abdomen touches mother's abdomen, (ii) Baby's entire body faces toward the mother, (iii) Baby's head, neck, and body are kept in same plane, and (iv) Baby' s body is well supported
- *Good attachment* of baby's mouth on mother's breast during breastfeeding should be ensured for effective suckling and prevention of breastfeeding problems. The important signs of good attachment are: (i) baby's mouth is wide open, (ii) baby's lower lip turned outwards, (iii) baby's chin touches mother's breast, and (iv) majority of areola of mother's breast is inside the baby's mouth
- *Effective suckling* is identified when the infant shows slow deep sucks with pause for sometimes. The infant should have rooting reflex, and coordinated sucking - swallowing reflex with breathing actions to help the infant to take milk secreted from the breast
- *Prolactin reflex* in mother is responsible for milk secretion and production. Its secretion increases at night, so night time breastfeeding must be continued for more prolactin secretion. Suckling of breast for sensory stimulation and empty breast after feeding stimulates prolactin reflex and promotes milk secretion
- *Oxytocin reflex* in mother is responsible for ejection or flow of milk from mother's breast. Oxytocin secretion increases by sensory impulses from the breast when the infant is suckling it. This secretion is also enhanced by the touch, sound and smell of the infant. Its secretion also increases when the mother is relaxed, stress free and calm. Back massage to the mother also stimulates for more secretion of oxytocin hormone
- *Both foremilk and hindmilk* should be given to the infant during breastfeeding to maintain sufficient intake of nutrients. Foremilk is secreted at starting of regular breastfeeding. It is more watery and contains more proteins, sugar, vitamins, and minerals. Hindmilk is secreted toward the end of regular breastfeeding and contains more fat and energy. Mother should feed the infant allowing one breast to empty to provide both foremilk and hindmilk, before offering other breast. For optimum growth and to fulfill adequate fluid and nutritional requirements, both foremilk and hindmilk are needed for the infant.
- *Technique of breastfeeding (Refer Unit – 2, Procedure – 4: Assisting in Breastfeeding)*
- *Counseling for breastfeeding* is most important for establishment of successful breastfeeding for the infants. Antenatal counseling, supporting the mother for early initiation of breastfeeding in delivery room, supporting for continuation of breastfeeding in postnatal period and management of breastfeeding problems

are essential for effective and optimal breastfeeding. Lactating mother needs postnatal diet with extra calorie, extra water intake, privacy, physical rest, comfort, exercise, and emotional support for successful breastfeeding to her baby.

- *Special support required to mothers having preterm/low birth weight or sick neonates* for prevention of lactation failure, continuation of breast milk feeding with expressed breast milk (EBM) and methods of expression of breast milk and paladai feeding.
- *Management of breastfeeding problems* helps in the promotion of successful breastfeeding by early identification and treatment of flat or inverted nipples, sore nipples, breast engorgement, breast abscess, and reduced milk supply. Mother should be taught about the technique of breast milk expression and storing of EBM, whenever needed *(Refer Unit - 2, Procedure - 22: Expression of Breast Milk)*.
- *Management of lactation failure* and relactation can be done and is possible by managing the causes of lactation failure. Prevention of lactation failure is more easy by continuous supporting the mother for successful breastfeeding and managing breastfeeding problems
- *Adequacy of breastfeeding* and intake of sufficient amount of milk by the baby can be assessed by counting passage of urine 6–8 times per day and average weight gain 1–1.5% of body weight daily or 20–30 g daily in first 3–4 months of life, after regaining birth weight of the neonates. Baby should sleep for 2–3 hours in between feeds. Mother should feel let down sensation during breastfeeding and softness of the breast afterward
- Initiate complementary foods after 6 months of age of the infant

Complementary Feeding (Weaning from Breastfeeding)

Complementary feeding or weaning from breastfeeding is the process of gradual and progressive transfer of the infant from breastfeeding to usual family diet. During this process the infant get accustomed to food items other than mother's milk. Breastfeeding only is not sufficient for growing infant after 6 months of age to maintain nutritional requirements.

Complementary feeding should be started after 6 months of age of the infants. Complementary feeding does not indicate the discontinuity of breastfeeding. Breastfeeding should be continued up to 2 years of age or beyond especially at night along with weaning foods. Delayed introduction of complementary feeding in infants leads to malnutrition, iron-deficiency anemia, and failure of growth and development.

Principles of Complementary Feeding

Following principles should be remembered during introduction of complementary feeding;

- Introduce liquid food first then gradually give semisolid and solid food items
- Food items should be clean, fresh, safe and hygienic to prevent infections
- Complementary foods should be easily digestible, easily acceptable, palatable, homemade, well-balanced, nourishing, age-appropriate, and suitable for the infants.
- Weaning foods should be high in energy density and low in bulk viscosity. It should contain all nutrients necessary for the infants.
- Selection of food items should be done based on cultural practices and traditional beliefs of the family but with good quality of foods.
- A small amount of new foods to be given in the beginning and gradually the amount of food to be increased during the course of a week. A single new food is added at a time. Additional food should be given at day time. New food should be given when the infant is hungry. New food should be given on tongue of the infant to get taste of the feed. Baby may spit the food out, but with patience the feed to be given again.
- Complementary feeding should be gradually increased in frequency, amount,

texture, variety of food items, with active feeding and hygienic practices.

- Never force the infant to take feeds, avoid force-feeding.
- Infant should be placed on mother lap during feeding. Mother should wash her hands every time before preparation of feeds and during feeding the infant.
- Observe the infant for problems related to new food. The infant may have indigestion, pain abdomen, diarrhea, skin rash especially in case of food allergy, and psychological upset due to withdrawn from mother's breast and suckling.
- Parent should consult health care providers and follow their advice to manage the problems carefully related to complementary feeding.

Complementary Feeding at Different Ages

At 6 months of age:

- Initiate complementary or weaning feed with fruit juices. Within 1 or 2 weeks new food item should be introduces such as vegetable soup, mashed and boiled potato, mashed banana, etc. Each food should be given with one or two teaspoons initially for 2 to three times per day. Within 3–4 weeks of time, amount of feed should be increases to half a cup. Breastfeeding should be continued on demand.

At 6–9 months of age:

- In this age, infants can have soft mixture of rice and dal, *khichri*, mashed and boiled potato, roti/chapatti or bread soaked in dal, mashed fruits such as banana, mango, papaya, stewed apple, etc. Fish and egg yolk can be added in this period (7 months onward) depending upon the infant's tolerance. Curd and *khir* can also be introduced from 8 months onward. By the age of 8–9 months with eruption of teeth, infant can enjoy to bite biscuit, piece of carrot and cucumber. This infant can have these added foods 3–4 times per day and amount of food should be increased gradually. Breastfeeding should be continued.

At 9–12 months of age:

- More variety of homemade foods can be added. Fish or egg should be given daily to increase protein intake and chicken can be introduced in this period. The infant can eat all foods cooked at home but spices must be avoided. Feeds should be well cooked and soft. Added food can be given 4 to 6 times per day. Breastfeeding should be continued.

At 12–18 months of age:

- The child can take all foods cooked in the family and need about half of mother's diet. Number of feeds 5–6 times according to the child's need. Breastfeeding should be continued especially at night.

Balanced Diet for Children

Balanced diet contains a variety of foods in such quantities and proportions that the need for energy, proteins, vitamins, minerals, fats, carbohydrates, and other nutrients are adequately available for maintaining health, vitality and general well-being of the individual. It is essential to protect the children from nutritional deficiencies and to overcome the short duration of lack of food or starvation. Balanced diet should be consumed by children to ensure proper growth and development and to stay healthy and free from diseases.

Following principles should be practiced for planning for balanced diet for the children:

- Balanced diet must be nutritionally adequate with appropriate intake of food items
- Daily requirement of protein intake should be given as 15–20% of daily energy intake
- Fat requirement should be limited to 20–30% of daily energy intake
- Carbohydrates should constitute the remaining food energy about 55–60% and should contain natural fibers
- Requirements of vitamins, minerals and all micronutrients must be fulfilled
- Food habit, taste, family food culture (vegetarian or non-vegetarian), religious beliefs, taboos, economical ability,

availability of foods and climate should be considered during selection of food items for balanced diet
- Age of the child should be considered for selection of dietary amounts
- Overfeeding and underfeeding should be avoided
- Balanced diet should contain age-appropriate adequate amount of cereals, pulses, green leafy and other vegetables, roots and tubers, fruits, milk and milk products, fats and oils, nuts, fish, egg, chicken, meat, sugar and jaggery

Assessment of Nutritional Status of Children

Assessment of nutritional status of children should be done using various techniques. These include: (a) detailed dietary history of the children, (b) clinical assessment for nutritional status (head to foot examination to detect clinical features of nutritional deficiency conditions), (c) anthropometry, (d) biochemical evaluation (e.g., serum protein, serum iron, enzyme level,) and laboratory tests (e.g., hemoglobin, stool, urine,), (e) functional assessment (e.g., nerve function, working capacity of heart and lungs), and (f) radiological examination for bone age and bony or other abnormalities and deformities.

Nutritional Counseling

Nutritional counseling and guidance to the parents and to the children in age-appropriate approach is the important responsibility of the nursing professionals to achieve the optimum nutritional status throughout the period of growth and development. Optimal nutritional status is required for promotion and maintenance of health, prevention of diseases and restoration of health in illness and injury. Adequacy of recommended dietary intake is essential for healthy survival and quality of life.

Nutritional counseling and guidance should be provided for all children, considering their feeding patterns, dietary habit, food fads, cultural beliefs, religion, and economical condition of the family, availability of food items, education, and understanding level.

Different aspects of age-appropriate nutritional counseling should include breastfeeding and related issues, complementary feeding, balanced diet, variety of food items, hand hygiene, food hygiene, food handling, healthy food preparation methods, and cooking process.

Discussion should be done regarding common nutritional deficiency conditions, their causes, signs and symptoms, preventive measures of nutritional problems, need for health checkup at regular interval and medical assistance.

Counseling should be done for utilization of available nutritional support from Integrated Child Development Services (ICDS) centers, Mid-day Meal Programme at school, Village Health and Nutrition D (VHND) and NGO services.

PRINCIPLES OF PHARMACOLOGIC MANAGEMENT IN CHILDREN

Medication administration is one of the most challenging and critical aspects of nursing interventions in child health. In adult, medication administration in which "one-dose-fits-all" principles generally applies, but in children dosing must be individualized. Medication administration to the children must focus on age-related developmental considerations. Because the pharmacokinetic and pharmacodynamics drug effects are less predictable in children, especially in preterm and young infants, because of their much smaller body size and immaturity of their organ system.

Therefore, close monitoring is very important during medications to the children. Likewise, safe administration of the right medication with right dose, to the right patient, at right time, through right route, and in right approach is a critical issue because children are at highest risk for medication errors. Children are more vulnerable to potential side effects and overdose.

Ensuring safe administration of medications is multidisciplinary responsibility that involves the physician, pharmacist, and nurse who serve as check and balance team. Appropriate education of the nursing professionals is the key element to ensure reliable administration of medications.

Developmental Pharmacokinetics

Children's size can vary greatly, from 500 gram preterm neonate to 100 kg overweight teenager. Thus size and age are the key factors that affect the child's ability to handle the absorption, distribution, metabolism and elimination of drugs. All four pharmacokinetic functions are important considerations in the choice of medications and selecting dosages that can be safely prescribed for a child.

A. *Factors that Affect Absorption of Drugs:*
- Gastrointestinal: Gastric pH is high in neonates. It becomes same as with adult values by 2 years of age of the child. Acidic drugs are more bioavailable, and basic drugs have decreased bioavailability. Gastric and intestinal motility (transit time) is decreased in neonates and infants but increased in older infants and children. The bile acid pool and biliary function are diminished in the neonates and reach full capacity over the first several months of life.
- Rectal: Only selected drugs are suitable for rectal administration. In addition, length of exposure to the rectal mucosa affects absorption.
- Intramuscular: Absorption from intramuscular administration is variable in the pediatric age group secondary to—(a) blood flow and vasomotor instabilities, (b) insufficient muscle tone and contraction, and (c) decreased muscle oxygenation.
- Percutaneous: Absorption of drugs from skin decreased with increased thickness of the stratum corneum and directly related to skin hydration. Neonates and infants have increased skin permeability, allowing greater penetration of medication and a greater surface area-to-body weight ratio with potential for toxicity.
- Intraocular: Ophthalmic eye medication can cause systemic effects in infants and young children because the eye membranes of infant and neonates are particularly thin.

B. *Factors that Affect Distribution of Drugs:*
- Neonates have higher proportion of total body water that rapidly reduces during the first year of life. Adult values are gradually reached by 12 years of age. This factor is an important consideration related to the water solubility of a drug.
- Children have a lower proportion of body fat than do adults.
- Protein binding of drugs is age dependent. Total protein concentration at birth is only 80% of adult values, which leads to more free, or active drug circulation and potential for drug toxicity.
- Fetal albumin in the newborn period has limited drug-binding ability.
- An immature blood-brain barrier during the newborn period can lead to higher concentration of drugs in the brain than at other ages.

C. *Factors that Affect Metabolism of Drugs:*
- The newborn's enzymatic microsomal system is less effective.
- Liver maturation varies among individuals. Each liver enzyme becomes functional at a different rate.

D. *Factors that Affect Elimination of Drugs:*
- Glomerular filtration and tubular secretion are reduced at birth.
- There is gradual increase in renal function, with adult values reached by the first 1–2 years of life.

Pharmacodynamics is the study of drugs and their actions on living organisms. It refers to the physiological and biochemical effects of the drugs on the human body. Most of the drugs interact with cellular component to initiate a series of physiological and biochemical effects which can be found as local or systemic presentations. Effects of administered medication are evaluated by patient's clinical condition and using laboratory investigations.

The child will manifest clinical improvement if therapeutic effects of medications are optimal, otherwise the child can have deterioration of health status. There may be changes in the laboratory findings along with improvement of clinical conditions. Basic understanding of pharmacodynamics is essential for nurses to evaluate therapeutic effects and adverse effects of medications.

"Ten Rights" of Medications Administrations

"Ten rights" should be followed during administration of medications to prevent medication errors. Ten rights include—right patient, right medication/drug, right dose, right route, right time, right approach, right assessment, right information/explanation and education, right evaluation and right documentation.

Another "six rights" can be followed for safe medication practices which include—right prescription/order, right preparation/handling, right process of administration, right storage, right expiration date, right universal precautions and right discard of medications.

Selection of medication is based on child's need for pharmacologic therapy and the ability of the child's body to handle the drug; that is to absorb, distribute, metabolize and to eliminate the drug. Nursing responsibility in administering the "*right medication*" should be viewed as multistep process.

To administer "*right medication*", the nurse should do the following:

- Know the medication to be administered: its indications, action, contraindications, and potential side effects
- Understand the connection between the child's health status, related illness or disease and use of particular medication. If such linkage is not present, clarify the medication order
- Read the prescription/medication order correctly, if not clear, consult physician
- Be careful of look-alike drugs and sound-alike name of drugs
- Look for unusual characteristics, i.e., color, odor and consistency of the drugs
- Select the correct medication for the particular child. Be familiar with generic name and trade name of the drugs. Do not administer outdated medicines
- Verify the medication label with child's medication administration record (MAR). Administer medication from clearly labeled container only
- Triple verification of label can help to prevent medication identification errors
- Check the label when first obtaining the drug, then when preparing the dose and when returning the container to the patient's medication box or storage area or discarding it.

To administer "*right dose*" of medications, the nurse must practice the following:

- Remember there are "*two rights in dosing of medication*". Prescribing the correct dose for the child and dispensing the correct dose to the child
- Pediatric dosages are usually calculated based on body weight of the child in kilogram or using body surface area (BSA)
- BSA is primarily used when calculating doses of cancer chemotherapeutic drugs
- BSA can be calculated using by Nomogram for estimation of BSA or by.

  Mosteller's formula,that is BSA (m^2)

  $$= \frac{\sqrt{\text{weight (kg)} \times \text{height (cm)}}}{3{,}600}$$

- Adult dose reference ranges may be used in children who weigh more than 50 kg, rather than body weight in kg (some physicians/prescribers are using 40 kg as the cut-off point)
- Always double-check the math calculations when preparing a medication. Double checking helps to prevent mathematical errors and ensure that correct amount of medication is given to the child
- Verify the right dose using body weight in kilogram and comparing it with standard pediatric dose reference. Read the physician's order to know the correct dose

- Age related metabolic changes and organ dysfunction may be factors in addition to body weight that are considered in determining an appropriate dose of medication for an individual child
- Draw up an individualized dose before administering the medication to the child. It is important to set up equations in consistent fashion when drawing up medication from a multi-dose container or from a single-dose container that contains more medication than the ordered dose. Always measure the accurate dose of medication at eye level
- Administer IV medication cautiously from powdered medication. Dilute the powdered drugs with sterile water for injection or with sterile normal saline and determine the final concentration of medication. Then calculate how much dissolved medicine is needed to obtain the prescribed amount and dose
- Know the abbreviations and symbol used for medication to avoid errors.

To ensure *"right patient"* the nurse should identify the child by an identification band attached to his or her body not according to the bed number. Identification band should include name, date of birth, sex, identification or registration number, and other information as per hospital policy. Take the patients MAR to the bedside to perform double identifier check. Parent or family member should identify an infant or younger child. Ask older child her or his name. Be careful with same name and same last-name of the child.

The *"right route of administration of medication"* affects absorption, effectiveness and speed of action of medications, especially in children. Read the physician's direction about route of the medication to be administered, know the abbreviations and technique of medication for the particular child in specific route correctly.

Medications at *"right time"* in correct interval can affect therapeutic blood levels. Each institution may have its own policy about scheduled times for medication. The general rule of practice is to administer medication within the time frame of one half hour before or after the scheduled time period. Some medications are given with meals, just before meals, on an empty stomach or at specific time as mentioned. Give the medication according to the action expected, e.g., diuretics are given in morning, so that child will have fewer disturbances.

The "right approach" for medication to the child with age-appropriate explanation and administration technique affects the success of administering medications in the least traumatic manner. Behavioral and developmental considerations of the child for medications should be a significant approach.

The important information should be obtained before medications for *"right assessment"* regarding child's health conditions by details history, physical examination and laboratory investigations including diet and fluid intake. History of drug allergy, altered vital signs and laboratory findings are important for continuation or discontinuation of medications.

The *"right information or explanation and education"* is a significant nursing responsibility during medications to the child regarding reason of drug therapy, its adverse effects, and duration of treatment, precautions to be followed and for drug compliance.

The *"right evaluation"* should be done after administration of medication to note the desired therapeutic outcome, presence or absence of side effects, improvement or deterioration the child's health condition and any dependence or tolerance of the medication.

The *"right documentation"* must be done in the child's record sheet/chart to note the administration of medications in details (date, time, name of drugs, dose, route, time interval), and to avoid repetition of dose as a medicolegal record for the child's treatment. If patient/child/parent refuses medication, document the event on child's chart and notify the physician responsible for the patient at that time. If any medication error occurs, report it immediately and implement appropriate patient protection procedure.

Prevention of Medication Errors

Medication errors indicate administering wrong medicine, administering an incorrect dose of medicine, failing to administer a prescribed medicine, or administering the medicine either at the incorrect time or via the incorrect route. Every effort should be made to prevent errors in medications. Following "rights of medications" helps to prevent medication errors.

Common errors in medication administrations are: (a) prescribing and transcription errors, and (b) dispensing and administration errors.

Prescribing and transcription errors: Medication errors related to prescribing are generally grouped into four categories: (1) poor hand writing, (2) decimal errors, (3) misused abbreviations, and (4) incorrect calculations. These can be avoided by following practices:

- Computerized or typed prescription can prevent prescribing errors which helps to eliminate problems of incorrect interpretation of handwriting.
- When typed medication orders are not common practice, then nurse must carefully interpret handwritten prescription and clarify the orders that are not clearly written, to avoid transcription errors.
- Decimal errors are most common error in pediatric calculations. These errors can be avoided by never placing a decimal and a zero after a whole number (called the trailing zero) because the decimal point might not be read correctly (e.g., 6.0 mL might be read as 60 mL. So it should be written as 6 mL). A zero should be placed before fractions (called the leading zero) that are less than 1 (e.g., it should be 0.6 mL not .6 mL, which might be confused with 6 mL, if the decimal is inadvertently missed)
- Avoid use of abbreviations (e.g., HS can be considered as "half strength" or at bedtime")
- Calculations of medication doses should be done on correct and present body weight.

Dispensing and administration errors: Nurses are involved in these errors when there is wrong calculations and incorrect drawn up of medications. Avoid these errors by following practices:

- Double check all math calculations of drug doses
- Double check amounts that are drawn up for dispensing
- Clarify medication orders whenever any confusion occurs
- Follow standard technique of administration of medication as per guidelines
- When a child/patient or parent questions whether a medication should be administered, then answer questions and double check the medication order and discuss the concern.

Administering Medications to Children

Administering medication to infants and children can be a challenge for the nurse. Behavioral and developmental considerations should always be emphasized. Explanation about reason and procedure of administration of medications should be simple and appropriate to the child's cognitive level. A child may cooperate more with the procedure if he or she understands why it is being done. Following "*Tips for Medication Administration*" to children should be practiced.

For neonates and young infants:

- Use oral syringe (without needle) to administer medication for accurate measurement
- Mix the medication with a small amount of milk (3–5 mL), especially if bitter tasting
- Hold the infant in an upright position while delivering oral medication, unless contraindicated
- Administer medication either before a feeding or when the infant is not sleeping deeply after a feeding
- Instill the medication in the side of the infant's mouth slowly
- Allow the infant to swallow the medication between sucking
- Gently stroke the infant's cheek to elicit the sucking reflex.

For toddlers:

- Use oral syringe (without needle) to administer medication for accurate measurement
- Mix the medication with a small amount of milk (3–5 mL), especially if bitter tasting
- Pills/tablets can be crushed and mixed with compatible syrup or milk. Enteric-coated pills should not be crushed
- If the toddler is not able to cooperate in taking medications, place the toddler on the lap and hold legs and arms firmly. Do not force during administration of medication. This is two-person procedure; second person can give the medication into child's mouth slowly in small amount. Check the child has swallowed the medicine and keep the toddler's cheeks together to prevent the medication to spit out
- Praise the toddlers after the medication has been taken.

For preschool-aged children:

- Give a simple explanation for why the medication is being given (e.g., cough will reduce)
- Never lie to a child that an injection will not hurt
- Give realistic choices, that will allow the child to control fear and anxiety
- Praise the child for his or her own efforts after taking medications
- If the child refuses to take medication, hold the child as for toddler and give medication

For school-aged children and adolescent:

- Explain the reason and specific instructions as appropriate to the child's cognitive level
- Be alert about taking of medication by the child. Some children of these age groups may hide their medication and pretend they have taken the drug
- Teach the children about importance of medications in chronic illness, potential side effects and need for necessary medical help
- Help the child to develop sense of responsibility for their own health care
- Prepare these children for discharge from health care setting by educating them about safe self-medication as per prescription and advice

Additional tips for administration of *medication to children:*

- Never leave medications at the child's bedside unless permitted by specific instructions
- When checking medication labels, pay close attention to the spelling of the medication because many drugs have similar name. Check the expiration date of the drugs always
- Prepare medications in a quite well lighted area
- Ensure about written prescription before preparation and administration of medications in the patient's treatment sheet.
- Follow the institutional policy and protocol about verbal orders for administration of medications. This should be practiced only in emergency and unusual circumstances. The nurse who takes such orders should listen to what the physician says, write the order down, and then read the order back to the prescribers. Verbal order must be written by the physician later and to be recorded in the treatment sheet afterward
- Check drugs for discoloration or unusual precipitates
- Use a calculator to check drug doses and be sure to calculate doses two times
- Do not administer a drug that another nurse has prepared
- If medications are prepared in a syringe beforehand, always label the syringe with the name of the drug, its concentration, date and time of drawing and initial signature
- Remember to remove syringe (and needle, needle cap, if used), from the child's bedside and place in an appropriate waste disposal containers
- Be aware of drug incompatibilities with other medications or fluids. This is especially important when administering multiple IV medications or when the

patient is receiving total parenteral nutrition or lipid

- Check the time interval between medication administrations for all drugs to ensure that enough time has elapsed
- Label and store the medications *"for external use only"* separately from other medications
- Record the amount of IV medications in the child's intake and output chart
- Follow strict aseptic techniques for administration of injectable medications
- Be aware of potential drug-drug and drug-food interactions
- The use of topical anesthetic before intramuscular injection may help to reduce child's pain. Institutional policy should be followed for pain prevention and management
- Take a careful drug allergy history and be sure that an "Allergy Alert" is maintained in the child's chart or treatment sheet
- Be especially careful when administering medications that are potentially toxic, such as antineoplastic drugs, digoxin, or insulin. Medications delivered by parenteral route also demand vigilance both in preparation and while infusing

PREVENTION OF INFECTIONS IN CHILD HEALTH CARE

Prevention of Infections in Hospitalized Children

Health care-associated infections (HCAIs) or nosocomial infections or hospital-acquired infections (HAIs) are those infections which developed within the hospital or produced during hospital stay by cross infections from one patient to another or from doctors, nurses, visitors, and attendant or other hospital staff. This infection was not present or incubating at the time of hospitalization.

Nosocomial infections are widespread and important public health problem with increasing economic and human impact because of overcrowding of people, more frequent impaired immunity (due to age, illness, and treatments), new microorganisms and increasing bacterial resistance to antibiotics.

The common nosocomial infections occurring in health care settings include urinary tract infections (UTIs), surgical site infections (SSIs), pneumonia/lower respiratory tracts infections [RTIs, ventilator associated pneumonias (VAPs)], and bloodstream infections/bacteremia (mainly related to vascular device infections). Other HCAIs include skin and soft tissue infections, upper respiratory infections, eye and ENT infections, etc.

Health care associated infections are significant problems in NICU, SNCU, PICU, pediatric high dependency units, pediatric surgical wards and pediatric operation theaters (OTs). Common risk factors related to HCAIs are severity of underlying diseases, frequent invasive procedures, prolonged intravenous fluid therapy, repeated needle pricks, use of various devices, poor nutritional status, malpractices and non-compliance with infection control practices and protocols.

Standard Precautions for Infection Control in Healthcare Settings

In healthcare settings many infections can be prevented and controlled by practicing basic precautions which are needed to be followed by each health care professionals for all patients at all times, regardless of age, diagnosis and infection status. These practices help to reduce the risk of transmission of blood borne and other pathogens from both recognized and unrecognized source of infections.

These precautions are termed as "Standard Precautions" and include the following practices:

- Hand hygiene by soap-water hand wash and use of antiseptic hand rub.
- Use of personal protective equipment (PPEs).
- Safe handling of biomedical waste (BMW) and hazardous waste.
- Appropriate handling of patient care equipment, instruments and linen.

- Environment cleaning and disinfection including spill management.
- Additional precautions including airborne precautions, droplet precautions, and contact precautions.

Beside these precautions other practices should be promoted to prevent HCAIs, such as patents cohorting and screening, placement of sick patients in all health care settings and hospitals, management of occupational exposure, evidence-based infection control practices, antibiotic stewardship, patient safety program, vaccination and surveillance.

Strategies to Prevent Health Care-Associated Infections in Hospitalized Children

- Meticulous hand hygiene practices with soap and water hand washing and use of antiseptic hand rubs as appropriate *(Refer Unit - 2, Procedure - 2, Hand Hygiene in Health Care Settings)*
- Appropriate use of PPEs, i.e., gloves, gown, cap, mask, eye shield, protective plastic apron, shoe cover or separate shoe for the designated area (such as NICU, SNCU, neonatal ward, PICU, OTs)
- Maintenance of "standard precautions and additional precautions of infection control"
- Aseptic precautions during invasive procedures (e.g., during parenteral medications, fluid therapy, intubation, PICC lines preparation and use, surgical interventions, wound care, dialysis, etc.) with appropriate use of sterilized supplies and standard precautions of infection control
- Safe injection practices (use sterile syringe and sterile needle, one syringe and one needle at one time, use of auto-disable syringes, skin antisepsis during IV cannulation, antiseptic cleaning of IV cannula hub and port with 70% alcohol swab, precautions for prevention of sharp injury, hand hygiene, etc.)
- Adherence with procedure-specific guidelines for prevention of common nosocomial infections (such as UTIs, SSIs, VAPs, nosocomial pneumonia, upper respiratory infections, bloodstream infections, vascular catheter-associated infections, soft tissue or skin infections, etc.)
- Barrier nursing and practice of isolation techniques for infected patients (such as children with communicable diseases, infected neonates and children)
- Promotion of hygienic practices of the sick hospitalized children, family members and visitors, such as hand hygiene, daily bath/sponge, skin care, oral hygiene, dental care, care of hair, use of shoes, clean bed and bed linen, clean clothing, clean surrounding at bed side, safe water intake, food hygiene, regular bowel and bladder habit, use of toilets, waste disposal and elimination of bad habits (such as nail biting, thumb sucking, spitting, smoking, substance abuse, etc.)
- Maintenance of appropriate nutritional and dietary intake with age appropriate and disease appropriate diet for the infant/child by oral or enteral route or whenever indicated in parenteral route
- Provision and availability of safe drinking water supply
- Rational use of antibiotics and periodic review of antibiotic policies and prescriptions
- Appropriate use and disposal of single-use disposable supplies
- Sterilization and disinfections with decontamination and appropriate cleaning of equipment and reusable care items. Use of autoclaving, use chemical sterilizing, and disinfecting agents must be done as per standard recommended instructions. Appropriate use of concurrent and terminal disinfection and sterilization methods
- Strict maintenance of "Waste Management Protocol" for general waste and BMW by segregation, handling, storage, transport and disposal of waste
- Adherence to "Sharp management protocol" and "Spill management Protocol"
- Safe handling of laboratory specimens, body fluids, blood and blood products

- Adherence to the management of accidental exposure of body fluids and post exposure prophylaxis protocol
- Improvement of hospital environment with good ventilation, cleanliness, soothing light, safe water supply, mosquito control, pest and animal control, appropriate drainage and sewage management, avoidance of overcrowding, etc.
- Adequate water sanitation, linen management, laundry services and kitchen services
- Strict adherence to house-keeping protocol with house-keeping team, supervisors, and house-keeping supplies. Maintenance of cleanliness of floor, walls, wash basins, furniture, toilets, care equipment such as bed pan, urinal, etc. Promotion of practice of wet mopping, damp dusting and no use of brooms inside the units/hospital wards
- Adherence to entry guidelines and restriction of visitors in special care units and general wards to prevent overcrowding in care areas
- Maximizing space and staff pattern in health care facilities
- Dealing of outbreaks of infections in health facility. Identifying the outbreak, investigating the outbreaks, describing the outbreaks, immediate interventions of control measures for outbreak management, communications with local administrations and higher authorities and follow-up
- Completion of "immunization as per schedule" to the children to protect the children from vaccine preventable infections.
- Health checkup, screening of susceptible staff and immunization to all health care providers as per institutional policy
- Assigned " Infection Control Nurse" and good coordinated infection control team
- Regular training and awareness program on infection control practices for healthcare professional, family members and visitors
- Implementation of "infection control surveillance program" in all healthcare institutions
- Well-functioning "infection control committee" for implementation of infection control program in each health facility

Prevention of Infections among Children in Community and Home

- Meticulous hand hygiene with soap and water hand washing before food intake and after use of toilet or handling of any dirty and contaminated objects. Use of hand sanitizer or antiseptic hand rubs when hand washing is not possible
- Maintenance of personal hygiene—daily bath, skin care, care of hair, oral hygiene, clean clothing, respiratory etiquette during coughing and sneezing and wearing of shoes
- Adequate rest, sleep and physical exercise
- Environmental hygiene—general cleanliness of surroundings, fresh air, dust control, water sanitation, safe drinking water, pest and animal control, mosquito control and use of mosquito nets
- Promotion of nutritional status with exclusive breastfeeding, introduction of complementary feeding after 6 months of age, balanced diet, adequate safe water intake, food hygiene for optimal nutrition
- Compliance with health instructions the "infection control practices" (e.g., use of mask, safe distance with people, hand washing or sanitization, and respiratory etiquette for prevention of COVID-19)
- Awareness generation programs and community involvement for hygiene promotion and promotion of environmental sanitation (water, air, soil).
- Behavior change communication using different media for removal of bad habits and promotion of good healthy habits should be organized in community (at home, schools, clinics, ICDS centers, etc.)

PRINCIPLES OF PAIN MANAGEMENT IN CHILDREN

Children experience pain just as much as adults. Children of all ages experience pain; preterm infants likely experience even more pain than an adult when subjected to same stimulus. Although management of pain has improved over last few decades, particularly for predictable pain problems (such as postoperative pain), but underestimation and under-treatment of pain in children remain problems till now. Untreated pain may have significant and lifelong physiologic and psychological consequences like altered pain sensitivity.

Pain has been defined as an unpleasant sensory and emotional experience associated with actual or potential tissue damage or described in terms of such damage (Defined by International Association for the Study of Pain, 1979).

Acute (nociceptive) pain is a common adverse stimulus that occurs as a result of injury, surgery, or illness. The severity of the physical damage and physiological response may play a role in the child's overall perception of pain. Acute pain experience generally resolves as the body heals.

Chronic pain may develop from or as consequence of acute pain, if the pain experience extends beyond the normal trajectory of healing for the amount of tissue damaged sustained. Chronic nociceptive pain stimulation may alter excitability in the peripheral and central nervous systems, resulting in sustained and recurrent pain having neuropathic qualities.

Clinical characteristics of neuropathic pain include dysesthesia (impaired sensitivity to touch such as paresthesia and cutaneous hypoesthesia), hyperalgesia (i.e., excessive sensation from pain), and allodynia (i.e., non-painful stimuli such as light touch, is perceived as painful), motor abnormalities and autonomic disturbances. Differing from acute pain, neuropathic pain involves the erroneous generation and transmission of information in the nervous system that often persists and even intensified over time.

The problems of untreated pain in children have been recognized by the professionals. They recommend the need for effective pain management in neonates and older children. They also address on special needs in pediatric pain assessment, management, research and education. Effective pain management is an essential component of child health care that encompasses initial pain assessment, therapeutic interventions, monitoring and reassessment or evaluation.

Pain Assessment in Children

Many factors including anger, fear, loneliness, strange hospital environment, separation from parents, emotions of anxiety, depression, and fear of body intrusion can alter perception and expression of pain. The followings must be considered when assessing pain in children as important components and guidelines for pain assessment and management.

- *Biological factors:* Age, gender, genetic characteristic and previous pain experiences
- *Type of pain:* Acute, chronic, recurrent, extensive, traumatic, surgical or due to treatment
- *Psychological factors:* Child's pain perception, present coping style, and previous coping techniques, perception of pain control and temperament (ability to adapt to the situation, negative versus positive in mood and reactions)
- *Cognitive factors:* Cognitive level or ability to describe pain and understanding of the pain experience
- *Cultural and social factors:* Standard by behavior, e.g., expression and acceptance of pain
- *Parental influence:* Parental reaction to the situation, separation from parents often intensified child's pain experience
- Subjective reporting by the child (e.g., children have words for pain)
- Behavioral observations (e.g., crying, facial expression motor response, clench fists, lie rigid or curled in fetal position)
- Physiological monitoring (e.g., tachycardia, variation in respiratory rate, pupil

dilation, peripheral vasoconstriction and increased blood pressure)
- Availability of "Pain assessment tools" for children.

Commonly Used Pain Assessment Tools for Children

Pain assessment tools should be selected based on age of the child and type of pain situation. The commonly used pain assessment tools are:

- ***Subjective Rating Scales***
  - Direct questioning: For children of more than 2 years with adequate cognitive abilities
  - Faces pain scale—Revised: For children having age 5 years or more
  - FACES: For children of 3–18 years
  - Visual analog scale: For children having age 5 years or more.
- ***Procedural Pain***
  - Neonatal facial coding system: For preterm and term infants aged 4 months or less
  - Neonatal infant pain scale (NIPS): For preterm and term infants
  - Premature Infant Pain Profile (PIPP): For preterm and term neonates.
- ***Postoperative Pain***
  - Premature Infant Pain Profile (PIPP): For preterm and term neonates
  - CRIES scale (Crying, Requires oxygen administration, Increased heart rate and blood pressure, Expression, Sleeplessness): For term neonates
  - FLACC scale (Face, Legs, Activity, Cry, Consolability): For children aged 2 months to 7 years (Willis, Merkel et al. 2003)
  - Toddler-Preschooler postoperative pain scale: For children aged 1–5 years.
- ***Chronic and Recurrent Pain***
  - Gauvain-Piquard rating scale: For long-term pain in cancer patients of 2–6 years age
  - Varni-Thompson pediatric pain questionnaire: For children aged 8 years or more
  - Pain diary: For the child who is able to write and record pain events.
- ***Nonverbal and Cognitive Tools***
  - Pain assessment tool (PAT): For preterm and term infants
  - COMFORT behavior scale: For 0–3 years age group
  - Pediatric pain profile (PPP): For children aged 1–18 years
  - Non-communicating children's pain checklist-Revised (vocal, sleeping, eating, social, facial, activity, body/limbs, physiologic signs): For children aged 3–18 years
  - Non-communicating children's pain checklist-Postoperative version (vocal, social, facial, activity, body and limbs, physiologic signs): For children aged 3–19 years
  - FLACC scale (Malviya et al. 2006): For children aged 4–19 years.

Therapeutic Interventions for Pain Management

Assessment of comfort level for pain is the first step in the process of pain management. Once the presence of pain is identified then interventions must be implemented to treat or to manage the pain. Pain management process consists of explanation and teaching about the pain relief techniques by pharmacological and non-pharmacological interventions. It is important to discuss the expectation of the child and the family regarding pain relief measure according to their level of understanding. Health care provider must develop a realistic goal for pain management based on coping behavior of the child and family believes.

Pharmacologic Interventions for Pain Management

Pain is best managed by proactive approach. It is much more effective to anticipate pain and treat it adequately, rather than to treat pain when it is present. Medications must be administered to manage moderate to severe pain. Biobehavioral techniques should be used to enhance the effectiveness of medications. Mild pain may be effectively managed by the use of biobehavioral methods alone or in conjunction with nonopioid analgesics.

Medication must be administered on an around the clock basis, if pain is present for most of the time. But if pain is present on an episodic basis, medication should be given as needed. Pain assessment must always be done before administration of medications. If the child can take oral medications and pain is controlled, then this is optimum method. Intravenous administration of medication is the method of choice in severe pain. Avoid intramuscular injections whenever possible as this route is more painful and children are usually fearful of needles.

Pharmacologic medications for pain relief include nonopioid analgesics, opioid analgesics, coanalgesics and local anesthetics.

Nonopioid analgesics include acetaminophen and nonsteroidal anti-inflammatory drugs (NSAIDs) and salicylates. They are most effective for treatment of mild to moderate pain. They can be used as a component of multimodal approach for severe pain (e.g., in conjunction with opioid analgesics).

Opioid analgesics include morphine, fentanyl, hydromorphone, methadone and meperidine. The effects of these drugs are mediated by different receptors in the central nervous system, therefore when one is not very effective, another may be useful. Concern over addiction is a common misunderstanding and may result in reluctance to administer opioids. It is important to distinguish between tolerance and physical dependence and psychological dependence. Addiction is extremely rare in children. Opioids may be administered by many routes including oral, sublingual, transdermal, IV (bolus, continuous infusion) or regional analgesia (e.g., peripheral nerve block). Injections are not recommended and are especially considered unacceptable for administration of pain medications to children.

Coanalgesics are drugs that play a role in pain management because of their effects of enhancing analgesia of other drugs, reducing anxiety or exerting an analgesic effect of their own. Coanalgesics drugs include tricyclic antidepressants, antihistamines, anticonvulsants (gabapentin), alpha-agonists (clonidine) and membrane stabilizers (lidocaine, mexiletine).

These medications are used depending on the type of pain, cause of pain, severity of pain, past pain experience and tolerance. Dosage of analgesics required to relieve pain usually vary by child's age, weight, route, frequency and techniques of administration. Always monitor the child for side effects associated with analgesics used and intervene accordingly.

Local anesthetics should be used to alleviate pain associated with procedures such as lumbar puncture, venipuncture, injections, wound repair and accessing implanted ports. Injectable local anesthetics (e.g., lidocaine, procaine) are administered subcutaneously around the area to be manipulated, 5–10 minutes before the procedure. A small needle should be used for administration of local anesthetics. The area should be tested for sensitivity before performing the procedure.

Topical (transdermal) anesthetics can be used alone or to reduce the pain of local infiltration. Lidocaine-prilocaine cream [e.g., eutectic mixture of local anesthetics (EMLA)] must be applied to intact skin at least 30–60 before the procedure. Skin refrigerants or vapocoolants such as Frigiderm, Fluoromethane and ethyl chloride are effective in reducing brief procedural pain such as injections and lumbar puncture. Lidocaine iontophoresis over intact skin has been demonstrated to reduce pain with venipuncture.

Lidocaine, epinephrine, and tetracaine (LET), is an anesthetic used for laceration repair. It is available as liquid or gel that is applied directly on the wound and on a cotton ball or swab and held firmly for 10–30 minutes.

Lidocaine jelly (2% water-soluble lubricant) can be used to minimize pain associated with urethral and enteral tube insertion. It should not be used over damaged skin or mucous membranes and having history of allergy to amide-type anesthetics. For urethral catheterization, insert lidocaine into the urethra 3–5 minutes before the procedure to allow anesthesia to occur. Use caution not to introduce lubricant into the lumen of the enteral catheter when coating the tube before insertion.

Nonpharmacologic Interventions for Pain Management

Nonpharmacological or biobehavioral techniques are used to manage mild pain and augment efficacy of medications in patients with moderate to severe pain. These interventions are now termed as complementary or alternative therapies. Some of these methods may result in an actual reduction in pain intensity but they are probably most effective as coping strategies. These techniques allow the child to play an active role and control over the pain response thus reduce distress, anxiety and pain perception.

Nonpharmacological and comfort interventions for pain management include biobehavioral and biophysical strategies. *Biobehavioral methods* include cognitive-behavioral interventions such as distraction, relaxation, biofeedback, imagery, auditory stimuli, controlled breathing, and hypnosis. *Biophysical management techniques* include swaddling, containment, holding, touching, rocking, positioning, non-nutritive suckling, sweet solutions, kangaroo care, traditional massage, transcutaneous electric nerve stimulation (TENS), environmental modification, application of heat or cold, acupuncture and acupressure.

Implementation of these interventions should be done in developmentally appropriate manner. Some biobehavioral interventions are not appropriate for certain age group or require a degree of cognitive development. For example, cutaneous stimulation may provide too much stimulus to preterm neonates, toddlers and preschoolers may not tolerate TENS, but preschoolers may cooperate well with imagery.

Parental involvement is an important component of pain management in children during both assessment and interventions. Therefore carefully preparing the parents to support the child to cope with painful procedures must be emphasized. Reinforce on parents role to help the child by giving specific, concrete and developmentally appropriate suggestions such as holding the child, speaking in low and soothing voice, maintaining eye contact and distracting the child. Sometimes parents may feel tired or scared when helping their child during procedures. Support from the nursing personnel typically helps the parents to recover from their own stress and anxiety and to continue as an effective support to the child for pain reduction.

Cognitive-Behavioral Interventions

The goal of cognitive-behavioral interventions is to teach patients to identify, evaluate and to change sensory patterns and thought process to facilitate coping behaviors. These techniques are designed to change either child's own behavior or the behaviors of the adults (parents, doctors, nurses), who interact with him or her. These strategies typically include combinations of the followings:

- *Preparation for the procedure:* Providing developmentally appropriate information to the child and family helps to develop realistic expectation of the pain and to reduce fear for the procedure.
- *Distraction:* Obtaining active involvement of the child according to the developmental level and preference, such as manipulating play materials, reading books, playing games, etc. Use of distraction remains a dominant strategy for reducing behavioral distress and relieving pain, despite the lack of evidence that distraction is effective at reducing or relieving pain in children. This technique should be used with pharmacologic interventions.
- *Biofeedback:* This gives information to the child about a physiologic function (heart rate, skin temperature, muscle tension) often through a visual display

or audible tone. The child is instructed to use mental imagery to increase or decrease response in the system being monitored. Reinforcement occurs when the child effects change in the system. This technique requires specialized training and equipment.

- *Modeling and rehearsal:* These are performed to demonstrate positive coping behaviors (through an adult or on stuffed animal or by video tape) to provide opportunity to practice the situation thus to reduce the stress and anxiety for better coping.
- *Controlled breathing:* This can focus the child's attention and help to induce relaxation. The child must be monitored for hyperventilation. This method can be done by the older children as deep breath-in through nose and exhale through pursed lips. It can also be done by counting 1 to 10 while inhaling and then saying the number with each exhalation.
- *Relaxation:* This can help to reduce anxiety and muscle tension to decrease the pain perception. Controlled breathing is frequently a component of relaxation. Imagery and hypnosis also able to induce relaxation. Children often require help to implement relaxation techniques under stressful condition. Practicing this technique before the painful events increases its success. It should be done in quiet environment with comfortable position and speaking in low, calm and measured tone. There is no evidence to indicate that relaxation alone is effective in lessening chronic, cancer, surgical or procedural pain. Therefore this should be combined with analgesics, distraction, imagery or hypnosis.
- *Imagery:* Typically, the more senses one involves in the imagery. The child is actively involved in visualizing a situation as image (imaging feeling, seeing, hearing a situation). Imagery begins with achieving a relaxed state. Guide the child to choose a favorite place. Cue the child to experience this familiar surrounding by exploring the sights, sounds, smells and his or her feelings when in special place.
- *Hypnosis:* During hypnosis, the child enters in an altered state of consciousness characterized by focused attention and profound relaxation. Hypnotic state induction should be performed under supervision of an experienced practitioner and requires practice by the child.

Biophysical Interventions

Biophysical techniques attempt to affect physiologic responses directly during pain experience. These strategies used to reduce pain in older children and adolescents. These are usually contraindicated in the high risk neonates. These interventions include the following strategies:

- *Environmental modification:* Reduce noxious stimuli by decreasing noise and light intensity. Provide periods of undisturbed rest and sleep. Care environment should be modified to reduce bad stimuli to help the child to cope with the situation.
- *Positioning:* Therapeutic positioning provides support for body alignment and reduces muscle tension over painful areas (e.g., knee flexed position can reduce pain with an abdominal incision). For infants, swaddling and containment provides boundaries and limit excessive motor response facilitating self-regulation in preterm infants. Containment can be provided by tucking blanket rolls or nesting around the infant or by holding with hands during painful procedures as hand containment. Holding is comforting for children of all ages and limits uncontrolled movement but might exacerbate pain. Infants older than 3–6 months often fight with swaddling, which may intensify pain and anxiety.
- *Interpersonal contact:* Skin to skin contact or kangaroo care with mother and holding with sucking during painful procedures reduces infant's pain response. The comforting benefits of holding are dependent on the child's temperament

and pain situation. Preterm infants respond more positively to firm pressure given by the caregiver on their head or heels than on the trunk.

- *Sucking:* Sucking during painful procedures in addition to other analgesia, attenuates pain distress and has pacifying effect for preterm infants and neonates. Sucking a pacifier at a rate at least 30 sucks per minute provide an analgesic effect. No short-term and long-term negative effects of non-nutritive sucking have been identified in the studies. Offering of pacifier or breast sucking or encouraging hand-to-mouth behaviors in infants during painful procedure help to reduce pain responses.
- *Use of sucrose:* Ingestion of sucrose decreases pain behaviors in both term and preterm infants. A systematic review of the research found that 24% solution of sucrose was effective in alleviating procedural pain in neonates. Other sweet-tasting solutions such as 12.5% dextrose, 30% glucose and 30% fructose reduce pain behaviors in newborns. Breast milk and breastfeeding are also having analgesic effect. Sucrose should be used with caution in any neonate having unstable blood glucose levels. A pacifier can be dipped in sucrose and offer to the infant or sucrose can be instilled into the baby's mouth by syringe followed by use of pacifier. Use of sweet-solution and sucking may reduce pain through multisensorial pathways, thus being more effective in combination rather than alone. They should be offered to the infant during painful procedure, either alone or to augment pharmacologic methods for moderate to severe pain.
- *Rocking:* Rocking by caregivers decrease recovery time from painful procedures in term neonates, but stimulated rocking using air mattress is not effective in decreasing pain response. Rocking may relax young children and reduce tension, but if there is overstimulation then it may contribute to increase pain perception.
- *Cutaneous stimulation and massage:* Stimulation of the skin and underlying tissues may provide sensory input to reduce or block transmission of painful stimuli. Cutaneous stimulation may be performed over painful areas, on localized areas or by total-body massage. If direct cutaneous stimulation is not possible or tolerated, it may be applied adjacent to the painful area. It should be used cautiously in preterm infants.

  Massage may be performed using hands or a vibrator, with constant rhythmic movement of moderate intensity. Light pressure is often perceived as a tickle and heavy pressure may induce more pain.
- *Thermal application:* This may involve application of heat, cold or ice. For trauma-associated pain, cold may decrease inflammation and muscle spasms. Ice massage is effective for headaches, musculoskeletal pain, pain due to injection and in brief procedures. Wrap cold and hot packs so that the pack feels cool or warm but not uncomfortable. Heat and cold application is not recommended for use in infants, who are more prone to thermal injury because of their immature skin structure. These interventions should be avoided in children with altered skin sensations and in non-verbal children.
- *TENS:* This method may interfere with pain signal transmission by use of a small electrical current applied to the skin through conductive pads attached to a battery-operated generator. It causes a tingling sensation that can make the child fearful. Demonstration of the equipment on parent and then applying on the non-painful area on the child followed by moving to painful area help to reduce fear in the child.
- *Acupuncture and acupressure:* Inserting fine needles at the acupuncture points reduces pain. Acupressure is a noninvasive form of acupuncture, whereby manual pressure is applied to the skin at acupuncture points. Acupressure may be

more readily accepted by children than acupuncture due to fear of needles.

Management of pain is typically more successful by using multimodal approach. Specific pain situations (procedural pain, acute pain, chronic pain) require different methods and approaches for optimal pain management. Severe pain is always a medical emergency and should be managed accordingly.

Effective management of pain in any situation requires maintaining a high index of suspicion for the presence of pain, assessment of pain with valid and reliable tools, use of nonpharmacologic interventions and to augment pharmacologic interventions when indicated, followed by reassessment of pain to evaluate the adequacy of interventions. Pain management must be individualized for the child, family and the pain situation. Adequate pain management is an ethical imperative. All members of the health care team must advocate for the patients and work as a team with the family members to achieve effective management of pain in children.

PRINCIPLES AND GENERAL GUIDELINES FOR PEDIATRIC PROCEDURES

Scientific principles must be followed during performance of pediatric nursing procedures in holistic and comprehensive approaches. Related anatomy and physiology of the system including all organs must be reviewed to understand the pathophysiology of the medical or surgical illnesses or clinical conditions. Microbiology is important to relate with disease pathology and infections control measures. Pharmacology should be reviewed to make treatment modalities clear with the use of medications. Psychology and sociology should be correlated to the children and family members and priority needs to be considered for family centered care. Fundamentals of nursing sciences and principles of advance nursing procedures should be included during performance of procedures on the children. Procedures for children need to be performed in both facility and community (home, clinic, school) settings, so principles of community health nursing should also be incorporated. Birth-related history or obstetrical information should be reviewed for the neonates, infants, and young children to understand their health problems, diseases and congenital anomalies.

Childhood disease conditions should be explained and discussed before performing procedures related to particular clinical situations. Childhood health problems should not be considered as miniature form of adult diseases, so special understanding for the childhood diseases and disorders is required for better performances of procedures. Neonatal health problems are different than older children in all aspects including pathophysiology and types of illness (such as congenital anomalies, prematurity, perinatal asphyxia, etc.), so special approaches are required for optimum outcome after any interventions.

Strategies to be followed for Performing Procedure on Children

The following strategies need to be emphasized to perform any procedure for the children:

1. *Clinical guidelines:* All procedures should be performed following clinical practice guidelines with evidence-based standard protocol. During performance of procedure scientific principles should be followed with developmental considerations. The institutional policy must give importance on infection control protocol and biomedical waste management. For performing any intervention, available "Standard Operating Protocol (SOP)' and "Standard Treatment Protocol (STP)" should be consulted and followed as feasible and possible.
2. *Equipment and supplies required* should be agc-appropriate for the child and specific for the particular procedure. Prevention of cross-contaminations and transmission of microorganisms must be

avoided through the used supplies and equipment. Ensure all equipment and supplies are functioning properly and available as required.

3. *Assessment of child's health status* before each procedure should be done (detailed related history, physical examination, laboratory values, and investigation findings) to identify the severity of illness and to plan for interventions. Assess child's anxiety, level of understanding and ability to perform self-care to provide necessary support to the child. Assessment of family members should also be done for their anxiety, understanding and previous adverse experience of hospitalization.
4. *Preparation for procedures:* Before performing the procedure healthcare professional should do self-preparation and prepare assistant, whenever needed. Preparation is also required for arrangement of necessary supplies and working environment. Preparation of the child and the parents or family members must be done with appropriate explanation and discussion about their concern. Specific instructions before initiation of the procedure (e.g., NPO, pain medication) should be followed.
5. *Performing the specific procedure for the child* should be done with rationale following scientific principles and point of emphasis. Special points to remember or care reminder and handling of unexpected situations must be emphasized and followed during performance of the procedure. Individualized approach should be followed considering the age specific growth and development of the child. Performance of all procedures should always be skillful and competency based.
6. *Post-procedure evaluation of the child and family:* Evaluate child's health status as appropriate to the procedure, ability of self-care and child's tolerance. Evaluate family members response to and coping with the procedure. Effectiveness of the procedure and occurrence of any untoward situation or problems related to the procedure should be evaluated promptly.
7. *Documentation of the procedure* with all related findings in medical records: Document followings in child's case sheet/ record—date and time of procedure, medications administered, type and size of supplies, findings of vital signs or hemodynamic monitoring, presence of any adverse effects, number of attempts at procedure, presence of parents during procedure and their response, child's response and tolerance of procedure, name of the person performing procedure and any assistant, etc.
8. *Communication with family and child* with age-appropriate simple language about post-procedure health status and plan of further management is also very important. Discuss about importance and technique of procedure performed, potential therapeutic and adverse effects and about any concern of the child and family members.
9. *Teaching and related instructions* for community and home-based care should be provided to the parents and to the child in developmental appropriate approach. Teaching can be given as incidental teaching or planned health teaching or educational program.
   Discuss about hygienic practices including hand hygiene, age appropriate diet and water intake, rest and sleep, exercise and activity of daily living, continuation of medications at home, immunizations and health checkup, prevention of accidents and injury, signs and symptoms of complications and new problems, need for medical help, assistance of community healthcare workers, need for transportation and its precautions, nearest referral facility, follow-up schedule and questions as asked by the family members.

General Guidelines for Performing Procedures on Children

- Perform hand hygiene. Don gloves as indicated (sterile or nonsterile) for the specific procedure. This helps to reduce transmission of microorganisms.

- Administer pain medication before procedure, as needed or prescribed, to manage pain and discomfort in the child. This will decrease fear and anxiety and promotes self-control of the child for better coping and cooperation during procedure.
- Collect and arrange all necessary supplies near the child's bed or in procedure room. Obtain extra supplies, if appropriate (e.g., extra syringe, needle, gloves, and catheter). This will promote efficient time management and provide an organized approach to the procedure. Having extra supplies in hand avoids prolonging procedure.
  Avoid delay to perform procedure after arrangement of supplies near the child; it can cause increased anxiety to the child and parents/family members due to waiting for procedure or looking equipment.
- Allow family members to accompany the child and healthcare personnel to the location where the procedure will be performed (if feasible), or allow them to wait in waiting area. Family presence and participation of family members during the procedures for their child has been demonstrated to be beneficial as better coping behavior for both the child and family.
  Remember, family members perceive themselves as active participants, caring for the child with the staff. Family presence has been viewed by the families as their right, obligation, and natural event. Family members also need emotional and psychosocial support from healthcare professionals.
- Move the child to treatment room or procedure room to perform painful procedure, whenever possible. If painful or traumatic procedures are performed in the child's bed or room, he or she might be fearful during the entire hospital stay with that experience in the particular bed or room. Other children and their families may be traumatized witnessing other children receiving painful procedures.
- Monitor the child's health status before, during and after the procedure, as indicated. Some procedures or medications may have adverse effects on the child's hemodynamic status. Continuous monitoring is essential.
- Perform the procedure or assist the physician or surgeon during the procedure following scientific principles, and standard precautions of infection control and considering developmental variations of the individual child. Complete the required task confidently, skillfully and promptly.
- Make the child comfortable in bed after the procedure and provide feeling of safety.
- Discard biohazards, single use disposable supplies and trash in appropriate containers to prevent injury and biohazards exposure to the staff members and others.
- Take care of reusable items by decontamination, cleaning, disinfection, sterilization and appropriate storage for next use to economize the time, energy and materials.
- Remove gloves and perform hand hygiene to prevent cross-contaminations and infections.
- Evaluate child's vital signs and health condition, as appropriate for the procedure. This ensures prompt detection of adverse effects resulting from procedure or medications, if administered.
- Provide period of debriefing for family members. Address family's concern and other psychosocial needs identified during the intervention. This provides consistent support to the family members.

UNIT 2

Neonatal Nursing Procedures

INTRODUCTION

Neonatal nursing is a specialized area of professional nursing services concerning care of the neonates during first 28 days of life. It includes care and nurturing of healthy, preterm, low birth weight (LBW) and sick neonates, individually or in groups in health care institutions or in communities.

Neonatal nursing procedures should be performed following same principles of the procedures for the older children or adults. Some special considerations must be emphasized for the neonates, as their problems including signs and symptoms of disease process are different from older children and adult.

General principles and guidelines for neonatal nursing procedures:

- Procedure should be performed based on priority need, individualized and cue based
- Clustering of care activities should be performed to prevent frequent handling of the small infants and to provide maximum rest with sleep.
- Gentle handling with developmental supportive care must be practiced for all neonates
- Mother should be allowed and involved for the care of sick neonates, unless mother is sick and unable to participate
- Clinical guidelines for the procedure must be followed, as per recommendations
- All necessary equipment, articles and supplies should be available ready near the infants
- Assessment of the neonates' vital signs and presence of any abnormal features should be done before performance of any procedure to identify hemodynamic stability of the neonates and feasibility of the procedure
- Preparation for the procedure should include self-preparation of the neonatal nurse/performer of the procedure and assistant (if required), environmental preparation, preparation of necessary equipment and supplies, preparation of parents and the neonate
- Performing the procedure in steps considering the rationale with scientific principles for each action
- Evaluation of the procedure should be done comparing with pre-procedural condition of the neonates and expected outcome
- Documentation must be done in details in neonates' case sheet and hospital records about the performed activity and observational findings during procedure
- Communication to the parents and other family members must be done regarding infant's condition, plan of management, possible outcome and complications
- Teaching to the parents (incidental or planned) should be organized about participation in neonatal care at hospital, continuation of care at home after discharge, danger signs, emergency medical help and follow-up care
- Infection control practices including standard precautions must be followed to prevent nosocomial infections of the infants. Waste management and handling of disposable items should be practiced as per institutional policy. Reusable

instruments, linens and other items should be taken care with decontamination, cleaning, disinfection and sterilization

- Standard treatment protocol (STP) and standard operating protocol (SOP) must be available in neonatal care units, [neonatal intensive care unit (NICU), special newborn care units (SNCU), neonatal ward, kangaroo mother care (KMC) ward] for the optimal care and treatment of the infants.

PROCEDURE–1: IMMEDIATE CARE OF STABLE NEONATES AT BIRTH IN DELIVERY ROOM

Clinical Guidelines for Immediate Care of Stable Neonates

The healthy stable newborn infant born at term between 38 and 42 weeks of gestation and cries immediately at birth with establishment of effective independent rhythmic respiration having an average birth weight and no congenital anomalies. The infant quickly adapts with extrauterine environment.

First minute of life (i.e., *first golden minute*) after birth is very significant for establishment of satisfactory and effective respiration. The first hour of life (i.e., *first golden hour*) is also very important as it has major influence on survival, future health, and well-being of the infants. So, immediate essential routine care of newly born infant after birth is prime importance for prevention of neonatal morbidity and mortality.

Intranatal assessment of fetal and maternal condition, using antenatal history, USG, partograph, obstetrical examination, etc., helps to identify the at-risk condition of the neonates. Initial assessment of fetal condition before birth must be done for gestational age, meconium stained amniotic fluid, high risk pregnancy and maternal health condition, and fetal anomalies on USG, fetal distress, prolonged labor, etc., those will help to anticipate the necessary care required for the infant after birth.

The basic and primary needs of the stable healthy neonates include establishment of breathing for air, warmth for prevention of hypothermia, own mother's milk for nutrition, prevention of infections by hygienic measures and identification of danger signs with initiation of prompt management.

Immediate routine care guidelines at birth for the newborn baby include:

- Announce the time of birth loudly to record the time and to make others alert
- Receive the baby on mother's abdomen on prewarm clean towel
- Assess breathing/crying to identify the need for resuscitation immediately. Heart rate and muscle tone should be assessed before initiation of neonatal resuscitation
- Check for clear airway, if required remove secretions using mouth wipes or suctioning
- Dry the stable baby having effective respiration thoroughly and remove the wet linen
- Place the baby in skin to skin contact between mother's breasts for uninterrupted one hour at least. Cover the neonate's head with a cap. Wrap both mother and baby together with warm cloth
- Follow "Zero separation" protocol. Observe the mother and neonates for 2 hours
- Apply identification tag/band and inform the mother about the baby
- Clamp and cut the umbilical cord after one minute of birth (between 1 and 3 minutes) using sterile scissors. Place sterile clamp/tie about 2–3 cm away from the abdominal skin. Apply nothing on the umbilical stump. Keep the cord open and dry. Observe for bleeding during initial hours
- Record APGAR scoring of the newlyborn stable baby at 1 minute and at 5 minutes of life
- Assess respiration rate, apical heart rate, body temperature and color at birth, then every 30 minutes during first 2 hours after birth, then every 3–4 hours for next 24 hours or as indicated to identify the physiological status

- Record all findings as baseline data for future reference
- Initiate breastfeeding within 1 hour of birth or as early as possible irrespective of mode of delivery, if both the mother and the baby are having no problems or not sick
- Assess birth weight, length, and chest circumference of the stable newborn baby within 2 hours of birth at delivery room. Head circumference is measured after 24 hours of birth
- Assess the newborn infant for gestational age using Ballard scoring and for presence of any life threatening congenital anomalies and birth injuries by head to foot examination
- Identify "at risk" neonates requiring admission in SNCU/NICU. "At risk" neonates are—(a) birth weight less than 1,800 gram, (b) gestation less than 34 weeks, (c) asphyxia needing post resuscitation care, (d) breathing difficulty, (e) major congenital anomalies and any illness
- Administer injection Vitamin "K-1" and hepatitis -"B" vaccine aseptically and keep record
- Provide prophylactic eye care to the neonates within 2 hours of birth, as per hospital policy. Routine eye care is not recommended in all institutions
- Communicate with the family members about mother's and baby's condition, sex of the baby, birth weight, identification number/tag and answer to their questions
- Arrange to send the baby with mother to postnatal ward with all documents after 2 hours, or as per instructions, if both the baby and mother are having no problems
- Document all necessary information in record book or delivery log book as per hospital policy. Standard "Log book" should be maintained with details information of birth event.

Equipment Required

- Hand hygiene articles and personal protective equipment (PPE) for care providers as standard precautions
- Prewarm towels or cloths to receive and cover the newborn baby
- Identification tag or band for mother and baby or footprint supplies
- Sterile mouth wipes in sterile covered bowl to clear the secretions or suction devices and sterile disposable supplies for suctioning of mouth and nose
- Sterile umbilical cord cutting instruments
- Thermometer and stethoscope to assess vital signs of the baby
- Clothing for the baby including cap and socks
- Weighing scale to measure baby's weight, preferably digital scale
- Tape measure to note length, head and chest circumference
- Supplies for intramuscular (IM) administration of vitamin "K-1" and Hepatitis -"B"
- Eye care articles and eye drops, as per hospital policy for prophylactic treatment
- Color coded waste disposal buckets to segregate and dispose all wastes
- Record book for documentation of birth and condition of mother and baby

Assessment and Preparation

- Assess fetal and maternal conditions and anticipate about any problems which may arise
- Assess the newly born infant quickly for satisfactory breathing and to decide for routine care at birth
- Explain to the mother about immediate routine care required for the neonate and all other procedures to be performed and ask for cooperation
- Involve other care providers or birth companion during birthing process and required care. One person for mother and one person for neonatal care must be present during birth. Communicate with other family members
- Perform hand hygiene and maintain strict aseptic techniques during delivery process and immediate neonatal care. Six clean practices should be practiced in the delivery room to prevent nosocomial

infections and to prevent early onset sepsis
- Arrange all necessary equipment and supplies ready in hand for care of the neonate
- Keep the delivery room temperature at 26–28°C.

Performing the Steps of Procedure with Rationale/Point of Emphasis

1. Perform hand hygiene and wear PPE including gloves to prevent cross infections.
2. Receive the newborn infant on mother's abdomen and cover with prewarm towel or cloth to prevent hypothermia.
3. Assess the baby for breathing/crying. If baby is breathing/crying well, then provide routine essential care.
   But if the baby is having no breathing/crying, then resuscitate the neonates after immediate cord clamping and placing the baby under radiant warmer *(Refer Procedure – 3: Neonatal Resuscitation of this Unit – 2).*
4. Remove the secretions to clear airway of the baby using mouth wipes or by suctioning.
5. Dry the baby thoroughly immediate after birth, remove wet cloth.
6. Place the neonate in skin to skin contact with mother in between her breasts. Keep the baby in skin to skin contact for at least 1 hour to maintain warmth. Cover the baby's head with cap and cover both mother and baby with prewarm cloth to prevent hypothermia.
7. Apply identification tag/band to the infant and also to the mother for security/legal purpose and show the baby to the mother. Identification tag/band should have the name of the mother, and hospital registration number, gender and birth weight of the infant.
8. Once the infant is stable, take footprint of the baby, as per institutional policy.
9. Assess APGAR score of the neonate to identify the baby's condition at 1 and 5 minutes.
10. Clamp and cut the umbilical cord after one minute (in between 1 and 3 minutes). Follow strict aseptic techniques during cord cutting to prevent cord infection/umbilical sepsis. Cord should be cut at 2–3 cm from the abdominal skin, so that the stump is away from the genitalia. Assess for any cord bleeding during initial hours after delivery. Do not apply anything on cord and keep it dry and open. Check vessels of the umbilical cord (two arteries and one vein), presence of one artery may be indicative of congenital anomalies.
11. Initiate breastfeeding early within 1 hour of birth to provide colostrum feeding. Support the mother and baby during early initiation of breastfeeding as breast crawl. Assess feeding behavior, sucking reflex and swallowing reflex of the neonate.
12. Measure the baby's birth weight, length, and chest circumference to identify at-risk conditions such as LBW, small for gestational age, and intrauterine growth retardation. Measure head circumference after 24 hours of birth to identify microcephaly and macrocephaly. Keep record of all findings. Ensure the baby is warm during anthropometric measurements.
13. Maintain general cleanliness for the baby. Gently clean off blood, mucus and meconium from the baby's body. No bath should be given to prevent hypothermia and infections. No vigorous attempts should be made to remove vernix caseosa from the baby skin. Wrap and dress the baby with clean cloths, when not in skin to skin contact with mother.
14. Administer injection vitamin "K-1" IM aseptically in anterolateral aspect of thigh using 26 gauge needle and one mL syringe. Dose is 0.5 mg for babies weighing less than 1,000 gram and 1.0 mg for babies weighing more than 1,000 gram. It is given to prevent hemorrhagic diseases of the newborn within 2 hours of birth.
15. Administer hepatitis B vaccine 0.5 mL IM "birth dose" at the delivery room or as per hospital policy within 24 hours of birth to prevent transmission of hepatitis B virus.

16. Give prophylactic eye care, as per institutional/hospital policy and if the mother is having genital tract infections and the baby is having infected eye.
17. Perform clinical screening to identify birth injuries and presence of any life threatening congenital anomalies such as cleft palate, tracheoesophageal fistula, congenital diaphragmatic hernia, umbilical cord anomalies, anorectal malformations/abnormal anal opening, meningocele, meningomyelocele, etc.
18. Monitor the baby's condition for at least two hours to detect any abnormalities and to initiate prompt management.
19. Document all necessary information in standard record book of birthing process.
20. Communicate with the mother, team members and family members about mother's and neonate's condition. Show the baby to the family members.
21. Plan and send the mother and baby together to the postnatal ward with all documents and hand over with all information.
22. Provide psychological support to the mother and teach about postnatal care.
23. Identify "at risk" neonates and arrange for admission in SNCU/NICU or refer.
24. Dispose the waste and used PPE. Take care of reusable articles and equipment by decontamination, cleaning, disinfection or sterilization. Re-set the equipment and articles for next use.
25. Do hand hygiene. Check for completion of the procedure and documentation.

Evaluation and Documentation

- Evaluate the mother-baby interaction, neonate's condition, and mother's conditions in details, at least for 2 hours in the delivery room. Evaluate father's and other family member's anxiety and level of understanding and need for support
- Document respiration rate, heart rate, temperature, SpO_2, capillary refill time (CRT), color, APGAR score, feeding behavior, birth weight, length, head and chest circumference, gestational age (GA), appropriate for GA (AGA)/small for GA (SGA)/ large for GA (LGA), presence of any congenital anomalies and birth injuries, time of initiation of breastfeeding, administration time of vitamin K 1 and Hepatitis B, passage of meconium and urine, condition of umbilical cord and eyes and time of sending out to postnatal ward/unit.

Communication and Teaching for Homecare

- Communicate with parents and family members to assess home environment for safety of the neonates and to identify the availability of supplies and support person for home care of mother and baby. Inform them about condition of the mother and baby. Explain about care at postnatal ward, discharge planning and home care.
- Teach the parents about care in postnatal ward and care of the baby at home with maintenance of warmth, continuation of exclusive breastfeeding, practice of hygienic measures (hand hygiene, care of cord, care of eyes, bathing, skin care, diapering, clean clothing, clean environment, avoiding overcrowding), identification of danger signs, date of immunization and follow-up visit, need for medical help for danger signs or whenever necessary and communication with community health workers [accredited social health activist (ASHA), anganwadi worker (AWW), auxiliary nurse midwife (ANM), community health officer (CHO)] and nearest health facility.

PROCEDURE–2: HAND HYGIENE IN HEALTH CARE SETTINGS

Clinical Guidelines

Hand hygiene is one of the most important aspects of standard precautions to prevent health care associated infections. Hands are the main pathways of transmission of microorganisms during health care. Any health care professionals, care givers or person involved in direct or indirect patient/

child care required to be concerned about hand hygiene and should be able to perform it correctly and at the right time.

Hand hygiene must be performed as contact precautions between caring of two children/patients to prevent cross infections. It is also important to perform hand hygiene between tasks on the same child/patient to prevent cross contamination of different body sites. Maintenance of hand hygiene is inexpensive and easy approach for prevention of infections in health care.

Special attention should be given to the neglected areas or missed areas during maintenance of hand hygiene. Common missed areas are nail beds, tip of the fingers, web space between two fingers and base of the thumbs.

Hand hygiene in health care settings is maintained: (a) by washing hands with soap and water when hands are visibly dirty or visibly soiled, and (b) by rubbing with alcohol based formulation, before and after all contacts with patients, if hands are not visibly soiled.

Hand washing with soap and water should not be done immediately before and after using of alcohol-based handrub solution. Health care professionals should take care of hands by regularly using protective hand cream or lotion daily to prevent dryness of the skin.

Use of gloves does not replace the need for cleaning hands. Hand hygiene must be performed when appropriate, regardless of indications for use of gloves. Use gloves only when indicated according to standard and contact precautions as per "World Health Organization (WHO)—The Glove Pyramid".

"Five moments of Hand Hygiene" include: (i) Before touching patient, (ii) Before clean or aseptic procedure, (iii) After body fluid exposure risk, (iv) After touching patient and (v) After touching patient's surroundings.

Hand Washing with Soap and Water

- Hand washing with soap and water is the simplest and most effective method of infection control in health care settings
- Purposes of soap water and hand washing include: (a) it helps to remove dirt and debris from hands, (b) it reduces the transmission of microorganisms from contaminated hands of care givers and health professionals and (c) it interrupts feco-oral route of disease transmission.
- Hand washing with soap and water must be done before entering the ward or unit or operation room, after handling of infected materials, blood and other body fluids, before and after use of sterile gloves, after use of toilets and when hands are visibly soiled. Otherwise use handrub with alcohol based formulation.
- Duration of hand washing procedure recommended by WHO is 40–60 seconds. For medical asepsis in neonatal care units, soap and water hand washing should be done for 2 minutes and for surgical asepsis it should be 3–5 minutes. The length of hand scrub varies based on need and the activity to be performed.
- It is better to use antimicrobial or medicated or antiseptic liquid soap for hand wash for better result and reduction of transmission of microorganisms.

Use of Antiseptic Alcohol-based Handrub

- Rinsing hands with alcohol based handrub is not a substitute for proper soap and water hand washing
- Duration of the entire procedure for antiseptic handrub is 20–30 seconds
- Use palmful of handrub solution 5–7 mL for hands and forearms
- Use of handrub is faster, more effective, better tolerated and easy to practice. It is preferred means for routine hygienic hand antisepsis.

Equipment Required

- Antimicrobial or plain liquid soap for hand washing, as available
- Running water with elbow/foot operated tap with wash basin
- Single use sterile towel or paper to dry hands

- Antiseptic alcohol-based handrub solution
- Waste disposal containers to dispose towel or paper, if used for drying of hands.

Assessment and Preparation

- Assess the need for hand wash or use of alcohol-based handrub depending upon the nature of the procedure
- Self-preparation should be done to perform hand hygiene in right time and in right technique for right purpose
- Environment should be clean and well lighted
- All essential requirements should be available. Hand washing articles should be arranged near the wash basin. Alcohol-based handrub solution should be available at the bed side near each child/patient, in the procedure room, at examination room or at any work place.

Performing the Steps of Procedure with Rationale/Point of Emphasis

Hand Washing with Soap and Water

1. Remove all ornaments, wrist band, wrist watch and sacred thread from hands.
2. Ensure nails are short and without nail polish and artificial nails.
3. Roll up both sleeves 2–3 cm above elbow.
4. Ensure all hand washing items are near the wash basin.
5. Wet hands and forearms with running water using elbow or foot operated tap. Do not use hot water to rinse hands.
6. Take adequate amount of liquid soap (5–7 mL) on the palm from the soap container with dispenser.
7. Apply the liquid soap over all hands surface, wrists, forearms and elbows.
8. First step of rubbing—rub hands palm to palm.
9. Second step of rubbing—rub right palm over left dorsum with interlaced fingers and rub left palm over right dorsum with interlaced fingers.
10. Third step of rubbing—rub palm to palm with fingers interlaced *(Note: this step can be done along with first step).*
11. Fourth step of rubbing—rub backs of the fingers to opposing palms with fingers interlocked as knuckle. Rub for both hands.
12. Fifth step of rubbing—rub left thumb clasped in right palm in rotational movement and rub right thumb clasped in left palm in rotational movement.
13. Sixth step of rubbing—rotational rubbing, backward and forward with clasped fingers of right hand in left palm and vice versa.
14. Seventh step of rubbing—rub left forearm from wrist to elbow with right hand and rub right forearm from wrist to elbow with left hand *(Note: Rubbing and cleaning of wrists and forearms are important for prevention of cross infections in the neonatal care units because neonates are handled using both hands and forearms. It is also necessary in critical areas, in ICU and in Operation rooms).*
15. Rinse both hands with running water thoroughly.
16. Keep the hands little higher so that water trickles down from hands to forearms to elbows.
17. Turn off the water tap using elbow or foot. In case of simple water tap, use towel/paper to turn off the faucet after drying hands.
18. Dry hands and forearms with single use sterile towel/paper or do air dry. Dry hands first then forearms and elbow. Avoid coming back from elbows to hands with the same towel/paper as it may touch non-washed area near elbows.
19. Discard the towel or paper in the appropriate bin.
20. Ensure hands are clean, dry and safe.
21. Do not touch anything after hand washing, except the procedure for which it is done.

Use of Antiseptic Handrub

1. Remove all ornaments, wrist band, wrist watch and sacred thread from hands.
2. Ensure nails are short and without nail polish and artificial nails.

3. Roll up both sleeves 2–3 cm above elbow.
4. Ensure sufficient amount of handrub solutions is present in the container.
5. Take adequate amount of antiseptic handrub solution (5–7 mL) on the palm from the container.
6. Apply the handrub solution over all hands surface, wrists, forearms up to elbows.
7. First step of rubbing—rub hands palm to palm.
8. Second step of rubbing—rub right palm over left dorsum with interlaced fingers and rub left palm over right dorsum with interlaced fingers.
9. Third step of rubbing—rub palm to palm with fingers interlaced *(Note: This step can be done along with first step).*
10. Fourth step of rubbing—rub backs of the fingers to opposing palms with fingers interlocked as knuckle. Rub for both hands.
11. Fifth step of rubbing—rub left thumb clasped in right palm in rotational movement and rub right thumb clasped in left palm in rotational movement.
12. Sixth step of rubbing—rotational rubbing, backwards and forwards with clasped fingers of right hand in left palm and vice versa.
13. Seventh step of rubbing—rub left forearm from wrist to elbow with right hand and rub right forearm from wrist to elbow with left hand *(Note: Rubbing and cleaning of wrists and forearms are important for prevention of cross infections in the neonatal care units because neonates are handled using both hands and forearms. It is also necessary in critical areas, in ICU and in Operation rooms).*
14. Ensure hands and forearms are dry and safe.
15. Do not touch anything after use of handrub, except the procedure for which it is done.

(Refer WHO Recommendation for Hand Hygiene as Appendix – IV for 'Five Moments of Hand Hygiene,' Appendix – V for 'Steps of Hand Wash,' Appendix – VI for 'Steps of Hand Rub' and Appendix – VII for 'Glove Pyramid').

Evaluation and Documentation

- Evaluate the practice of hand hygiene among all health care professionals, parents and other supportive persons. Evaluate the understanding level of parents and supportive persons regarding practice of hand hygiene and its importance.
- Document about teaching provided for improvement of hand hygiene practices.

Communication and Teaching for Homecare

- Communicate with the parents and family members about importance of hand hygiene
- Teach the parents and supportive persons about purpose, technique and duration of hand hygiene in hospital and home.

PROCEDURE–3: NEONATAL RESUSCITATION

Clinical Guidelines

- Approximately 10% of the newly born infants need some assistance to establish respiration at birth and only 1% of these neonates need advance resuscitative measures, i.e., endotracheal (ET) intubation, chest compression and medications.
- Aims of neonatal resuscitation include: (i) to assist the newly born infant to take satisfactory respiration within one minute of life, i.e., in "first golden minute" of age, (ii) to prevent neonatal morbidity and long-term complications related to hypoxic damage of the brain and other vital organs of the infant, and (iii) to reduce neonatal mortality due to complications of asphyxia neonatorum or perinatal asphyxia.
- Steps of neonatal resuscitation are: (a) initial steps of resuscitation, (b) positive pressure ventilation (PPV), (c) endotracheal intubation, if indicated, (d) chest compression and (e) medications.
- The most important and effective action in neonatal resuscitation is to ventilate the newly born baby's lungs. PPV must

be started within 60 seconds/ 1 minute of birth

- About 90% neonates take spontaneous respiration and another 9% neonates takes respiration with basic resuscitative support, i.e., initial steps and positive pressure ventilation, which can be done by the skilled nursing professionals only.
- Assessment of antepartum or intrapartum risk factors (preterm delivery, pregnancy. induced hypertension, antepartum hemorrhage, meconium-stained amniotic fluid, maternal anemia and diseases, prolonged labor, fetal distress, etc.) can help to identify the neonates who may need additional steps of resuscitation.
- Anticipation of need for resuscitation and identification of risk factors are very important. Continuous fetal monitoring in labor and partograph are very important that helps to identify the at-risk neonates with problems.
- All neonates at birth must be initially assessed to determine the need of resuscitation and for gestational age, meconium stained liquor, breathing/ crying and muscle tone. "Vigorous neonate" will have strong respiratory efforts, heart rate more than 100 beats per minute and good muscle tone.
- Evaluation and decision making for resuscitative measures are based primarily on respiration, heart rate and oxygenation.
- Every birth should be attended by someone who is trained and skilled in initiating neonatal resuscitation. Additional personnel should be available, when further advance resuscitation is required.
- Team briefing, antenatal counseling, adequate preparation, and equipment check must be done before birth of the newborn baby. Neonatal Resuscitation Algorithm should be made available and displayed near Newborn Care Corner (NBCC) at all delivery rooms *(Refer Appendix – IX: Neonatal Resuscitation Algorithm).*

Equipment Required

- Hand hygiene supplies and PPE including sterile gloves for all team members
- Radiant warmer with bassinet, sterile baby sheets/towels for the newborn infant
- Sterile single use shoulder roll (3/4th – 1 inch thick) for positioning the baby
- Suction devices: De Lee's disposable sterile mucus extractors, meconium aspirator, sterile disposable suction catheters (6 F, 8 F, 10 F, 12 F, and 14 F), suction tube and mechanical suction machine. For suctioning of meconium-stained secretion 12 F or 14 F suction catheter is used
- Pediatric stethoscope and clock with seconds hand to assess apical heart rate
- Sterile self-inflating neonatal resuscitation bag (250 mL, 500 mL, 750 mL) with oxygen tube and oxygen reservoir to provide positive pressure ventilation (PPV)
- Sterile neonatal resuscitation masks (round shaped - size 0 and 1) to provide PPV
- Source of oxygen with oxygen tube, humidifier, flow meter and regulator
- Sterile laryngoscope and straight blades (size 00, 0 and 1) with extra batteries and bulbs
- Sterile endotracheal (ET) tube (size 2.5 mm, 3 mm, 3.5 mm)
- Adhesive tape and scissors for fixation of ET tube, if ET intubation is needed
- Sterile umbilical catheters (size – 3.5 F, 5 F) to perform umbilical venous catheterization and three-way stopcock to administer medications
- Sterile intravenous (IV) neonatal size cannula for fluid therapy and medications
- Orogastric feeding tube: 8 F to deflate to stomach of the neonates
- Medications: Epinephrine, Normal saline
- Syringe: 1 mL, 2 mL, 3 mL, 5 mL, 10 mL, 20 mL
- Waste disposal containers to dispose all waste
- Neonatal case sheet and monitoring sheet for documentation.

Assessment and Preparation

- Assess gestational age (preterm or term), antenatal risk factors (multiple gestation, IUGR, maternal medical problems, etc.) and intranatal risk factors (fetal distress, meconium-stained amniotic fluid, prolonged labor >24 hours, premature labor, malpresentations, etc.). Check the "Partograph" findings for fetal condition, maternal condition and progress of labor.
- Self-preparation should be done with meticulous hand washing and use of PPE with sterile gloves. Resuscitation team must be present in delivery room before the birth of the baby. Team briefing must be arranged and done before delivery of the neonate
- Environment should be clean, calm, quiet, well lighted and well ventilated. Delivery room temperature should be within 26–28°C. Radiant warmer should be "switched on" 20–30 minutes before the birth of the neonate
- Neonatal Resuscitation Algorithm must be available at NBCC
- All necessary equipment and supplies should be arranged before birth of the newborn baby for easy access. Ensure intactness of disposable sterile articles. Reusable articles must be made sterile before use. Assemble sterile articles in a sterile container.
  Check the equipment for their working condition especially the self-inflating neonatal resuscitation bag and mask. Strict infection control practices and standard precautions must be followed to prevent neonatal infections
- Preparation of mother and father and other family members: Inform the mother gently about the need for resuscitation. Explain to father and other family members about risk factors and possible neonatal complications and plan of management
- Preparation of neonate: Fetal condition should be assessed before delivery to anticipate the need for resuscitation. Assess the partograph findings. After delivery of the baby, note the time of birth, announce the birth loudly, receive the baby in dry prewarm linen, and assess baby's breathing/crying and muscle tone. If the baby is taking spontaneous breathing/crying provide "Routine Care". If there is no breathing/crying, cut the umbilical cord immediately and place the baby under prewarmed radiant warmer and start steps of resuscitation.

Performing the Steps of Procedure with Rationale/Point of Emphasis

1. Perform hand hygiene and arrange all equipment and articles conveniently at NBCC.
2. Switch "ON" the radiant warmer 20–30 minutes before the birth of the baby to receive the baby on prewarm environment. Place two baby sheets/towels on the bassinet to make them warm and to receive the baby on prewarm sheets/towels.
3. Perform hand washing and wear PPE with sterile gloves to be ready to receive the newborn baby for resuscitation.
4. Assemble and check the "self-inflating bag and mask" for functioning.
5. Check the time of birth of newborn baby and announce the birth of the baby loudly.
6. Receive the baby in dry prewarm linen and assess breathing and muscle tone.
7. If there is "no breathing", cut the umbilical cord immediately, separate the baby from mother, inform mother gently about need for resuscitation.
8. Place the baby under prewarm radiant warmer and start initial steps of resuscitation. Remember, initial step of resuscitation should be completed within "30 seconds of birth".
9. Position the neonate on back with slightly neck extended in sniffing position using a shoulder roll.
10. Clear secretions from airways by suctioning, if needed. Suction the mouth first then nose. Introduce suction catheter 4–5 cm in mouth and 1–2 cm in nose. Suction pressure should be less than 100 mm of Hg. In case of meconium-stained

amniotic fluid and "non-vigorous" baby, ET tube suctioning should be done.

11. Dry the baby quickly after clearing airways, then discard wet linen and place the baby on dry warm linen.
12. Provide tactile stimulation to help the baby to breath/cry. The safe method of providing tactile stimulation is gently rubbing the back, trunk and extremities of the baby.
13. Reposition the neonate in sniffing position using shoulder roll.
14. Evaluate respiration and heart rate of the baby. Check apical heart rate using stethoscope for "6 seconds" only and multiply by 10 to get heart rate beats per minute (bpm). For example, if the neonate's "6 seconds" heart rate is 8, it indicates the baby is having heart rate 80 beats per minute.
15. Attach pulse oximeter to assess heart rate and oxygen saturation. During neonatal resuscitation, apply pulse oximeter sensor probe to the infant before connecting to the pulse oximeter that leads in quickest acquisition of accurate heart rate and oxygen saturation. Attach the probe in right hand of the baby to assess preductal saturation.
16. If the neonate is having spontaneous breathing/crying after initial steps and "no apnea or no gasping and heart rate more than 100 bpm" then provide "routine care" to the baby in skin to skin contact with the mother, uninterruptedly for at least 1 hour.
17. If the neonate is having "labored breathing or persistent cyanosis" then monitor SpO_2, provide supplementary oxygen therapy, and consider CPAP in preterm baby. This neonate needs to be admitted in SNCU/NICU.
18. If the neonate is having "apnea or gasping or heart rate less than 100 bpm" after 30 seconds of effective initial steps of resuscitation, then initiate PPV using bag and mask. Bag mask ventilation must be started within 60 seconds/1 minute of birth.
    Remember, the contraindication of bag-mask ventilation is "congenital diaphragmatic hernia (CDH)". So, assess the presence of clinical features of CDH in the neonate.
19. Provide PPV with room air using appropriate size sterile self-inflating resuscitation bag and mask [i.e., Bag Mask Ventilation (BMV)]. Mask on the baby's face should be placed from tip of the chin, then mouth and then nose but not covering the eyes.
20. Look for adequate chest rise during BMV in first 5–10 inflations. If there is "No chest rise", do corrective measures following "MRSOPA". (M – mask adjustment, R – reposition of baby's head, S – suction the airway, O – Open baby's mouth, P – increase pressure during squeezing the bag, A – alternative airway like ET intubation or laryngeal mask airway).
21. Continue PPV using bag and mask with effective chest rise for 30 seconds at the rate of 40–60 breaths per minute. Count as "Breath-two-three, Breath-two-three, and so on. Assess for respiration and heart rate for every 30 seconds during PPV.
22. Monitor SpO_2 using pulse oximeter. Attach the probe in right hand or wrist to assess preductal saturation. Consider ECG monitoring, if available.
23. Evaluate baby's respiration and heart rate after every 30 second of PPV/BMV and take decision for further action or steps of resuscitation.
24. Call for help from expert, if the neonate is not improving with PPV/BMV.
25. Examine the baby for presence of CDH, especially if there is no improvement during PPV. Arrange for ET intubation, as CDH is the contraindication of BMV. Then PPV should be provided using ET tube and self-inflating bag.
26. Assist during "ET intubation" and maintain strict aseptic technique. Four critical points requiring ET intubation during neonatal resuscitation are: (a) to perform tracheal suctioning, if the neonate is non-vigorous with meconium-

stained amniotic fluid, (b) if the baby is not improving with PPV using bag and mask, (c) if there is need of PPV for more than few minutes, and (d) if the baby requires chest compression along with PPV to improve the efficacy of ventilation and heart rate.

27. Start "chest compressions" along with PPV and 100% oxygen, if after 30 seconds of effective PPV, the baby's heart rate remain below 60 beats per minute. To provide 100% oxygen, attach oxygen reservoir and oxygen tube to the resuscitation bag and to oxygen source. Chest compressions are given usually by "thumb technique" on the lower third of the sternum in midline. Sternum is depressed to a depth of approximately one-third of anterior-posterior diameter of the chest. Chest compressions and PPV is given at the ratio of 3:1. In 1 minute, 90 chest compressions and 30 PPV, i.e., total 120 events are performed. For these counting sequence is "One and Two and Three and Breathe and". ("Breathe and" is for squeezing the bag for ventilation, whereas "One and Two and Three and" for chest compressions)
28. Administer "Medications" as indicated. (i) Epinephrine, a cardiac stimulant, is indicated when heart rate remains below 60 bpm, after 30 seconds of effective PPV followed by another 30 seconds of coordinated chest compressions and PPV with 100% oxygen, (ii) Normal saline as volume expander is indicated if the baby is not responding to resuscitative measures or in shock or there is history of fetal blood loss.
29. Administer injection Epinephrine in 1:10,000 concentrations through intravenous (IV) or umbilical vein or ET tube route. It should be given rapidly as quickly as possible. Dose for IV route is 0.1–0.3 mL/kg and in ET tube dose is 0.5–1 mL/kg.
30. Administer normal saline in umbilical vein or in IV route with dose 10 mL/kg over 5–10 minutes.
31. Decide for endpoints of resuscitative measures in neonates as follows:
    i. When heart rate remains less than 60 bpm, continue chest compressions and PPV with 100% oxygen. If the neonate is not improved, consider special situations
    ii. When heart rate is more than 60 bpm, then stop chest compressions but continue PPV
    iii. When heart rate is more than 100 bpm and baby is breathing well, then stop PPV
32. Assess neonate's respiratory rate, heart rate, SpO_2, CRT, air entry, body temperature, birth weight, problems in respiration (i.e., chest indrawing, grunting, persistent cyanosis, nasal flaring) and presence of any other problems and congenital anomalies.
33. Evaluate "Apgar Score" at every 5 minutes to assess the effectiveness of the resuscitative measures and monitor baby's condition continuously.
34. Provide "post-resuscitation care", if the neonate requires more than one minute PPV. Admit the baby in SNCU/NICU and do team debriefing.
35. Decide to discontinue resuscitative efforts, after providing optimum technique of resuscitation for a minimum of 10 minutes or more, when there is no signs of life, no respiration, no heart rate, and no progress is being made in certain conditions, such as extreme prematurity and lethal congenital malformations *(Refer Appendix - VIII: Segregation of Bio-Medical Waste (BMW).*
36. Complete the procedure of resuscitation, as required.
37. Dispose the waste as per biomedical waste management (BMW) rules, clean and sterilize reusable articles and reset the NBCC with resuscitation items.
38. Documents details of the resuscitative measures required for the neonate.

Evaluation and Documentation

- Evaluate neonate's response to resuscitative efforts, Apgar score (at 5-minute, 10-minute, 15-minute and 20-minute),

vital signs, CRT, presence of respiratory distress, seizures and general condition. Evaluate parent's anxiety and understanding level to provide necessary support in relation to neonate's condition
- Document the following:
  - Date and time of birth, mode of delivery, gestational age, sex, birth weight
  - Resuscitative measures/steps performed and response of the neonate
  - Medications administered to the neonate, if required
  - Observational findings: Respiratory rate, heart rate SpO_2, CRT, air entry, body temperature and problems in respiration, Apgar Score, seizures, etc.
  - Parents' response regarding neonate's condition
  - Personnel present at delivery room during resuscitative measures.

Communication and Teaching for Homecare

- Communicate with mother and family members about the neonate's condition and further plan of treatment and care required at home
- Teach the parents about participation in neonatal care at hospital, continued care at home after discharge and need for follow-up care for better neurodevelopmental outcome.

PROCEDURE–4: ASSISTING IN BREASTFEEDING

Clinical Guidelines

- Breastfeeding provides optimal nutrition to the infant. It is estimated that over one million children die each year from diarrhea, respiratory infections and other infections due to inadequate breastfeeding
- Breastfeeding must be initiated soon after birth within 1 hour of life irrespective of mode of delivery, if mother and newborn baby are not sick or having no problems
- Colostrum feeding provides first immunization, as it contains anti-infective proteins. It has mild purgative effect, which helps to clear meconium from neonate's intestine and prevents hyperbilirubinemia
- Mother's own milk (MOM) is best for the infant nutritionally, immunologically and psychologically. It is easily digested and available at normal temperature. It protects the baby from allergies including eczema and asthma. Breastfeed babies have higher intelligence and less chance of developing hypertension, diabetes mellitus, coronary heart disease and even cancer in later life
- Avoid prelacteal feeding with honey, sweet water, *ghutti*, animal milk, etc., to reduce breast milk intake by the baby from the mother
- Exclusive breastfeeding must be continue up to 6 months of age (i.e., feeding only breast milk and allowing any medications only, if required)
- Initially breastfeeding can be given at 1–2 hours interval, then breastfeeding should be given on demand at least eight times or more in 24 hours. Night feed must be continued and not to be omitted
- Mother should allow the baby to take feed at one breast till the infant stops suckling and releases the breast. Then offer other breast, if the baby demands for more. This technique allow the infant to take both foremilk and hind milk
- Burping should be done gently. Incorrect positioning and poor attachment during breastfeeding allow air entry into infant's stomach, which requires burping
- Mother can position the infant during breastfeeding as cradle-hold, cross-cradle-hold or in clutch technique in sitting position comfortably or in side-lying position. Following lower uterine segment cesarean section (LUCS) delivery, mother can be lying flat with the infant on the chest to feed in "breast crawl" technique
- Adequacy of breastfeeding in infant can be assessed by counting passage of urine 6–8 times/day and daily weight gain 1–1.5% of body weight or about 20–30 gram in first 3–4 months after regaining birth weight.

The infant usually sleeps 2–3 hours in between effective and successful feeds

- Effective suckling, empty breast after feeding or expression of milk, correct positioning of the infant and good attachment of the baby's mouth with mother's breast are essentials for successful breastfeeding
- Mother should be calm, stress free and relaxed with touch, smell and sound of the baby to promote let-down or oxytocin reflex for better flow of milk
- Mother should be encouraged to take postnatal lactating mother's diet and sufficient water intake (4–5 liters) with adequate rest and sleep for adequate secretion of breast milk for her baby
- Breastfeeding problems related to abnormal breast conditions such as inverted or flat nipples, sore nipples, breast engorgement or breast abscess and reduced milk supply should be managed promptly to prevent lactation failure
- Mother requires extra support for establishing breastfeeding in preterm and LBW neonates. The coordination of suckling, swallowing, and breathing actions is seen at 32–35 weeks of gestation. Mother should be motivated to express breast milk when direct breastfeeding is not possible
- Complementary foods should be introduced after 6 months of age. But breastfeeding should be continued up to 2 years of age or beyond, especially at night time
- Advantages of breastfeeding include benefits to the infant, mother, family, and society. Mother needs teaching and physical support to practice breastfeeding effectively
- "Ten steps to successful breastfeeding" must be followed by every health facility to promote breastfeeding practices by the mother with support from health care providers and family members.

Equipment Required

- Hand hygiene articles for cleaning hands
- Drinking water for mother to maintain good hydration
- Pillow or blanket roll for comfort of the mother during breastfeeding
- Extra clothing for mother and baby, if required
- Waste disposal container.

Assessment and Preparation

- Assess mother's knowledge and preparation for early initiation of breastfeeding and exclusive breastfeeding. Check mother is having no illness and ready to feed the baby
- Ensure that the infant is alert and clinically stable with normal vital signs
- Check and confirm about effective suckling and swallowing reflex in the neonate
- Ensure that the infant is warm, dry and clean
- Perform hand hygiene and arrange necessary articles at mother's side
- Provide comfortable position to the mother to make her relaxed during feeding
- Allow the mother to drink glass of water.

Performing the Steps of Procedure with Rationale/Point of Emphasis

1. Perform hand hygiene and ensure mother also has done hand hygiene.
2. Assist mother to drink a glass of water before breastfeeding or in between.
3. Maintain privacy of the mother during breastfeeding. Do minimum exposure.
4. Position the infant close to the mother with head slightly elevated and abdomen turned in contact with mother's body. The infant should be well supported by the mother's forearm with head, neck, and body in same plane having baby's face toward mother's breast. Baby's abdomen should touch mother's abdomen. Correct positioning promotes good attachment during breastfeeding and it helps by making milk flow better.
5. Provide pillow or blanket roll to make the mother comfortable.
6. Teach the mother to do "tickling" the infant's cheek with the nipple of the breast. This elicits the rooting reflex and encourages the infant to open mouth wider for good latching.

7. Check for good attachment/latching of infant's mouth to the mother's breast **(Fig. 2.1)**. Signs of good attachment are wide open mouth of the infant with lower lip turned outward and chin touches the mother's breast having majority of the areola inside baby's mouth.
   Poor attachment leads to pain and sore nipples, breast engorgement, poor milk supply, dissatisfaction and frustration of the infant and poor weight gain of the baby.
8. Assess infant's feeding behavior. Infant takes several deep sucks followed by swallowing of milk and then pause.
9. Encourage the mother to feed the infant at least for 10 minutes from one side. When baby needs more, then opposite side breast can be offered. Initially the infant can feed for less time. The baby leaves the breast spontaneously after full feeding. Total feeding time may require 20–30 minutes, in older infant.
10. Do burping to remove swallowed air by the infant in between feeding and at the end of feeding. Correct positioning and good attachment prevent swallowing of air by the baby. Then burping may not be required if the breastfeeding technique is done correctly.
11. Teach the mother to break the suction, if required, while infant is feeding. Mother should insert the tip of her little finger between the breast and the corner of infant's mouth and pull slightly downward to break the seal and prevent nipple injury.
12. Observe for any discomfort of the mother during feeding and promote comfort, if needed.
13. Place the infant in side lying comfortable position safely after feeding. Baby can also be placed in supine position with continuous supervision.
14. Assist the mother to redress and assume comfortable position.
15. Perform hand hygiene and document the event of breastfeeding.

Evaluation and Documentation

- Evaluate the adequacy of breastfeeding, passage of urine and meconium/stool, feeding behaviors of the infant, presence of any problems of mother and the infant, infant's daily weight, mother-infant interaction, parents concern and level of understanding
- All abnormalities should be reported to neonatologist/health care prescriber for continuation of management
- Document the length of time of breastfeeding and any problems encountered.

Communication and Teaching for Homecare

- Communicate with mother and family members to inform about the conditions

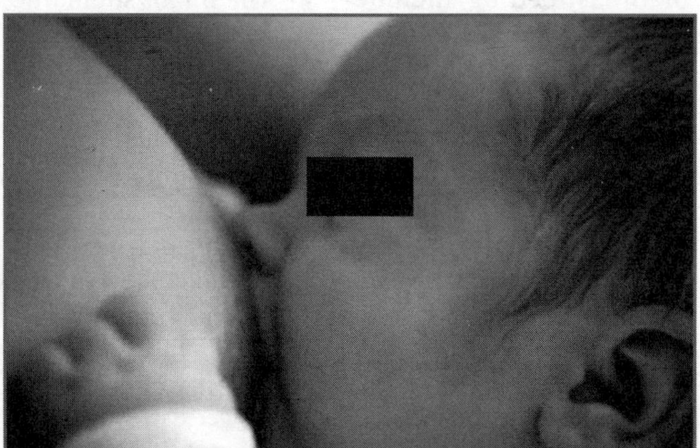

Fig. 2.1: Good attachment in breastfeeding *(For color version, see Plate 1)*.

of both mother and infant. Explain about the success or problems of breastfeeding
- Teach the parents about the following:
  - Exclusive breastfeeding up to 6 months and demand feeding for the infant
  - Benefits and continuation of breastfeeding up to 2 years of child's age
  - Assess adequacy of breastfeeding by counting wet diapers, at least 6–8 times in 24 hours and weight gain after first week of life
  - Give no pacifiers or teats or mixed feeding with other milk (animal milk or formula milk) to the infant to prevent confusion with breastfeeding
  - Initiate complementary foods after 6 months, but to continue breastfeeding up to 2 years or more especially at night along with top feeds
  - Clean mother's breasts during bath and to wear clean dress
  - Maintain good personal hygiene for both mother and infant
  - Practice of "bedding-in/rooming-in" to allow mother and infant together
  - Maintain warmth and environmental cleanliness
  - Allow lactational diet to the mother with extra calorie and avoiding highly spiced food
  - Contact health care providers for any emergency problems (poor feeding or refusal to suck/feed, yellow urine, watery stool, irritable infant with excessive crying, difficulty in respiration) or for regular health check-up of both mother and infant.

PROCEDURE–5: ASSESSMENT OF VITAL SIGNS OF NEONATES

Clinical Guidelines

- Vital signs are considered to those physical signs concerning functions essential to life. These signs are objectively measurable and verifiable
- Measurement of vital signs helps to assess normal or abnormal condition of the patients thus helps in diagnosis. It also helps to detect whether the patient is improving or deteriorating during the course of treatment.
- Important vital signs of the neonates are respiration, heart rate, and body temperature. Other vital signs for neonates include SpO_2, and CRT. Blood pressure is also a significant vital sign usually measured with precautions, when indicated
- Pain is considered also as an important vital sign, but it depends on various factors and difficult to measure objectively. Assessment and management of pain in neonates should also be emphasized in neonatal care practices
- In neonates, normal respiration is 40–60 breaths/minute, normal heart rate is 140–160 beats/minute and normal body temperature at axillae is 36.5–37.5 degree centigrade. The normal SpO_2 is 90% - 94% and CRT is less than 3 seconds in newborn baby
- Respiration of neonate at birth is assessed by observation to identify the presence of effective breathing to initiate resuscitation. Afterwards full one minute counting of respiration rate and assessment of presence of chest indrawing and grunting or any abnormal sound is very important
- Apical heart rate is counted using pediatric stethoscope for 6 seconds at birth and thereafter for full one minute. Heart rate assessment can be done along with SpO2 using pulse oximeter or multipara monitor. Peripheral pulse rate can be checked in all four limbs by feeling to detect any abnormalities
- Temperature assessment in neonates can be done by recording of axillary temperature using digital thermometer or by recording skin temperature using thermistor probe of radiant warmer or with reasonable precision using human touch by trained person. Mercury thermometer is not recommended to prevent environmental pollution by mercury. Rectal temperature measurement can lead to infection and injury in neonates
- Blood pressure is usually checked using noninvasive method with multipara

monitor and appropriate size blood pressure cuff for the neonates, whenever indicated. Mean arterial pressure is roughly equal to gestation age of the neonates.

Equipment Required

- Hand hygiene articles for cleaning hands to prevent cross infections
- Pediatric stethoscope to auscult the heart sound
- Digital thermometer to measure the temperature
- Digital clock with second hand to check time
- Pulse oximeter to check heart rate and SpO_2
- Multipara monitor, if available to measure heart rate, SpO_2 and blood pressure, etc.
- Alcohol 70% to clean the thermometer and stethoscope before and after each use
- Cotton swabs in a small bowl to clean the thermometer and stethoscope
- Baby clothing, sheet and diaper to change, if soiled
- Buckets to dispose waste
- Record sheet to note the findings.

Assessment and Preparation

- Assess the neonate for any abnormalities by observation or palpation or manipulation
- Check for color as it is also an important sign. Normal color is pink and non-mottled. Central cyanosis is abnormal and indicative of respiratory and cardiac problems. Peripheral cyanosis of hand and feet may normally present immediate after birth but persistent cyanosis indicates hypothermia or ineffective breathing. Yellow discoloration indicates hyperbilirubinemia. Plethoric or reddish color indicates dehydration or hyperthermia. Pallor indicates neonatal shock or anemia in neonates
- Self-preparation should be done by hand hygiene
- Environment must be calm, quiet, well lighted and clean
- All necessary articles or supplies should be kept ready near the neonate
- Explain to the mother about the procedure and ask for her involvement
- Check and change the diaper, if needed and place the baby in warm comfortable position.

Performing the Steps of Procedure with Rationale/Point of Emphasis

1. Perform hand hygiene. Dry and warm hands before touching the infant.
2. Place the baby in supine position for easy observation and manipulation.
3. Observe the *respiration* pattern as rise and fall of both chest and abdomen. Count respiration rate for full one minute. Look for any abnormal features such as tachypnea, chest indrawing, grunting, nasal flaring, etc. Note all findings.
4. Disinfect the pediatric stethoscope using alcohol swab and make it dry and warm before auscultation of the apical heart rate of the neonate.
5. Place the stethoscope on infant's chest on the apex area at point of maximum impulse. Count the apical *heart rate* for full one minute, noting irregularities of rhythm and any murmurs. Infant should have strong regular heart rate without 'murmurs'. Many infants have "innocent murmurs", with no implication of pathologic conditions. All murmurs should be reported to doctor/health care prescriber for further evaluation. Note findings.
6. Feel peripheral pulse in all four limbs and note the presence of any abnormalities.
7. Clean the digital thermometer using alcohol (70%) swab from bulb to stem and dry it.
8. Dry the infant's axillae with dry cotton swab to make it free from moisture.
9. Place the bulb of the digital thermometer at the apex/roof of the dry axillae to measure infant's *body temperature*. Keep the thermometer parallel to the baby's arm. Baby's arm is held close to the body to keep the thermometer in place. Wait for beep sound, take out the thermometer and then read the infant's body temperature. Note the finding.

10. Clean the thermometer again with alcohol swab from stem to bulb after use and keep the thermometer in dry container gently to prevent accidental breakage.
11. Place the infant in comfortable position and maintain warmth
12. Check *SpO_2, CRT* and *blood pressure,* whenever required *(Refer details of SpO2 assessment in Procedure - 14 and CRT assessment in Procedure - 16 of this Unit - 2).*
13. Inform the mother about infant's condition and answer to her questions.
14. Take care all articles used and keep ready for next use.
15. Perform hand hygiene and document all findings of vital signs assessment.

Evaluation and Documentation

- *Evaluate:* Always check vital signs on admission in any unit, then hourly for first 4 hours and then once every 3–4 hours for next 24 hours and then as indicated. Evaluate mother's reaction, interaction and involvement during the procedure
- *Document:* Record all findings of respiration, heart rate, pulse, temperature in details in neonate's case sheet and in hospital recording system and report the abnormalities.

Communication and Teaching for Homecare

- *Communicate with family:* Inform the mother and family members about the infant's condition and plan of further management with expected date of discharge
- Teach the parents about the following:
  - Abnormal respiratory pattern, fast breathing, chest indrawing, abnormal sound in respiration, bluish or any other abnormal color or discoloration, etc.
  - Measurement of infant's temperature by human touch technique (with clean, dry and warm dorsum of the hand) and by using thermometer.
    By human touch, tactile assessment of infant's temperature can be done. If the infant is having warm and pink feet, then it indicates that the baby is in normal body temperature. But when feet are cold and abdomen is warm, then it indicates that the baby is in cold stress/mild hypothermia. When both feet and abdomen are cold, then the infant is hypothermic
  - Infant is hypothermic when body temperature is less than 36.5°C and hyperthermic when it is more than 37.5°C by thermometer. So, it is important to teach the parent to measure infant's body temperature using thermometer also
  - Identification of danger signs, like infant is cold to touch or hot to touch, poor suckling/feeding, lethargic, difficulty in breathing, abnormal movements or seizures, no passage of urine or meconium/stool, excessive crying, persistent vomiting, watery stool, any discoloration of skin (blue, yellow, reddish, pale), superficial infections (like umbilical sepsis, skin pustules, oral thrush and eye infections/conjunctivitis), etc.

PROCEDURE–6: WEIGHT RECORDING OF NEONATES

Clinical Guidelines

- Birth weight of the newborn infant should be measured within 2 hours of birth after stabilization of the condition and then every 24 hours daily during hospital stay, using same digital weighing scale at same time each day
- Average birth weight of the Indian neonate is 2,500–3,800 gram. Birth weight below 2,500 gram is termed as low birth weight. These LBW infants require special care in neonatal period. Neonates having birth weight less than 1,800 gram require admission in special newborn care units (SNCU), as they are at risk of various health problems and complications
- Measuring birth weight helps to identify the required level of care for the neonate
- Daily weight measurement of the hospitalized neonates is necessary to

monitor the adequacy of feeding (i.e., for adequacy of nutrition and fluid balance) and loss of weight pattern
- Healthy term neonates have weight loss during first 2–3 days of life and it remains stationary during next 1–2 days. Birth weight usually regains in healthy infant by the end of first week of life. An initial weight loss can be up to 5–10% of birth weight in first few days of life in normal neonate and it is considered as normal
- Preterm neonates have 2–3% weight loss daily, up to maximum of 10–15%. Any weight loss more than 5% in 24 hours is abnormal. Preterm neonates should regain birth weight by 10–14 days of age
- So, all infants should regain birth weight by the 2 weeks of age. The term neonate regains birth weight within 10 days of life and the preterm neonates within 15 days of life
- If initial weight loss is more than 10%, then infant's feeding or nutrition and hydration must be reassessed. Delayed feeding and unsatisfactory feeding may be associated with excessive weight loss
- Neonate's body weight must be measured and recorded on discharge from hospital.

Equipment Required

- Hand hygiene articles for hand wash and antiseptic handrub
- Weighing scale to measure baby's weight, preferably digital weighing scale
- Small mackintosh and clean warm sheet or single use paper drape to cover the weighing scale tray/pan to prevent soiling
- Baby clothing and diaper to dress up the infant
- Diaper changing articles such as dry and wet cotton swabs
- Buckets to discard soiled diaper and clothing
- Disinfectant solution for cleaning of weighing machine, as per unit protocol
- Cotton swabs in a bowl to disinfect the tray/pan of weighing machine
- Waste disposal containers
- Record sheet to note the infants body weight.

Assessment and Preparation

- Perform hand hygiene before touching the infant
- Assess and ensure that the infant is stable and warm before recording birth weight
- Ensure that the environment is clean, warm, free from draught and having good light
- Check that the weighing scale is placed on a firm flat surface near the baby
- Digital weighing scale should be calibrated weekly
- Clean the weighing scale with soap and water. Disinfect the tray/pan of the scale with disinfectant solution and allow drying. Ensure weighing scale tray/pan is centrally placed
- Collect all necessary supplies and articles at work table/NBCC/bedside of the infant for easy access during the procedure
- Explain the procedure to the mother before measuring the infant's weight.

Performing the Steps of Procedure with Rationale/Point of Emphasis

1. Perform hand hygiene to prevent transmission infections.
2. Ensure the weighing machine is clean and disinfected.
3. Place the mackintosh and sheet or single use paper drape or waterproof sheet on the tray/pan of the weighing scale to prevent soiling by the infant with urine or meconium.
4. Set the digital weighing scale at "Zero". If facility for making "Zero" is not available, then weight of the mackintosh and sheet or waterproof sheet or single use paper drape should be deducted from total weight recorded.
5. Check and change the diaper (if it is soiled), to provide comfort to the infant.
6. Undress the infant completely. Minimum clothing can be allowed, but weight must be deducted. For sick infant, detach as many tubes as possible.
7. Place the baby centrally on the weighing scale to measure the accurate body weight.

8. Keep/hold one hand slightly above the infant, while on scale, to provide support and to prevent fall of the infant. Keep the baby on the middle of the tray/pan.
9. Note and record infant's body weight, when the baby is still, not moving and unsupported by anyone to get measurement of actual weight in gram.
10. Remove the infant from the scale carefully and dress up with clothing, cap and diaper.
11. Place the infant on the bassinet or with mother either skin to skin contact or in same bed (bedding-in) with good wrapping to provide warm and to promote breastfeeding.
12. Inform the mother about infant's body weight and explain about presence of any abnormalities.
13. Dispose all wastes and disinfect the weighing scale.
14. Reset the supplies and equipment for weight recording to keep ready for next use.
15. Perform hand hygiene and document the body weight of the infant in record sheet.

Evaluation and Documentation

- Evaluate the infant's weight as normal or LBW, AGA or SGA or LGA as per gestational age. All abnormalities should be reported to doctor/health care prescriber for future management.
- Document infants weight in delivery record/Logbook, infant's case sheet and in mother's case sheet for future reference.

Communication and Teaching for Homecare

- Communicate with parents and family members about the neonate's body weight and regarding any variations of infant's weight. Answer to any questions as appropriate to the level of understanding
- Teach the parents about weight loss, time of regaining of birth weight, weight gain pattern (20–30 g/day) in neonatal period, exclusive breastfeeding to promote weight gain, hygienic measures and follow-up visit date in well baby clinic.

PROCEDURE–7: PHYSICAL EXAMINATION OF NEONATES

Clinical Guidelines

- Physical examination of neonates is an important part of neonatal assessment. Neonatal assessment includes detail history collection (antenatal, intranatal, family, and genetic), physical examination of neonate, review of maternal investigations and neonatal screening along with related laboratory and radiological investigations of neonate
- Initial assessment of the neonate is done at delivery room to identify the need of resuscitation, to ascertain the gestational age and to detect presence of any congenital anomalies. Subsequent or follow-up assessment in neonatal period must be done to detect danger signs, congenital anomalies and presence of any physical or physiological abnormalities for prompt management
- Assessment of neonate in postnatal ward/unit should be done at least three times or more depending upon the neonate's condition. Mother and the baby should be routinely observed daily at least twice a day or more in case of any problem arise in the hospital. Routine assessment on first day of life within 24 hours and at the time of discharge is very important. Second assessment should be done at the age of 2 weeks of age and third assessment between 4 and 6 weeks of age of the infant
- All methods of physical examination, i.e., inspection, palpation, manipulation, percussion and auscultation must be followed wherever and whenever appropriate for the neonate. Examination should be done as convenient for the neonate. Rigid sequence of examination can be difficult to follow in some situations for infants.

Equipment Required

- Hand washing supplies and antiseptic handrub for maintenance of hand hygiene

- Articles for vital signs assessment and weight measurement of the neonate
- Tape measure for anthropometric measurement (length, head and chest circumference, abdominal girth)
- Infantometer for measuring length of the baby, if available
- Examination light or torch for better visualization
- Baby sheets to wrap the infant and molly sheet or mackintosh with sheet to protect examination table or bassinet from soiling
- Ballard Scoring Sheet and Neonatal Assessment Record sheet
- Diaper changing articles to change the soil diaper
- Waste disposal containers
- Documentation sheet for keeping record of findings of physical examination

Assessment and Preparation

- Assess for presence of any emergency or priority signs of the neonate and manage immediately. Then perform routine physical examination in stable baby
- Assess the parents' anxiety and level of understanding about neonate's health status
- Self-preparation should be done with adequate hand hygiene and following standard precautions whenever required
- Environment should be made clean, warm, well lighted and free from overcrowding
- All supplies and necessary items should be arranged near the neonate
- Preparation of mother: Explain the mother about the importance of physical examination. Encourage her to participate or to help during the procedure if she is not sick. Head to foot examination can be done on mother's lap
- Preparation of neonate: Make the baby clean and comfortable. Examination can be done under radiant warmer, on mother's bed or mother's lap or in examination table.

Performing the Steps of Procedure with Rationale/Point of Emphasis

1. Perform hand hygiene initially with soap water hand wash then use handrub in between examination of different parts of the body.
2. Collect and arrange all articles near the neonate. Ensure infection control measures.
3. Assess vital signs *(Refer Procedure-5 of this Unit)*.
4. Measure neonate's body weight *(Refer Procedure-6 of this Unit)*.
5. Perform Anthropometric measurements:
   - *Measure of length* using tape measure or Infantometer for assessing crown-heel length. Place the baby on hard surface or on Infantometer in supine position with extended legs. Length is measured at delivery room or on first day of life and before discharge from hospital and also in the clinic at regular interval
   - *Measure head circumference (HC)* using ordinary tape measure, by placing it just over the supraorbital ridges in front, above the ears on the sides and over the occipital protuberance at the back. Measure the points of highest circumference. Take HC measurement after 24 hours of birth, when molding and caput are disappeared and before discharge from hospital for all neonates. For preterm, LBW and sick hospitalized infants measure occipito-frontal circumference (OFC) once a week during hospital stay
   - *Measure chest circumference (CC)* using tape measure, by placing it around the chest at the level of nipples in between inspiration and expiration. Take CC measurement at birth or on the first day of life or as indicated in case of any chest problems
   - *Measure abdominal circumference (AC)* using tape measure, by placing it around the abdomen at the level just above the umbilical cord or over the umbilicus, when umbilical cord fallen off. Take AC measurement at birth, on admission at NICU/SNCU, before giving gavage feeding and in case of suspected abdominal distension of the baby.

6. Examine head to foot of the neonate:
   - *General appearance, posture, muscle tone and movements* - for any abnormalities
   - *Examine head and hair:* For presence of caput succedaneum, cephalohematoma, molding, injury, asymmetry, encephalocele and any other abnormalities. Check fontanels (depressed or elevated or flat) and sutures (widely separated or closed). Examine shape of the skull, condition of the scalp and hair for any abnormalities
   - *Examine the baby's face:* For shape, asymmetry, swelling, paralysis, dysmorphic look, cleft lip, presence of any abnormal movements and facial expression indicating pain
   - *Examine eyes:* For symmetry, discharge, edema, subconjunctival hemorrhage, and color of the sclera, presence of congenital cataract and features of conjunctivitis. Check with ophthalmoscope for red reflex
   - *Examine nose:* For shape, symmetry, patency of nasal passage, any nasal discharge, nasal flaring and flat nasal bridge
   - *Examine mouth:* For cleft palate (in soft palate or in hard palate), natal teeth, tongue tie, oral infections, and oral thrush. Check for cyanosis of tongue and oral mucosa
   - *Examine ears:* For size, shape, cartilage formation, skin tag, preauricular sinus, any discharge and position of ears (low set ear)
   - *Examine neck:* For fracture clavicle, mobility, stiffness, retractions, congenital cyst or mass, excessive skin folds, shortness and webbing,
   - *Examine chest:* For shape and size of chest, breast tissue formation, nipple size, mastitis neonatorum, rate and rhythm of respiration, abnormalities of respiration (such as chest indrawing, grunting) and rate, rhythm and apex position of heart sound
   - *Examine abdomen:* For shape, synchronous movement with chest during respiration, condition of umbilicus (cord fallen off or not, redness of surrounding skin, foul smell, features of sepsis, bleeding), bowel sound and presence of abdominal distension, or any mass or any congenital abnormalities (such as omphalocele, umbilical hernia, exstrophy of urinary bladder). Liver is usually palpable 1 – 2 cm below costal margin
   - *Examine hips:* For developmental dysplasia of hips/congenital dislocation of hip with features of asymmetrical gluteal folds and positive Ortolani's sign. Check for femoral pulses and it's any abnormality
   - *Examine extremities:* For fracture, range of motion, paralysis, irregular shape and size, abnormal fingers and toes (missing digit, syndactyly, extra digit/polydactyly), club foot/talipes, edema and abnormalities of nails. Check for palmer creases and color of palms and soles
   - *Examine back:* For abnormal spinal curvature, tuft of hair, spina bifida occulta, and spina bifida cystica (meningocele, meningomyelocele)
   - *Examine buttocks:* For any mass (sacrococcygeal teratoma) or injury and in perianal area for anal opening or presence of any other abnormalities (imperforate anus, fistula, polyp)
   - *Examine skin:* For abnormal color (cyanosis, jaundice, pallor, plethoric), lanugo hair, vernix, Mongolian spots, erythema, milia, dryness, peeling, abrasion, laceration, injury, skin turgor, and hemangioma or any other abnormalities
   - *Examine genitalia:* In female baby look for labia majora covers labia minora and clitoris or not, presence of white mucoid discharge or pink-red mucoid discharge, hymenal tag and imperforate hymen. In boy baby look for testes in scrotal sac, pigmentation and rugae of scrotum and presence of hypospadias, epispadias, hydrocele, inguinal hernia or any other abnor-

malities. Confirm about identification of external sex organs or difficulty in sex determination (DSD).

7. Assess gestational age at delivery room or on first day using New Ballard Scoring for assessment of neuromuscular maturity and physical maturity. Gestational age initially assessed before delivery from LMP and EDD of mother and from the ultrasound findings *(Refer Appendix - X: New Ballard Score)*.
8. Assess general behavior: Look for baby's abnormal crying, response to stimulation, alertness, activity pattern, posture, position, movements of limbs, asymmetry in movements, presence of pain and sleep pattern.
9. Examine feeding behavior: Assess sucking, swallowing and rooting reflex, presence of vomiting, excessive frothy secretions from mouth (tracheoesophageal fistula, esophageal atresia), chocking and poor sucking with lethargy.
10. Check pattern of elimination: Confirm passage of meconium within 24 hours and passage of urine within 48 hours or not. Look for presence of transitional stool on 3–4 days of life and typical stool at one week of age. Check for any abnormalities in elimination pattern.
11. Assess neurological status: Examine for muscle tone, posture, movements, level of consciousness (with simple "AVPU" scale - **A**lert, response to **V**oice, response to **P**ain only, and **U**nresponsive), behavior and reflexes (mainly sucking reflex, swallowing reflex and Moro reflex are assessed in neonates). Usually other primitive and protective reflexes are examined when indicated only.
12. Assess special sense: Examine the baby for presence of sensation of touch, taste and smell (with mother's milk), hearing (response to sound) and visual sensations (with mother's face, in late neonatal period).
13. Check for danger signs: Look for presence of any danger signs of the baby such as poor feeding, lethargy, cold or hot to touch especially periphery, fast or rapid breathing (more than 60 breaths/minute), difficulty in respiration, chest indrawing, apnea, cyanosis, excessive crying, abnormal movements/seizures, persistent vomiting, watery stool, bleeding from any site or opening and superficial infections like umbilical sepsis, skin pustules, oral thrush and conjunctivitis.
14. Examine for congenital anomalies: Look for presence of any structural abnormalities and systemic dysfunctions, present at birth or thereafter. Early identification of congenital anomalies is essential for prompt initiation of management to prevent neonatal mortality and morbidity of the infants.
15. Make the neonate comfortable during and after the physical examination and allow the mother for breastfeeding.
16. Involve mother during examination. Answer to mother's questions as appropriate.
17. Terminate the procedure, dispose waste and take care of reusable items.
18. Documents the procedure and all findings of the neonatal examination record.

Evaluation and Documentation

- Evaluate the examination findings and compare with previous assessments and note the alterations, if physical examination already done. Evaluate parent's response and reactions related to examination findings
- Document all findings of the physical examination in neonatal assessment standard recording proforma, as per institutional policy.

Communication and Teaching for Homecare

- Communicate with mother, father and the family members about the findings of the examination in details according to their level of understanding. Discuss about plan of management and discharge plan from the hospital
- Teach the parents about involvement in routine neonatal care at hospital,

continued care at home after discharge, danger signs, importance of medical help, communication with community health workers, and schedule of follow-up visits.

PROCEDURE–8: CARE OF NEONATES AT POSTNATAL WARD/UNIT WITH DAILY MONITORING

Clinical Guidelines

- Essential and routine care of the normal stable term newborn baby at postnatal ward/unit is important for prevention of neonatal morbidity and promotion of neonatal survival
- Assessment of normal healthy stable neonates suitable for routine care with mother should be done at delivery room. Identification of "At Risk Neonates" and hospitalization at SNCU/NICU for appropriate management should also be done at birth for prevention of long-term complications and reduction of neonatal mortality
- At risk neonatal condition requiring hospitalization are: (i) birth weight less than 1,800 gram, (ii) gestational age less than 34 weeks, (iii) asphyxia neonatorum requiring post-resuscitation care, (iv) presence of major congenital anomalies and (v) respiratory difficulty/distress
- In postnatal ward, mother and baby should be allowed to stay in bedding-in/rooming-in to promote "Zero Separation" between mother and newborn infant
- Majority of the complications and death in neonatal period occur in first week of life. So, observational and supportive care for both mother and baby is very essential
- Daily essential and routine neonatal care includes maintenance of warmth, exclusive breastfeeding, prevention of infections, maintenance of hygienic measures (care of umbilical cord, eyes, skin, and clothing), monitoring of neonate's condition and immunization
- Daily monitoring of neonates should be done for vital signs, activity pattern, feeding behavior, skin color for jaundice, cyanosis, pallor and reddish, passage of urine and meconium/ stool, body weight and danger signs. Identification of abnormal features should be done immediately and prompt management must be initiated
- Parents require special support, explanation and reassurance for minor neonatal problems (such as vomiting, hiccups, napkin rash, cradle cap, excessive sleepiness, excessive crying, etc.) and for developmental peculiarities (such as erythema toxicum, milia, Mongolian blue spots, mastitis neonatorum, vaginal bleeding, transitional stool, tongue tie, peeling skin, subconjunctival hemorrhage, nevus simplex, etc.)
- Few neonates require special attention and care at postnatal ward such as low birth weight baby (LBW) having weight between 1,800 and 2,499 gram and neonates requiring resuscitation with PPV less than one minute. Kangaroo mother care and feeding support should be provided to the LBW neonates of this group with monitoring for neonatal problems. Special observational care for neonates having PPV less than one minute should be arranged in postnatal care keeping the baby with mother
- Immunizations with birth dose of Hepatitis B, OPV and BCG must be administered before discharge from hospital, in case institutional delivery
- Discharge from the hospital should be planned according to the condition of the mother and baby. As per recommendation, normal spontaneous delivered mother and baby should be discharged after 48 hours of birth, if the mother and baby are having no illness. After LUCS delivery, discharge from hospital is planned on 5–7 days of delivery depending upon the condition of the mother and baby
- Discharge advice for care at home and follow-up care should be explained to the parents and family members. Printed copy of discharge certificate must be given to the parents as legal document with all detailed information of birth.

Equipment Required

- Hand hygiene supplies for hand wash and handrub for mother, caregiver and health professionals
- Articles for vital signs assessment of neonates
- Articles for physical examination of the newborn baby
- Articles for BCG immunization, if not given at delivery room
- Baby clothing, cap, socks, sheets, towels, diapers
- Routine baby care articles and supplies as needed
- Diaper changing articles
- Waste disposal containers
- Neonatal daily monitoring record sheet.

Assessment and Preparation

- Assess the mother's ability to take care of the baby and need for necessary support. Assess neonate's condition and need for care to be provide
- Self-preparation should be done by maintenance of hand hygiene
- Environment should be clean, well-lighted and free from overcrowding
- All necessary articles should be arranged near the neonate. Articles can be arranged for individual baby or for a group of neonates
- Preparation of the mother: Explain to the mother about the procedure and encourage her to participate during the procedure
- Preparation of neonate: Make the neonate comfortable for the procedure. Avoid undue exposure before and during care.

Performing Steps of Procedure with Rationale/Point of Emphasis

1. Perform hand washing initially then use handrub in between care and touch.
2. Ensure all articles are ready in hand for easy access.
3. Involve the mother and family members during observation and care of the baby.
4. Ensure the baby is warm with adequate clothing. Check the baby's temperature by human touch. Warm and pink feet of the baby indicates that baby's body temperature is normal.
5. Assist and support the mother during breastfeeding. Observe baby's feeding behavior, correct positioning of the baby, correct attachment during breastfeeding, adequacy of breastfeeding and breastfeeding problems of the mother (such as retracted/flat nipple, sore nipple, breast engorgement, not enough milk or reduced milk supply).
6. Ensure nothing is given as feed to the baby other than mother's own milk. Avoid prelacteal feeding like honey, gripe water, etc.
7. Manage mother's breastfeeding problems promptly to continue exclusive breastfeeding.
8. Check the diaper for passage of urine and meconium/stool. Change if it is soiled and teach the procedure to the mother.
9. Observe the neonate for respiration, heart rate, body temperature, CRT, feeding behavior, activity pattern, skin color especially for jaundice, urine output, and passage of meconium or stool. Observe the baby twice daily in postnatal ward to identify the problems early in time.
10. Ensure cleanliness of the baby and baby's care articles. Baby bath is usually given after umbilical cord is fallen off and baby's weight becomes more than 2,500 gram. In hospitalized baby, sponge bath should be given with lukewarm water. Tub bath during hospital stay can lead to infection to the baby.
11. Measure body weight with same weighing scale at same time every day (as per hospital policy), and before discharge to assess weight loss pattern.
12. Look for condition of umbilical cord, eyes and skin for features of infection and presence of other danger signs of neonates.
13. Ensure the umbilical cord is open and dry. No kajal is applied in baby's eyes.
14. Assess adequacy of breastfeeding by number of wet diaper (6–8 times in a day) and weight loss. Most healthy term baby's weight loss in first 2–3 days of life can be

5% to 10 % of the birth weight. Delayed feeding and unsatisfactory feeding may be associated with excessive weight loss.

15. Arrange to administer BCG immunization to the neonate before discharge, if not given at delivery room. BCG injection is given in intradermal route with the dose of 0.05 mL at left upper arm, just above the insertion of deltoid muscle. Cold chain must be maintained. Usually immunizations are administered with all precautions by the health professionals from post-partum unit or well-baby clinic, as per hospital policy
16. Explain and inform mother about the activities to be done for the baby
17. Make the neonate comfortable and allow the mother for breastfeeding
18. Discuss about plan of discharge. Check for fulfillment of discharge criteria. Inform about probable date, time and official procedure to be followed for discharge from the hospital
19. Complete the procedure, dispose waste and take care of reusable items
20. Document the procedure and all findings of observation during care.

Evaluation and Documentation

- Evaluate neonate's condition and compare with previous findings to identify problems in the neonate and for prompt management. Evaluate mother's ability to take care of the neonate and to identify the danger signs. Evaluate anxiety and level of understanding of the parents to provide necessary care of the infant at home
- Document the procedure done for the neonate and all observational findings in detail in the neonatal case sheet.

Communication and Teaching for Homecare

- Communicate with mother and the family members about condition of mother and baby, plan of discharge and continued care at home. Answer to the questions asked by parents
- Teach the parents about home-based neonatal care and follow-up care:
  - Demonstrate wrapping, dressing, putting cap and socks to maintain warmth
  - Teach assessment of baby's temperature by human touch or using thermometer
  - Inform and support for exclusive breastfeeding up to 6 months of age
  - Instruct the mother to keep the umbilical cord open and dry
  - Discuss about harmful traditional practices for the neonate such as feeding honey, application of kajal in the eyes, any applications on umbilical cord, etc.
  - Ensure KMC for LBW infants till their weight become 2,500 gram or more
  - Demonstrate hygienic practices to be continued at home such as hand washing, clean clothing and dress, clean linen, bathing and skin care, and diapering
  - Explain to the parents about immunization schedule, danger signs, parenting tips, family planning practices and growth and development of the infant, as per Maternal and Child Protection card (MCP card)
  - Discuss about importance of follow-up visits and medical help whenever necessary
  - Inform the date, time and place of immunization, and follow-up visit
  - Instruct and explain about preservation of all records of birth and immunization.

PROCEDURE–9: BATHING (SPONGE BATH) AND DIAPERING THE NEONATES

Clinical Guidelines

- Bathing and diapering the neonates are essential procedures for maintenance of personal hygiene and cleanliness. These procedures help to provide comfort and to prevent bad odors. Bathing promotes circulation and stimulation
- Sponge bath can be given as first bath after the infant's temperature has stabilized

in the normal range (36.5–37.5°C) and when appropriate care is taken to support thermal stability. It can be given after 24 hours of birth only, or as per hospital policy, if the baby is having no problems. Sponge bath is usually given for hospitalized neonates/young infants as there is risk of cross infections in the infants due to tub bath, if appropriate precautions are not taken

- The infant can have complete bath for two or three times in a week or more often, if necessary. Hair washing can be given with first newborn bath and as needed thereafter. Between complete baths, the infant's face, neck, hands, and genital areas can be washed, as required. Routine eye care may not require unless infected. Orbital area can be cleaned with sterile or clean cotton swab, as per unit policy
- Change of diaper, when it becomes wet or soiled is important to prevent skin excoriation around perianal area. It provides comfort and prevents sore buttocks and bad odor
- In neonates, tub bath/dip water bath should be given when the umbilical cord has fallen off, thus to prevent umbilical infection. Tub bath is not recommended in LBW baby, having birth weight less than 2,500 gram, as it can lead to hypothermia and infections. It is usually given at home to the young infants after discharge from hospital *(Refer details of the Procedure of 'Tub Bath' in the Procedure - 9: 'Bathing Infant and Young Child' of Unit - 3 of this Manual).*

Equipment Required for Sponge Bath

- Hand washing supplies and handrub
- Water proof apron for care provider to protect the dress
- Clean nonsterile gloves to prevent cross infections
- Baby dress/clothing: Frock, shirt, cap, socks, and diaper
- Baby sheet, linen, and dry blanket especially in winter season to remake the baby's bed
- Two bath towels—for wrapping and drying the baby
- Two wash cloths—to give sponge bath to the infant
- Sterile cotton balls/swabs in a covered sterile bowl, for cleaning of eyes/orbital area
- Basin with lukewarm water to be used for sponge bath. Water temperature for bathing should be 100°F or 37.8°C
- Two water jugs—one with hot water and another with water having normal temperature
- Bath thermometer to measure the water temperature
- Baby soap to clean the baby's skin, as recommended
- Baby oil to apply on baby's dry and rough skin, if required
- Baby powder, if recommended. Usually baby powder is used for perianal area to prevent bad odor. It should not be irritating to the baby's skin
- Soft bristle hair brush or fine toothed comb
- For change of diaper: (a) A bowl with wet cotton swabs to remove urine and meconium/stool and to clean the buttocks, (b) A bowl with dry cotton swabs to dry the buttocks after cleaning, (c) A covered bucket to discard the soiled diaper and cotton swabs, (d) Baby powder to apply on the buttocks to prevent bad odor and to smooth the skin, as per unit policy, (e) Vaseline or Barrier cream (such as zinc oxide paste) or non-irritating oil to apply on the perianal skin, (f) Ointment (such as antibiotic or antifungal), as prescribed, in case of perianal dermatitis or skin erosions, and (g) Disposable cleaning wipes, if available
- Waste disposal containers as per BMW rules for clothing and linen
- Procedure documentation sheet, as per unit policy.

Assessment and Preparation

- Assess the baby's vital signs and presence of any problems. Bath is not allowed for sick unstable baby. Assess mother's level of understanding to follow the procedure

of bathing and diapering that need to be performed at home
- Self-preparation should be done with hand washing
- Environment should be warm, clean, and well-lighted. Fans should be switched off
- Arrange all articles near the baby or in the procedure room
- Preparation of mother: Explain the procedure to the mother. Allow the mother to participate during the procedure
- Preparation of neonate: Avoid undue exposure during bathing and diapering. Change the diaper first before bathing, if soiled

Performing the Steps of Procedure with Rationale/Point of Emphasis

Giving Sponge Bath to the Neonate/Infant

1. Perform hand washing and wear protective apron.
2. Ensure all arrangements for bathing are ready around the baby for easy use.
3. Wrap the baby with a towel and place on the bath table/bassinet securely on supine position for easy observation.
4. Check the baby's diaper, change if it is wet/soiled (See the steps of "Diapering" in continuation of this procedure).
5. Perform hand hygiene. Wear clean gloves as per unit policy. Sponge bath can be given without wearing gloves, as clean procedure.
6. Fill the basin with lukewarm water for giving sponge bath.
7. Begin by bathing face using soft washcloth or cotton balls soaked in water.
8. Clean the orbital area from inner canthus to outer canthus using fresh cotton balls for each eye or using clean corner of washcloth.
9. Cleanse nose with corner of cloth or cotton ball. Remove secretions, incrustations from the nares gently.
10. Wash external ears and behind the ears by winding the damp washcloth around the little or index finger.
11. Dry the bathed area with the dry towel every time. Do not rub the skin surfaces.
12. Hold the wrapped baby's head over the basin by the left hand and wash head and hair with right hand. If soap is applied on head, then removal of soap and rinsing of head with hair should be done thoroughly followed by complete drying. Avoid water getting into the ears by covering ears with left thumb and finger
13. Discard the used water and use clean fresh water for cleaning baby's body.
14. Take off the baby's wrapping and dress to expose for sponge bathing.
15. Cleanse the neck, shoulder, chest, abdomen, and legs gently with clean washcloth. Then cleanse back and buttocks by placing the baby in prone position. Give special attention to the skin folds of neck, underarms and thighs.
16. Cleanse the groin, genital area and perianal area at last with special attention.
17. Apply soap in same sequence, when soap and water bath is given to remove dirt. Apply soap by hands gently over the baby's body and remove the soap with washcloth. Soap and water bath may be necessary to cleanse the baby thoroughly. Remove the soap with washcloth, rinse and dry after washing. Do not rub the skin.
18. Comb the infants hair with soft bristle brush or fine toothed comb.
19. Dress the baby and wrap appropriately and make the baby comfortable.
20. Remake the baby's bassinet or crib/bed with clean sheet and molly sheet.
21. Cleanse all used articles and reset for next use.
22. Dispose all waste in appropriate containers
23. Perform hand hygiene.
24. Document the procedure and observational findings.

Diapering the Neonate /Infant

- Instruct the mother about importance of prompt diaper changes to avoid skin irritation of the infant and about steps of the procedure
- Involve the mother and other care giver during diaper change of the infant

- Perform hand washing and arrange necessary items near the neonate.
- Wear clean nonsterile gloves, as per unit policy. This procedure can be done in nontouch technique without contamination of hands
- Place the infant on a firm clean surface such as diapering table, or crib or bed or bassinet securely
- Remove the soiled diaper and assess the contents of diaper for unusual or abnormal appearance or odor of urine and meconium/stool and discard in appropriate container
- Assess infant's perianal area for redness, excoriation, skin rash, diaper dermatitis or features of any other problems in diaper area at each diaper change. Fungal infection with *Candida albicans* is common in the infants, especially with unhealthy and broken skin
- Cleanse the perianal skin with disposable wipes or using wet warm cotton swabs and mild soap, if necessary. Clean the skin folds with precautions. Use one wet swab at a time. Dry the perianal area with dry cotton swabs immediately
- Apply barrier cream (such as zinc oxide paste) or medicated ointment on clean and dry perianal skin, as prescribed, if the baby is having diaper dermatitis
- Ensure umbilical cord/umbilicus is not contaminated with urine or meconium/stool
- Apply new clean diaper securely, folding front of the diaper to avoid irritation of umbilical cord/umbilicus. Fold the plastic part of the diaper away from the skin
- Collect the stool/urine specimen for examination, if required to detect any abnormalities
- Dispose the soiled diaper and all wastes in appropriate containers as per BMW rules
- Remove gloves, if used and perform hand washing
- Take care of clothing, linens, and other reusable items. Reset for next procedure
- Make the infant comfortable, wrap adequately and secure in the crib/bassinet/bed
- Document the procedure and record the observational findings in infant's record sheet

Evaluation and Documentation

- Evaluate parental participation during infant bathing and diapering. Evaluate abnormal findings noted during bathing and diapering
- Document the following: (a) general appearance of the infant, (b) skin condition including genital and perianal area, (c) infant's reaction during the procedure (d) characteristic of urine and meconium/stool, and any abnormalities observed.

Communication and Teaching for Homecare

- Communicate with parents/family about the infant's general condition and importance of the hygienic measures along with other care. Answer to the related questions
- Teach the parents about the following:
  - Special precautions during bathing and diapering such as avoidance of undue exposure, keeping the baby unattended and use of mixture of hot or cold water
  - Demonstrate the bathing and diapering steps that should be followed at home
  - Instruct about use of reusable cloth diaper which must be cleaned, washed, thoroughly dry, preferably in sunlight and made up of cotton material
  - Use of any powder should be done cautiously, especially on moist diaper area as it can lead to diaper dermatitis or skin rash
  - Discuss about home-based care of the infant for continued care
  - Inform about danger signs, need for medical help and follow-up visits.

PROCEDURE–10: CARE OF INFECTED UMBILICAL CORD OF THE NEONATES

Clinical Guidelines

- Normally umbilical cord falls off after 5–10 days of age, but it may take longer period to fall off especially when infected. For routine care, nothing to be applied on the umbilical cord. It must be kept open and dry without any dressing or application. Natural drying of the umbilical cord does not result in increased incidence of infection. But treatment with antiseptics prolongs time for cord separation and falling off

- The cord should be observed for any bleeding and clinical features of infection. Umbilical sepsis is a common superficial infection and can lead to septicemia and jaundice in neonates
- Infection of umbilical cord is clinically identified with the features as swollen and moist periumbilical tissues with redness and foul smelling. Other features include fever, serous or seropurulent discharge and delayed falling off the umbilical cord. Severe umbilical infection is considered if the redness extends more than 1 cm of surrounding tissue and other signs of sepsis present. In severe infection, local therapy and systemic antibiotic is required for the neonate.

Equipment Required

- Hand hygiene supplies for hand washing and handrub
- Sterile container/tray with sterile articles—gloves, cotton swabs, gauze pieces, three small bowls (one for swab, one for normal saline, one for antiseptic solution) and a small dressing forceps to clean the umbilical cord
- Transfer forceps or lifter in a sterile container to handle the sterile articles/items
- Treatment towel or molly sheet to protect the bed/bassinet
- Normal saline bottle, alcohol 70%, antiseptic solution and medication as prescribed
- Waste disposal containers as per BMW rules
- Neonatal care record sheet and procedure documentation sheet.

Assessment and Preparation

- Assess the neonate's vital signs, feeding behavior, clinical features of sepsis and any other abnormalities. Assess parents' anxiety and level of understanding
- Self-preparation should be done with hand hygiene. Strict aseptic technique should be maintained. Assistant may be arranged to perform the procedure aseptically
- Environment should be clean, well-lighted and free from overcrowding
- All necessary articles and supplies should be arranged near the neonate
- Preparation of mother: Explain the procedure to the mother, if she presents with the baby. Plan of management to be explained to both parents
- Preparation of neonate: Make the baby clean and comfortable. Check and change the diaper before the procedure, if it is soiled.

Performing the Steps of Procedure with Rationale/Point of Emphasis

1. Perform hand washing and arrange all articles/supplies near the neonate.
2. Explain the mother for participation during procedure, if possible.
3. Place the baby in supine position and expose the umbilical area.
4. Wash hands, dry and wear sterile gloves to prevent transmission of infection.
5. Take help for handling sterile articles or arrange all sterile articles before wearing gloves.
6. Clean the skin around the umbilical cord using sterile cotton swabs/gauze pieces soaked in normal saline. Lift the umbilical cord and clean the base. Cleaning should be done from the base of the cord and to 2–3 cm diameter circle around the base of the umbilical cord on infant's abdomen.
7. Clean the umbilical cord stump and then umbilical cord by longitudinal stroke with sterile cotton swabs/gauze pieces soaked normal saline or alcohol as per unit policy. Apply antiseptic solution or antibiotic ointment, if prescribed.
8. Remove gloves, and take care of used items.
9. Discard used cotton swabs/gauze pieces and gloves as per BMW rules.

10. Perform hand washing following six steps.
11. Administer antibiotic medications, as directed in case of severe umbilical cord infection.
12. Make the baby comfortable and allow the mother to take care of the baby.
13. Instruct the mother to keep the cord open and to prevent contamination from urine.
14. Documents the procedure and condition of the umbilical cord.

Evaluation and Documentation

- Evaluate the baby's vital signs, feeding behavior, and condition of umbilical cord and compare with previous findings. Evaluate parents' response and understanding
- Document the procedure and findings of vital signs and condition of the cord in the neonatal case/treatment record.

Communication and Teaching for Homecare

- Communicate with parents and family members about the problem of umbilical cord infection and plan of management. Answer to their questions
- Teach the parents about hand hygiene, general cleanliness, clean clothing, and clean environment and not to apply harmful traditional remedies or agents on the umbilical cord. Teach the mother about breastfeeding, warmth, immunization, danger signs, continued care of the baby at home and follow-up visits.

PROCEDURE–11: CARE OF NEONATES UNDER RADIANT WARMER

Clinical Guidelines

- Radiant warmer provides heat by an infrared energy source to keep the infant warm. It helps in the process of heat gain by radiation, conduction and convection. It prevents heat loss by the provision of warm micro-environment around the infant
- Radiant warmer and bassinet are considered as *open care system* for neonatal care and commonly used at NBCC in delivery room and in neonatal care units (NICU, SNCU) for sick, preterm/LBW neonates. Isolette/Incubator (*closed care System*) is used for preterm neonates, as per availability or as per hospital policy
- Place the radiant warmer away from air currents and maintain room temperature 22°C or more (25–28°C) for optimal functioning
- Clean and disinfect the warmer and mattress and use sterile/clean sheet, as needed
- Switch "ON" the warmer at least 20 minutes before placing the infant to provide prewarm environment
- Use "*Manual mode*" only for prewarming, during resuscitation and initial stabilization of the infant. Use maximum 100% heater output for rapid warming of bassinet in delivery room and in triage bed. After 10 minutes, reduce heater output to 25–75%. Never use 100% heater output unsupervised. Keep in mind, that there is risk of hyperthermia in neonates, if placed in manual mode without supervision
- In "*Servo mode*", set the "required temperature" at 36.5°C. Heater output will adjust automatically to keep the infant at set temperature. Attach the thermistor probe on the baby's skin over upper abdomen at right hypochondrium in supine position. In prone position, attach the probe in flank/loin area. The probe will sense the skin temperature and will display it on the panel as "infant's temperature"
- Parts of *open care system* include:
  - *Bassinet* with mattress on its platform to place the baby. Bassinet has side support/panel made up of plexiglass material, drawers/storage area to keep baby care articles, wheels for easy mobility and foot-operated lock to keep the bassinet in fixed position, whenever required
  - *Radiant warmer* is having the following parts:
    - » Body the radiant warmer with stand and heat source

- » Quartz rods as heat source in parabolic reflector
- » Examination light
- » Control panel with mode selector (Manual mode, or Servo mode), heater output control key/knob, heater output display, temperature selection key/knob, temperature display (required or set temperature, infant's actual temperature and air temperature), alarm display and key lock
- » Thermistor probe or skin probe that to be attached to infant's skin in servo mode
- » Air probe to measure air temperature of the bassinet (available in few model)
- » Metal stand to attach syringe pump or infusion pump and IV fluid bag or bottle
- » Small tray at one side to keep monitor, handrub solution, bottles of alcohol and povidone-iodine, small bowl with cotton swabs, thermometer, tape measure, etc.
- » Ports and switch for electric connections
- » Wheels and locks to keep the warmer fixed or to move when required

- Periodic preventive maintenance of the "open care system" must be done for optimal functioning, as per hospital policy and manufacturer guidelines. Calibration of the radiant warmer should be done every 4–6 months or as per manufacturer guidelines. Trouble shooting during use of warmer should be done based on problems identified
- *Cleaning and disinfection of the open care system* is very important to reduce transmission of microorganisms and to prevent cross infections. The recommended procedures should be followed as per guidelines:
  - For concurrent disinfection, clean the bassinet with soap and water or detergent and disinfect with disinfectant solution daily, as per hospital policy or as available
  - For terminal disinfection, every 7th day or after discharge or after death of the infant, thorough cleaning and disinfection of the bassinet must be done
  - Radiant warmer should be disinfected with disinfectant solution 2–3 times daily
  - Skin probe should be cleaned with 70% alcohol soaked swab before and after each use
  - Front panel/control panel should be cleaned with wet/damp cloth. If is contaminated, mild detergent water or soap and water can be used for cleaning. "No Chemical" should be used to clean the microcomputer control panel
  - Do not use alcohol to clean the bassinet and its side support to prevent it to be hazy.

Equipment Required

- Hand hygiene supplies for hand washing and handrub
- Radiant warmer with bassinet, mattress, sheets, shoulder roll to prepare the bed
- Extra sheet for preparation of nesting or boundaries
- Thermometer, 70% alcohol and cotton swab to record infant's body temperature
- Bottles of alcohol and povidone-iodine, small bowl with cotton swabs, tape measure and routine care articles for the neonate
- Diaper, diaper changing articles and baby clothing
- Pulse oximeter and oxygen delivery system and device, if required
- Neonatal case sheet, monitoring sheet and treatment sheet
- Waste disposal containers.

Assessment and Preparation

- Assess the following:
  - Before placing the infant under radiant warmer note the baseline parameters. Check respiration, temperature, heart rate, SpO_2, CRT, skin color, activity pattern, alertness, level of consciousness, present body weight and presence of abnormal clinical features

- Collect birth history including history of illness
- Assess parents level of understanding and anxiety about the infant's condition

- Self-preparation should be done with hand hygiene and other precautions
- Environment should be clean, warm, well ventilated and without overcrowding
- All required articles should be collected and arranged conveniently for the infant
- Explain to the mother and family members about the plan of management
- Preparation of neonate: For newly received neonate, quickly assess the infant's condition, classify as emergency case or priority case or non-urgent case and then arrange for necessary management and admission in neonatal care unit for continuation of care.

Performing Steps the Procedure with Rationale/Point of Emphasis

1. Perform hand hygiene and arranged all supplies and articles around the radiant warmer.
2. Check the cleaning and disinfection of the open care system is done appropriately.
3. Prepare the bassinet by covering the mattress with sterile/clean sheet.
4. Ensure the electric connection of the system to the mains and switch on the warmer.
5. Select manual mode and keep the heater output at 100% for 20–30 minutes to prewarm the system, if there is no emergency. Reduce the heater output after 10 minutes.
6. Clean the skin probe with 70% alcohol swab and allow to dry.
7. Place the infant under radiant warmer and attach the cleaned skin probe on the infant's skin over upper abdomen at right hypochondrium in supine position. In prone position, attach the cleaned skin probe on flank/loin area. The probe will sense the skin temperature and display it on the panel as "Infant's temperature".
8. Select servo mode and set the required skin temperature of the infant at 36.5°C.
9. Attach the skin probe/thermistor with transparent skin friendly adhesive tape. Do not place the probe on hollow organ or on bony area or on bruised skin. Check the sensor probe area at regular interval for its placement and skin condition. Change the probe position every 24 hours. Ensure the neonate is not lying on the probe wires. Do not reuse disposable probes.
10. Cover the baby's head with cap and feet with socks. Infant's body can be covered with dress exposing the chest and abdomen for observation. In case very sick neonates, infant's body should be kept uncovered for full visualization.
11. Use shoulder roll to position the baby with neck slightly extended to keep airway open.
12. Place a diaper to prevent soiling from urine and stool. Keep the infant dry and change the diaper when it is soiled.
13. Keep the infant within the "Nesting/Boundaries" to prevent postural deformity.
14. Apply "Transparent Cling Wrap" across the side support to prevent insensible water loss in extreme LBW neonate.
15. Measure infant's axillary temperature with digital thermometer every 2–4 hourly. In hypothermic baby, monitor axillary temperature every 30 minutes till it reaches 36.5°C, then hourly for next 4 hours and 2 hourly for 12 hours, thereafter 3 hourly as routine.
16. Do not leave the infant unsupervised in manual mode. In severe hypothermia, quick rewarming should be done up to 34°C, then gradual rewarming should be done till neonate's body temperature becomes normal.
17. Respond to "Alarm" immediately, identify the problem and solve promptly.
18. Observe for side effects or dangers of placing the neonate under radiant warmer such as hyperthermia, hypothermia and increased insensible water loss especially in preterms.
19. Prevent insensible water loss of the neonate under radiant warmer by following practices—(i) clothe the baby

and use cap and socks, (ii) apply oil to the baby's skin and (iii) maintain ambient temperature and humidity.

20. Allow the mother to see the baby and involve in care, if possible.
21. Provide all prescribed treatment and feeding to the infant in time with precautions.
22. Apply pulse oximeter for sick neonates to monitor continuously.
23. Measure admission weight for new baby after stabilization and daily morning weight at same time using same weighing scale.
24. Monitor the infant continuously and record the findings in monitoring sheet.
25. Perform hand hygiene and maintain strict infection control practices.
26. Take care of used articles and dispose the waste.
27. Documents the findings and communicate with the parents.

Evaluation and Documentation

- Evaluate the following:
  - Evaluate the infant's condition for presence of hypothermia and hyperthermia
  - Monitor respiration, temperature, heart rate, SpO_2, CRT, skin color, activity pattern, and alertness, level of consciousness, body weight, urine output and presence of abnormal clinical features. Check whether the baby is improving or not
  - Compare infant's axillary temperature with that of display at radiant warmer and with previous readings. Check infant's response under warmer
  - Evaluate mother's and family's anxiety and level of understanding
- Document infant's respiration, temperature, heart rate, SpO_2, CRT, skin color, activity pattern, and alertness, level of consciousness, body weight, urine output, and presence of abnormal clinical features on the monitoring sheet. Note the radiant warmer mode used for the neonate and rewarming process, if needed

Communication and Teaching for Homecare

- Communicate with the mother and the family members about infant's condition and plan of management. Encourage the mother to be present in the neonatal unit and to participate in infant's care
- Teach the parents about the following:
  - Assessment of temperature by human touch and using digital thermometer
  - Normal body temperature of the infant and its variations
  - Kangaroo mother care, when the baby become stable and as indicated
  - Breastfeeding or expression of breast milk to feed the baby by alternative methods
  - Hand hygiene, general cleanliness and measures for prevention of infections
  - Daily routine care of the infant, wrapping with cloth, dressing and clothing for the baby, feeding, danger signs, home-based care and follow-up visits.

PROCEDURE–12: CARE OF NEONATES DURING PHOTOTHERAPY

Clinical Guidelines

- Phototherapy is the treatment of neonatal jaundice in which the jaundiced baby is exposed to ultraviolet light to decrease the bilirubin levels in the bloodstream. Thereby it helps to reduce the risk of bilirubin deposition in the brain and to prevent bilirubin encephalopathy
- Phototherapy is an effective, inexpensive, noninvasive and easy to perform procedure to treat neonatal hyperbilirubinemia and to prevent related neurotoxicity
- The phototherapy light waves convert the unconjugated bilirubin to water soluble nontoxic forms which can be easily excreted through urine and stool
- Naked infant is placed under phototherapy light source having wave length 450–460 nm, using conventional fluorescent blue and white tube lights combination or using compact fluorescent light (CFL) bulbs or using light emitting diode (LED) bulbs.

Biliblanket can also be as light source for phototherapy
- Recommended irradiance for intensive phototherapy in blue-green spectrum should be at least 20-35 microwatt/cm^2/nm
- Infant's eyes and gonads should be kept covered during phototherapy to prevent retinal damage and gonadal damage in boy baby by the light source. Maximum exposure of neonate's skin to the phototherapy light should be ensured
- Light exposure must be done to as much of the infant's body surface area as possible
- Prophylactic phototherapy is not recommended as it has no clinical benefits
- Phototherapy has adverse effects like hypothermia, hyperthermia, increased insensible water loss, dehydration, irritability and excessive crying, skin rashes, loose green stool and Bronze-baby syndrome. These adverse effects are reversible when the phototherapy is discontinued. Early identification of these problems and prompt problem-based management during phototherapy helps to prevent further complications
- Bronze-baby syndrome occurs if the neonate has conjugated hyperbilirubinemia. If this condition is found, then discontinue phototherapy, as it requires different management based on the cause of this condition
- Discontinuation of phototherapy should be done once the bilirubin level is below the cut off value by 2–3 mg% as per postnatal age. In case of hemolytic jaundice, bilirubin level must be reassessed after 12 hours of discontinuation of phototherapy to identify the rebound increase of bilirubin level
- Phototherapy is initiated as per standard "nomogram" based on infant's postnatal age, birth weight and total serum bilirubin level. AAP guideline is mostly used, but it can be used for the neonate more than 35 weeks of gestational age. Other nomograms are also available, especially for preterm neonates and can be followed as per hospital policy.
- Decision to treat neonatal jaundice depends upon the severity and its cause. Continuous phototherapy is given with temporary interruptions for feeding or for any procedure only
- Ineffective phototherapy may occur due to low irradiance of the light source or the baby is frequently removed from phototherapy or baby's maximum skin surface is covered or recommended distance between phototherapy lights and baby's skin is not maintained
- Optimal irradiance of the phototherapy unit should be checked at regular interval.

Equipment Required

- Supplies for hand hygiene both for hand wash and handrub
- Overhead phototherapy light unit/source, as per availability and hospital policy
- Radiant warmer with bassinet to place the neonate
- Eye shades or eye pad or eye shield to cover the infant's eyes
- Diaper and diaper changing articles
- Thermometer, 70% alcohol and cotton swab to record infant's body temperature
- Weighing scale and other necessary items to measure the neonates body weight
- Feeding articles and milk, if mother is not available for breastfeeding
- Supplies for blood sampling for bilirubin estimation or transcutaneous bilirubinometer, as per unit policy
- Phototherapy nomogram to check and confirm the indication
- Waste disposal containers as per BMW rules
- Phototherapy record sheet and neonatal case sheet.

Assessment and Preparation

- Assess the infant for the following:
  - Collect history to determine the risk factors for hyperbilirubinemia (e.g., Rh or ABO incompatibility sepsis, prematurity, poor feeding, polycythemia, etc.). Detection of causes of

pathological neonatal jaundice is very important for prompt management
- Assess and divide jaundiced neonates into three groups (lower risk, medium risk and higher risk) to use AAP guidelines for phototherapy and exchange transfusion. Risk factors are isoimmune hemolytic disease, G6PD deficiency, asphyxia, significant lethargy, temperature instability, sepsis, acidosis and serum albumin <3.0 g/dL
- Look for gestational age, birth weight, postnatal age and clinical features of jaundice
- Check available blood values of the infant (bilirubin, hematocrit, hemoglobin, reticulocyte count, blood group, and Rh-type of mother and baby, Coomb's test, etc.)
- Identify baseline parameters such as respiration, heart rate, temperature, CRT, present body weight, level of hydration, passage of urine and stool pattern, skin condition and level of consciousness
- Examine for the extent of yellowish discoloration based on Kramer's criteria, and presence of cephalohematoma, ecchymosis, abrasions, injury, petechiae, hepatosplenomegaly to detect presence of complications
- Self-preparation should be done by meticulous hand hygiene
- Environment should be clean, warm, well-lighted and well-ventilated. Phototherapy is given inside the neonatal care units under radiant warmer
- All necessary articles, equipment and supplies should be cleaned and arranged around the radiant warmer. Clean the phototherapy lights with soap/detergent once daily. Disinfectant can be used once a week. Switch on the unit before placing the baby and check that all lamps are working
- Explain to the mother and the family members about the reason for phototherapy, possible adverse effects and about the technique of the phototherapy
- Preparation of neonate include the followings:
  - Check the cut off value of bilirubin level for phototherapy
  - Allow the mother to give breastfeeding to the baby before starting the procedure
  - Weigh the baby to measure current weight and to detect percentage of weight loss
  - Assess vital signs to ensure hemodynamic stability and normothermia
  - Position the infant comfortably under pre-warmed radiant warmer
  - Check the diaper and change it if soiled. Look for urine output and its amount. Observe for stool color, if it is white or clay color that indicate conjugated hyperbilirubinemia.

Performing the Steps of Procedure with Rationale/Point of Emphasis

1. Perform hand hygiene. Ensure all articles are clean and well arranged around the warmer.
2. Set up the bassinet with all necessary requirements.
3. Arrange the phototherapy light source around the bassinet. Ensure cleanliness of the machine and the bulbs/lights.
4. Ensure weight and vital signs are assessed and are within normal range.
5. Perform hand hygiene. Turn the radiant warmer "ON".
6. Place the infant under the prewarmed radiant warmer in supine position. Undress the infant to expose maximum skin surface to the lights.
7. Apply eye shades to prevent retinal damage of the infant.
8. Use shoulder roll to position the baby with neck slightly extended, if needed.
9. Place a diaper to prevent soiling from urine and stool and to protect gonads against chromatic radiant damage from the light exposure, especially in boy baby. Diaper should be folded to expose maximum body parts to the light source.

10. Switch on the phototherapy lights unit. Adjust the distance between the light source and infant's skin surface. For intensive phototherapy distance should be as low as 10 cm. For CFL or LED lights it can be about 35 cm. For conventional fluorescent tube lights it is 45 cm. When the neonate is placed in an isolette, the distance should be 38–45 cm. Distance is maintained as per manufacturer recommendations. Phototherapy machine/unit should not be placed directly under the radiant warmer to prevent heating of the unit.
11. Observe the infant for any untoward reactions. Make the baby comfortable.
12. Provide breast feed at 2–3 hours interval, if mother is available. Otherwise give artificial feed to provide nutrition and to prevent dehydration. Water supplements are not recommended. Monitor adequacy of feeding.
    If there is any evidence of dehydration, increase the fluid allowance for the neonate and if required intravenous fluid therapy may be initiated.
13. Change the infant's position every 2 hours, assess for skin integrity and eye pad position.
14. Check body temperature (2–3 hourly) to detect hypothermia or hyperthermia, urine output to identify dehydration and neurological status to detect encephalopathy, frequently at regular interval.
15. Ensure that bilirubin level monitoring is done as prescribed time (at 12 hours or 24 hours of starting the phototherapy or earlier) to determine the continuation or discontinuation of phototherapy and to identify the need for exchange blood transfusion.
16. Monitor infant's daily weight, feeding behavior and adverse effects of phototherapy.
17. Discontinue the phototherapy when bilirubin level falls below the cut off value by 2–3 mg% as per postnatal age and allow the infant to stay with the mother.
18. Follow infection control precautions and hand hygiene during entire course of treatment.
19. Inform the mother and family about the treatment and infant's condition.
20. Report and document the treatment in details, as per hospital policy.

Evaluation and Documentation

- Evaluate the following:
  - Infant's general condition, temperature, CRT, other vital signs, feeding reflex, passage of urine and stool, daily weight and bilirubin level to detect improvement or deterioration
  - Need for exchange blood transfusion
  - Level of understanding of the mother and the family members regarding hyperbilirubinemia and phototherapy
  - Intensity of the light source and optimal irradiance using flux-meter
- Document the following:
  - Date and time of bilirubin estimation and initiation of phototherapy
  - Findings of vital signs measurement, bilirubin level, daily weight, feeding behavior, urine and stool pattern, level of hydration, skin integrity, and level of alertness
  - Intensity of the light source and environmental temperature.

Communication and Teaching for Homecare

- Communicate with the mother and the family members about the effects of phototherapy and about infant's condition. Encourage the mother to participate in baby care and breastfeeding or feeding with EBM
- Teach the mother about hand hygiene, breastfeeding at 2 hours interval, temperature assessment by human touch, general cleanliness and about adverse effects of phototherapy and their preventive measures. Instruction should be given for post-discharge homecare, danger signs and follow-up visits for

neurodevelopmental assessment related to neonatal hyperbilirubenimia.

PROCEDURE–13: OXYGEN THERAPY FOR NEONATES

Clinical Guidelines

- Oxygen is one of the most commonly administered drugs to the sick neonates
- Oxygenation can be expressed as PaO_2 (partial pressure of oxygen) - pressure exerted by dissolved oxygen and as SpO_2 (% saturation of oxygen) which is percentage of Hb totally bound to oxygen
- Normal PaO_2 is 50–70 mm of Hg. Normal SpO_2 is 90–94%
- Both hypoxia (PaO_2 < 50 mm of Hg and SpO_2 < 90%) and hyperoxia (PaO_2 > 70 mm of Hg and SpO_2 > 95%) are harmful
- Oxygen should be used with precautions only in case of definite indications, as it is harmful to the infant's eyes, brain and lungs
- Indications of oxygen therapy include definite hypoxemia (oxygen saturation <90% in room air) and respiratory distress (respiratory rate > 60 breaths/minute, chest retractions, grunting and cyanosis). It prevents hypoxic damage of the vital organs
- The administration of supplemental oxygen is required to the sick neonates to maintain tissue oxygenation without any adverse effects of oxygen toxicity
- Adverse effects of recurrent hypoxia are pulmonary hypertension, increased risk of necrotizing enterocolitis, periventricular leukomalacia, neurodevelopmental impairment, and death. Hyperoxia leads to complications like retinopathy of prematurity, bronchopulmonary dysplasia and brain injury/damage
- Oxygen should be administered in neonates via nasal prongs and oxygen hood/head box
- Oxygen therapy is given at higher levels than are normally found in the atmosphere, i.e., more than 21%. Oxygen delivered to neonates is termed as fraction of inspired oxygen concentration or as FiO_2
- Pulse oximetry must be done for monitoring the baby during oxygen therapy to maintain target oxygen saturation level between 90 and 94% in neonates. Maintaining optimal oxygen saturation targets is essential to prevent harmful effects of hypoxia or hyperoxia
- Once the infant's oxygen saturation on pulse oximeter is within acceptable range, then gradually wean the baby from oxygen therapy. Reduce the flow rate by ½ liter/minute every few minutes and observe the saturation level. If the saturation remains in normal range, then gradually remove oxygen therapy
- Avoid use of nasopharyngeal catheter, partial rebreathing mask and non-rebreathing mask in neonates
- Infection control precautions should be followed. All necessary articles (oxygen humidifier, oxygen tube) must be changed daily including humidifier water

Equipment Required

- Hand hygiene articles to prevent infections
- Source of oxygen: It can be from centralized piped oxygen supply or from compressed gas cylinders or from oxygen cylinder or from oxygen concentrator
- Oxygen administration device for neonates, i.e., oxygen hood/head box or nasal prongs/cannula, oxygen tubing, oxygen flow meter, oxygen humidifier
- Adhesive for fixation of prongs, if needed
- Sterile water for humidifier
- Pulse oximeter monitor and probe to monitor oxygen saturation
- Cotton swab and 70% alcohol to clean the oximeter probe
- Waste disposal containers
- "No Smoking" sign in the area where oxygen is used
- Oxygen monitoring sheet to document the findings and neonate's case record.

Assessment and Preparation

- Assess the infant vital signs including SpO_2 to identify the definite indications of the oxygen therapy. Check the prescription for flow rate and any other directions

- Self-preparation should be done by hand hygiene to prevent cross infections
- Environment must be calm, well lighted, clean and with display of "No Smoking" sign
- All necessary articles and supplies should be clean and kept ready near the neonate
- Nasal prongs and oxygen tube must be sterile. Oxygen hood is used clean and dry
- Explain and counsel to the mother about the procedure and ask for involvement
- Place the baby in warm comfortable position. Check and change the diaper, if soiled.

Performing the Steps of Procedure with Rationale/Point of Emphasis

1. Perform hand hygiene and gather all necessary supplies to promote efficient and organized approach to the procedure.
2. Connect oxygen flow meter with the oxygen source to adjust the prescribed rate.
3. Connect the humidifier and oxygen tube. Fill humidifier with sterile water. Check the water level in humidifier. Humidified air is having less drying effect to nares and to lungs.
4. Apply the pulse oximeter probe to the neonate after cleaning the probe with 70% alcohol.
5. Switch on the pulse oximeter. Check the alarm limits of the machine.
6. Select proper size prongs/cannula to prevent nasal blanching or injury.
7. Connect the distal end of the oxygen tube to the oxygen delivery device (prongs or hood).
8. Apply the nasal prong with precautions or use oxygen hood, as available or as prescribed.
9. Ensure that neonate's head is within the hood or head box, even when the baby moves. The hood should not rest on the baby's neck.
10. Turn on the flow meter, adjust and check the flow of oxygen, as required. Feel the oxygen flow. Observe the bubbles in the humidifier.
11. Set the flow rate. For nasal prongs, flow of oxygen is 0.5–2 L/minute and for oxygen hood it is 3–5 L/minute to achieve the target saturation.
12. Ensure that the neonate is in midline and in neutral/sniffing position with shoulder roll. This position maintains proper alignment of mouth, pharynx and trachea.
13. Secure the nasal prongs. Use transparent adhesive on the cheek.
14. Monitor SpO_2 and assess the baby's condition for signs of improvement.
15. Report the findings and document the procedure.
16. Change the humidifier, oxygen tube, and water daily after use of 24 hours. Reuse all these articles after cleaning and sterilization.
17. Take care of the waste and perform hand hygiene.

Evaluation and Documentation

- Evaluate the respiratory status, SpO_2, temperature, heart rate, CRT and features of improvement or deterioration of the neonate. Evaluate the level of understanding of the parents and provide necessary support
- Document: Type of oxygen delivery system used, setting of the oxygen flow meter, time of initiation of oxygen therapy, SpO_2 level, temperature, heart, CRT, respiratory status (rate, retractions, grunting, cyanosis, nasal flaring), skin condition of the nares with any redness or irritation due to pressure of the prongs.

Communication and Teaching for Homecare

- Communicate with mother and family members about the infant's respiratory condition and effects of oxygen therapy. Answer to the questions asked by the family
- Teach the parents about purpose of oxygen therapy and its precautions. Instruct about fire safety and avoidance of use of synthetic materials and oils or oil-based product or petroleum products in the area around oxygen equipment. Instruct the mother

about hand hygiene, cleanliness, feeding and routine daily care of the infant. Post-discharge home care and follow-up visits should be explained and ensured for the infant with respiratory problems

PROCEDURE–14: PULSE OXIMETRY OF NEONATES

Clinical Guidelines

- Pulse oximeter is an electronic device that selectively measures oxygen saturation of "pulsed" (arterial) blood. It determines the percentage of hemoglobin in arterial blood saturated with oxygen
- Pulse oximetry is based on the physical principle of Beer Lambert Law
- It is a simple, convenient and noninvasive method for continuous monitoring of oxygen saturation and heart rate
- Indications of pulse oximetry include: (i) all sick neonates especially having respiratory difficulty or failure, (ii) in post-extubation period followed by mechanical ventilation support, (iii) in postoperative infants, and (iv) during supplemental oxygen therapy
- Pulse oximetry must be done for continuous monitoring during oxygen therapy to maintain target oxygen saturation level between 90 and 94% in neonates
- Clinical identification of hypoxia or hyperoxia is not possible
- Maintaining optimal oxygen saturation targets is important to avoid both hypoxia or hyperoxia and related complications in neonates
- The oximeter probe should not be so tight that it prevents circulation of the finger or toe
- Special precautions should be followed during use of pulse oximeter as—(a) change the site of the probe once per shift, (b) do not apply blood pressure cuff proximal to the limb where the probe is attached and (c) do not allow excess light exposure on the probe and cover the probe site with opaque material
- Pulse oximeter findings may not be reliable in presence of cold extremities, shock, excessive movements of limbs, exposure of probe to bright ambient light and electrical interference. Precautions should be followed for optimal functioning of the pulse oximeter and display of both numeric and graphic findings.

Equipment Required

- Hand hygiene supplies (both for hand wash and handrub)
- Pulse oximeter saturation monitor with power supply cord
- Pulse oximeter probe appropriate for the neonate
- Cotton swab and 70% alcohol to clean the probe
- Waste disposal container
- Fixation tape for probe
- Bedside oxygen delivery equipment
- Record/monitoring sheet to document the SpO_2 level.

Assessment and Preparation

- Assessment: Identify the neonate's respiratory problems and indications of pulse oximetry
- Self-preparation must be done with meticulous hand hygiene
- Environment preparation should be done for cleanliness, good light and ventilation
- Articles and supplies should be arranged conveniently near the neonate. Monitor panel should be cleaned with moist soft cloth only. Body of the oximeter can be cleaned with soft cloth dampened with soap water followed by cleaning with moist soft cloth
- Family members and mother should be explained about the procedure
- Preparation of neonate should be done with appropriate position, warm and diaper change

Performing the Steps of Procedure with Rationale/Point of Emphasis

1. Perform hand hygiene to prevent cross infections. Ensure all supplies ready in hand.
2. Clean the SpO_2 probe with 70% alcohol and allow to dry.

3. Apply the saturation probe to any extremity (palm of hand, wrist, ankle, and sole of foot below the toes with the cable extending toward the heel).
4. Ensure both sides of the probe are directly opposite to each other with the light source at one side and sensor at other side. Keep the sensor at the level of the heart, whenever possible.
   During neonatal resuscitation efforts, apply sensor at right hand or right palm of the infant to measure preductal saturation. Apply sensor probe before connecting to the pulse oximeter that leads in quickest acquisition of accurate heart rate and oxygen saturation. This allows measurement of the light transmitted through a pulsating arterial vascular bed to calculate the percentage of hemoglobin saturated with oxygen.
   Avoid placing the sensor probe over thick skin, extremities that are moved excessively by the baby and at areas where perfusion is known to be poor.
5. Apply the probe on a well-perfused site. Avoid bruised and edematous area.
6. Do not apply excessive pressure. Secure the probe loosely.
7. Ensure the connection of the probe with the pulse oximeter socket and connection of the power cord to the power supply. Turn the monitor "ON".
8. Check the alarm limits of the pulse oximeter. For SpO_2 it is 89–95% and for heart rate it is 100–160 bpm.
9. Wait for stable plethysmographic waveform or bar signal on the monitor.
10. Make the baby comfortable and observe for abnormal clinical features.
11. Take care of used articles and perform hand hygiene.
12. Document SpO_2 reading, heart rate and other findings.

Evaluation and Documentation

- Evaluate the following:
  - Count respiratory rate for full one minute and observe for any abnormalities
  - Check apical heart rate of the infant by stethoscope and compare with heart rate shown in the monitor
  - Inspect the probe site every 2–4 hours for any erythema or discoloration or blistering
- Document: SpO_2, heart rate, respiratory rate, temperature and other abnormal findings.

Communication and Teaching for Homecare

- Communicate with the mother and the family members to inform about neonate's condition. Answer to their questions to reduce their stress and anxiety
- Teach the mother and family about the importance of pulse oximetry and necessary precautions during the procedure. Explain about routine care and care at home after discharge from hospital. Discuss about danger signs, need from medical help and plan for follow-up visits for continuation of care.

PROCEDURE–15: BLOOD GLUCOSE ESTIMATION OF NEONATES

Clinical Guidelines

- Blood glucose estimation using glucometer is a common procedure. It is done to monitor blood glucose level of "at risk neonates" and to detect neonatal hypoglycemia
- Hypoglycemia in neonates is a most common problem due to various reasons. It is diagnosed when the blood glucose level is less than 45 mg/dL in all neonates with or without any clinical features
- Symptoms of hypoglycemia are very nonspecific and can mimic any illness in neonates. Hence, it is important to monitor blood glucose level of all at risk neonates
- Indications of blood glucose estimation include: (i) infants born to diabetic mothers, (ii) LBW and preterm neonates weighing less than 2,000 gram (iii) sick neonates having asphyxia, hypothermia,

respiratory distress, shock, sepsis, poor and/or delayed feeding, polycythemia, and (iv) those neonates having predominantly on IV fluid therapy
- Screening of hypoglycemia for "at risk neonates" after birth should be done at 2 hours, 6 hours, 12 hours, 24 hours, 48 hours and if indicated at 72 hours of age
- Heel prick is the commonly used method to obtain capillary blood sample for glucose estimation by glucometer. Venous blood can also be used to get blood sample for glucose estimation, especially during intravenous cannulation
- Heel prick is more painful. Ensure that the heel is not cold. Warm the neonate's heel that helps to get the blood drops easily
- Make needlestick puncture on the posterolateral aspect of heel. Avoid the making deep puncture and puncture on the middle portion of the heel
- Follow strict aseptic technique and standard precautions for infection control during the procedure to prevent infections at puncture sites
- Pain management especially non-pharmacological methods should be practiced before and during the procedure of blood sampling (such as breastfeeding, or drops of breast milk in neonate's mouth or holding the baby with hands, etc.).

Equipment Required

- Hand hygiene articles and supplies
- Glucometer and test strips
- Lancets, lancet device or 26 gauge needle
- Sterile cotton swabs, sterile gauze pieces in a sterile container
- Sterile gloves to prevent transmission of organisms
- 70% alcohol for skin preparation
- Waste disposal containers
- Procedure record sheet and neonate's case sheet.

Assessment and Preparation

- Assess the infant's body temperature, signs of poor perfusion, local edema and infection at the puncture site and clinical features of impaired blood coagulation
- Self-preparation should be done by hand hygiene and donning sterile gloves
- Environment should be clean, warm, well lighted and well ventilated
- Articles should be collected and arranged near the neonate for easy approach
- Preparation of the mother/family: Explain about the procedure and its purpose. Encourage the mother to hold the infant by hands to support during procedure and to minimize the stress
- Preparation of neonate:
  - Allow the mother to give breastfeeding before the procedure or give 2 mL EBM in the baby's mouth to reduce pain sensation
  - Pain management of the neonate can be done by oral glucose/sucrose drops, swaddling, holding by hands or by containment or by application of local anesthetics, as per policy
  - Check the baby's feet for warmth by touching with the dorsum of the clean, dry and warm hand. If it is cold, then warm the baby's heel by holding in the hands for few minutes or by wrapping with warm cloth or dipping in lukewarm water.

Performing the Steps of Procedure with Rationale/Point of Emphasis

1. Perform hand hygiene. Collect all necessary items near the neonate.
2. Ensure the neonate's feet is warm and the baby is in comfort.
3. Confirm about pain reduction measure is followed for the neonate.
4. Use handrub for hand hygiene. Wear sterile gloves.
5. Prepare the puncture site with sterile cotton swab soaked in 70% alcohol by scrubbing in circular and gentle motion. Allow the site to dry to avoid fallacious results.
6. Do not use povidone-iodine for skin preparation as it can contaminate the blood sample and may elevate blood glucose result.
7. Grasp the baby's heel firmly at arch and ankle with dorsiflexion of the foot using

index finger and thumb as circle. Place infant's extremity in dependent position.

8. Perform needlestick puncture of the heel at posterolateral aspect.
9. Avoid the middle portion of the heel and avoid deep puncture. Avoid puncturing through the previous puncture site that might be infected. Heel sticks should be done 2 mm apart.
10. Wipe out the first drop of blood using sterile dry cotton swab to prevent specimen contamination.
11. Allow the second drop of blood to fall on the test strip for examination.
12. Do not rub the strip against the skin.
13. Follow the instruction of the test strip bottle to obtain the result.
14. Note the blood glucose value on the glucometer.
15. Elevate extremity above the level of heart. Gently press the puncture site with sterile gauze/cotton swab for some time until bleeding stops.
16. Make the infant comfortable and allow the mother to hold or to care the baby.
17. Remove gloves. Wash hand.
18. Discard the needle and swab/gauze pieces as per waste disposal policy.
19. Rearrange all used items and keep the glucometer ready for next use.
20. Report and record the finding of blood glucose level.

Evaluation and Documentation

- Evaluate the blood glucose level (presence of hypo- or hyperglycemia) for further management. Assess the puncture sites for continued bleeding, bruising, scarring, and infection. Evaluate parents' reaction and level of understanding for continuation of treatment of the baby
- Document the date and time of blood glucose estimation, site of puncture, blood glucose level and presence of any problem.

Communication and Teaching for Homecare

- Communicate with the mother and the family members about the findings of the procedure, any deviations, and plan of further management.
- Teach the mother about feeding, warmth and danger signs to prevent further complications. Instruct about daily routine care, homecare and plan of follow-up care for neurodevelopmental status.

PROCEDURE–16: CAPILLARY REFILL TIME ESTIMATION OF NEONATES

Clinical Guidelines

- CRT indicates the adequacy of tissue perfusion. It is estimated by assessing the time required to refill the capillaries following emptying the blood supply by application of pressure and thereafter quickly releasing the pressure
- Estimation of CRT is very simple procedure to identify poor tissue perfusion and shock in neonates. It should be done for all sick and at-risk neonates for early detection of circulatory status
- Normal CRT is less than 3 seconds. Prolonged CRT of more than 3 seconds indicates poor circulation and poor peripheral tissue perfusion. Prolonged CRT is the early sign of neonatal shock along with unexplained tachycardia (heart rate >160 beats/minute)
- CRT can be prolonged in hypothermia due to peripheral vasoconstriction. If the infant is hypothermic, then CRT assessment should be done after rewarming the infant and improvement of the body temperature
- CRT is assessed on the central part of the neonate's chest at the body of the sternum.

Equipment Required

- Hand hygiene supplies and record/ monitoring sheet.

Assessment and Preparation

- Assess the infant's body temperature, heart rate, respiratory rate, SpO_2, color and presence of any other abnormalities. Assess parents' stress and level of understanding about the infant's condition

- Self-preparation should be done by hand washing or by using handrub, then drying and warming the hand before touching the neonate
- Environment should be clean, warm, well lighted and well ventilated
- Articles preparation: Only hand hygiene supplies needed, no extra articles are required
- Preparation of neonate: Place the neonate in supine position and ensure normal body temperature before doing the CRT estimation.

Performing the Steps of Procedure with Rationale/Point of Emphasis

1. Perform hand hygiene, make the hand dry and warm.
2. Ensure the baby is normothermic. Assess neonate's thermal state by human touch. Warm and pink feet of the baby indicates that the neonate is in thermal comfort.
3. Apply gentle pressure on the body of the sternum using thumb or index finger for 5 seconds (by slowly counting from 1001, 1002, 1003, 1004, 1005). This will result blanching of the underlying tissue.
4. Release the pressure from the skin surface by lifting the thumb/index finger.
5. Observe and note the time taken for return of color to refill the blanched area that becomes pink and the same color of the surrounding tissue.
6. Interpret the finding. Normal CRT is < 3 seconds. CRT more than 3 seconds indicates poor tissue perfusion that required prompt management.
7. Check *noninvasive blood pressure (NIBP)* using multi-parameter monitor, when indicated, especially to diagnose neonatal shock with clinical features of tachycardia, prolonged CRT, mottling of skin, pallor, poor peripheral pulses, cold extremities, lethargy and decreased urine output.
8. Place the baby in comfortable position and perform hand hygiene.
9. Document the findings of CRT estimation in neonate's monitor sheet.

Evaluation and Documentation

- Evaluate the infants' clinical state due to poor perfusion of the body tissues in case of shock, when demands of oxygen and nutrients are not met. Presence of tachycardia, poor peripheral pulses, pallor, mottling of skin, cold extremities, decreased urine output and low blood pressure along with prolonged CRT are diagnostic features of neonatal shock
- Document infants CRT, heart rate, body temperature, respiration rate, skin color, blood pressure and other abnormal findings with date and time of observation

Communication and Teaching for Homecare

- Communicate with the mother and the family about the infant's condition and plan of treatment
- Teach the mother/parents about care of the neonate, i.e., warmth, feeding, cleanliness and identification of abnormal symptoms or danger signs. Explain about daily care at hospital and home including follow-up care.

PROCEDURE–17: INTRAVENOUS FLUID THERAPY IN NEONATES

Clinical Guidelines

- Adequate breastfeeding is sufficient to maintain fluid balance in most clinically stable neonates who are taking feeds orally. But sick neonates require intravenous fluid and electrolytes therapy to sustain their life
- The goal of appropriate fluid and electrolyte management of sick neonates is to allow normal weight loss and to ensure physiological stability
- Indications of intravenous fluid therapy in neonates include: (a) any sick neonate not tolerating enteral feeds, (b) neonate with moderate to severe respiratory difficulty, (c) neonatal shock, (d) perinatal asphyxia, (e) neonatal seizures, (f) neonate with abdominal distension, and (g) neonates having birth weight less than 1,200 gram or

gestational age less than 30 weeks during initial period of life

- Recommended fluid therapy in first 48 hours of neonatal life is electrolyte-free fluid, i.e., 10% Dextrose. After 48 hours of age, when the neonate passed urine at least 5–6 times a day, then electrolyte is added in IV fluid therapy (commercial IV fluid with electrolyte is available for neonates as Isolyte P or Arolyte P)
- Appropriate glucose infusion rate (GIR) should be maintained based on day of life, birth weight and blood glucose level. Measure blood glucose every 8 hours for as long as the neonate is receiving IV fluid for any reason
- IV fluid therapy is given with calculated amount based on gestational age, birth weight, and day of life. Fluid therapy is administered using syringe/infusion pump with pressure monitoring (PM) line or micro-drip infusion set
- Strict intake and output chart should be maintained with hourly monitoring of the IV fluid therapy along with other intake and output of the neonate
- Serial weight recording and measuring urine output are useful for assessment of fluid balance in neonates. Normal urine output in neonates after 48 hours of age is about 1–5 mL/kg/hour
- Peripheral IV catheter is placed by cannulation of superficial veins of the neonates using appropriate size sterile disposable peripheral IV cannula/catheter (size 22–26 G). Common peripheral veins used for IV cannulation are cephalic vein and basilic vein in the arms, median marginal vein and lateral marginal vein in the feet
- Peripheral IV catheters are used for direct administration of primed IV fluids, intermittent use for medications and blood products, parenteral nutrition supplement and occasional venous blood drawing for laboratory tests
- Peripheral IV catheters in neonates may remain in place as long as there are no signs of complications and extravasation. They do not need to be changed on routine basis.

Equipment Required

- Supplies for hand hygiene as liquid antiseptic soap for hand washing and antiseptic handrub solution
- Sterile disposable IV cannula of appropriate size for the neonate
- Antiseptic solution—70% alcohol and povidone-iodine for skin preparation
- Sterile container with sterile gloves, sterile cotton swab, sterile gauze, sterile syringe with normal saline
- Transfer forceps or lifter to handle sterile items
- Transparent adhesive tape/dressing and scissors to fix the catheter
- Syringe/infusion pump, IV fluid infusion set with micro-drip, IV fluid tubing, PM line and IV fluid bag/bottle, as prescribed
- Intake and output chart and neonate's treatment sheet
- Waste disposal containers as per BMW rule.

Assessment and Preparation

- Assess the neonate's vital signs and body weight before calculation of fluid requirement. Fluid and GIR calculation should be counter-checked by two healthcare professionals to prevent incorrect calculation. Assess parents' level of anxiety and understanding for appropriate explanation
- Self-preparation should be done by hand hygiene and donning gloves. Help of assistant is required to maintain aseptic technique during IV cannulation
- Environment should be clean, calm, quiet, well lighted and well ventilated
- All necessary items and supplies should be arranged near the neonate. Maintain strict aseptic technique and non-touch technique to prevent nosocomial infections
- Preparation of the mother/parents: Discuss the purpose and risk of IV cannulation and fluid therapy. Explain about comfort measures for the neonate that can be provided by the mother. Teach

about hygienic practices and features of complications of fluid therapy

- Preparation of neonate: Make the neonate clean and comfortable.

Performing the Steps of Procedure with Rationale/Point of Emphasis

1. Perform hand washing and arrange all necessary items near the neonate.
2. Take assistance to hold the infant's extremities and to make the selected vein prominent and visible to do the cannulation easily. Be sure about the appropriate site.
3. Take assistance for maintenance of sterile technique during the cannulation.
4. Use non-pharmacological measures to reduce pain in neonate during insertion of cannula.
5. Wear sterile gloves before performing the IV cannulation.
6. Clean the skin over the chosen insertion site with antiseptic swab in circular motion, as per unit policy. Usually "alcohol–povidone iodine–alcohol" is used for skin preparation. Allow the alcohol to dry. Once the skin is prepared, the cannulation site should not be touched to prevent contamination of the insertion area.
7. Insert the cannula by picking at 30–45° to the skin surface. Look for blood in the hub of the needle then withdraw the trocar a bit and advance the cannula further. After inserting the cannula fully, then withdraw the needle. Cannula is then flushed with 0.5–1 mL normal saline. Then cover the outer end of the cannula with sterile cap.
8. Secure the cannula firmly with transparent tape (e.g., tegaderm) and dressing cautiously. Keep the cannula tip area visible to detect extravasation during fluid therapy.
9. Make the neonate comfortable after IV cannulation and allow mother, if she present.
10. Ensure IV fluid is prepared aseptically. Fill the tubing and PM line with the infusate to ensure rapid delivery of fluid. Attach tubing and PM line to the syringe or fluid container.
11. Wipe the cannula cap with 70% alcohol swab, remove the cannula cap and attach with IV fluid micro-drip set to the outer end of the cannula. When syringe infusion pump is used for IV fluid administration, prepare IV fluid in the appropriate size syringe and attach PM line then attach to the IV cannula of the neonate.
12. Adjust infusion flow rate and time and ensure patency of the IV line.
13. Monitor fluid leakage from the cannula site or connection, any blockage or kink in the tubing. Check for blood glucose level 8 hourly, daily weight, amount of urine output, oliguria (urine output <1 mL/kg/hour over a 6-hour period beyond 48 hours of age), signs of overhydration (puffiness of eyelids, excessive weight gain and respiratory distress) and signs of extravasation, during continuation fluid therapy.
14. Maintain strict intake-output chart. Check the volume of fluid infused and compared to the prescribed volume. Monitor urine output. Remember normal urine output in neonates is 1–5 mL/kg/hour. Note other fluid intake in the form of medications. Record other output such as vomiting and gastric aspiration. Calculate total intake and total output.
15. Adjust IV fluid requirement with the amount of enteral feeds. Initiate gavage feeding and paladai/spoon feeding as soon as the neonate's clinical condition is improved.
16. Change syringe, PM line, micro-drip infusion set and fluid bag/bottle every 24 hours to prevent contamination of IV fluids and for prevention of nosocomial infections.
17. Discard used syringe, tubing, PM line, gloves and used articles as per BMW policy.
18. Wash hand and document the IV cannulation and fluid therapy.

Evaluation and Documentation

- Evaluate the IV site, total fluid intake, total output, body weight, blood glucose

level and signs of extravasations such as redness, swelling, tenderness, leakage from IV site and signs of overhydration, and dehydration. Evaluate the parents concern to provide necessary support
- Document the date and time of IV cannulation, type and size of cannula used, number of attempts for insertion of cannula and amount of flush solution Record date and time of starting fluid therapy, type of fluid used, finding of vital signs assessment, present postnatal body weight, any other fluid intake, urine output and any other output. Note all findings accurately in intake-output chart of the neonate.

Communication and Teaching for Homecare

- Communicate with the mother and the family members about neonate's condition, whether improving or deteriorating. Encourage them to ask questions and answer appropriately
- Teach the parents about the involvement routine baby care during fluid therapy, hand washing, maintenance of cleanliness, signs of complications, continuation of care at home after discharge and plan of follow-up care.

PROCEDURE–18: INTRAVENOUS MEDICATIONS IN NEONATES

Clinical Guidelines

- Medications are administered by the intravenous (IV) route for rapid absorption. Intravenous route of medications is less traumatic for the infant than other routes, when already IV cannulation is in place
- Very sick neonates are mostly treated with IV medications rather than intramuscular or oral or other route
- Principles of IV medications in neonates are same as for older children such as checking of label of drugs and expiry date, calculations of exact dose, counter-checking of dose calculations before administration of drugs, strict asepsis, checking the patency of IV cannula, continuous monitoring and communicating with team members and parents
- Special precautions during IV administration of medications should be followed for the neonates, such as slow bolus for small volume of medication, use of syringe pump and pressure monitoring (PM) line for administration of large volume drugs, cleaning of IV cannula port/hub with alcohol swab and use of normal saline to keep the cannula patent if there is no continuous IV fluid therapy is running
- Small amount of medication doses are required for neonates. Single dose vial is useful to prevent incorrect dose. When single dose vial is not available the calculation of amount of drugs from multi-dose vials should be done very cautiously
- Strict asepsis and standard precautions for infection control must be followed
- "Ten Rights of Medications" and all principles of pharmacologic management should be practiced during administration of drugs. Presently 16 rights are recommended for administration of medications.

Equipment/Articles Required

- Hand hygiene supplies for hand washing and handrub
- Sterile gloves to prevent transmission of microorganisms
- Existing intravenous access with IV cannula ports for giving medications
- Sterile syringe to administer medications, size of the syringe is selected as per volume of the medication to be administered
- Sterile knife dish/small tray to carry the drug loaded syringe to the neonate
- Transfer forceps or lifter to handle sterile items
- Syringe pump, and sterile PM line
- Sterile cotton swabs and alcohol 70% to clean the medication port and hub
- Prescribed medications in ampule or vial
- Sterile water for injection to dissolve the drug and normal saline for further dilution
- Waste disposal container, puncture proof container, syringe hub and needle cutter
- Medication record sheet/card and treatment sheet of the neonate.

Assessment and Preparation

- Assess infant's vital signs, general condition. Check for signs of complications with IV line and patency of IV access. Assess level of understanding and anxiety of the mother
- Self-preparation should be done by hand washing and use of sterile gloves
- Environment of the medication room or treatment room or laminar flow and neonatal care area should be clean, well-lighted, and free from noise and free of overcrowding
- All necessary articles should be collected and arranged in medication room or treatment room or under laminar flow for preparation of medications. Assistant is required for handling of sterile items. If assistant is not available, packets of disposable items should be open and sterile articles must be placed on sterile field with precautions before wearing of gloves. Prevention of contamination is very important. After preparation of medication, it should be carried to the neonates in sterile container
- Preparation of mother: Explain to the mother about purpose of injections, precautions to be followed for medications, possible side effects and for necessary help as required
- Preparation of neonate: The infant should be made clean and comfortable.

Performing the Steps of Procedure with Rationale/Point of Emphasis

1. Verify the written prescription before preparation of the drug to avoid medication errors.
2. Counter-check the calculations of drug dose with the team members.
3. Wash hands and collect all necessary items in medication preparation area.
4. Check the label of the drug, date of expiry and amount of drug in the ampule or vial.
5. Follow the "Ten Rights of Medications" and infection control practices.
6. Ensure the drugs are in room temperature before preparation and administration, if it was preserved in refrigerator.
7. Wash hand following six steps for preparation of medications to prevent infections.
8. Dry hands and wear gloves. Prepare sterile field for medication preparation or use laminar flow, if available.
9. Take help of the assistant to open the syringe-needle and PM line packets. Assistant will clean and break the ampule with precautions after cleaning with alcohol swab or clean the vial top with alcohol swab before reconstituting and drawing the drug, as required. If assistant is not available, before donning gloves open all unsterile packets, take out sterile items and place on sterile field.
10. Draw up the medication in the syringe having attached needle with required dose. Syringe size depends upon the amount of medication. Dissolve/reconstitute the powder drugs and dilute the drugs to administer the small amount of exact dose. Follow the standard guidelines for dilution of drugs before administration.
11. Carry the prepare drugs in syringe, PM line (if needed) and sterile alcohol swabs to the neonate in sterile container.
12. Identify the neonate and counter check the identity with mother/caregiver present.
13. Explain to the mother about the procedure and ask for supporting the baby.
14. Take help from mother or any assistant to position and to comfort the infant.
15. Clean the IV cannula port/hub with cap using squeezed alcohol swab and allow it to dry.
16. Administer the very small amount of drug slowly and then push 0.5 mL of normal line and replace the cannula cap to cover the cannula port/hub.
17. Administer large amount of drug using syringe pump and PM line with recommended time following strict aseptic techniques.

18. Set the syringe pump, select the type of syringe (10 mL, 20 mL, and 50 mL) and flow rate.
19. Start the infusion of medication and check arrow indicator movement to confirm the flow.
20. Check the flow of drugs and IV site to assess any extravasations during administration.
21. Observe the infant's condition for any reaction during medication infusion.
22. Stop the infusion of drug when it completely delivered. Time required of IV infusion of medication using syringe pump depends upon amount of drugs. It may take 30 minutes or longer depending upon the nature of medications.
23. Comfort the neonate and allow mother to hold and care the baby, if she present.
24. Dispose the syringe, needle, PM line, swabs and gloves as per BMW rules of the hospital policy in different color coded container.
25. Wash hands and document the administration of IV medication to the neonate.

Evaluation and Documentation

- Evaluate the infant's response to the procedure and potential side effects. Evaluate parents concern and understanding level about the treatment to provide support
- Document: The type/name of the medication with date, time, dose, route of administration, presence of any side effects, appearance of IV access site, dilution and flush amount and infant's reactions.

Communication and Teaching for Homecare

- Communicate with mother and the family about the therapeutic effects of the medications, plan of further treatment and about infant's condition
- Teach the parents about participation in infant's care, maintenance of warmth and cleanliness, infant feeding, danger signs, continuation of care at home, necessary medical help and plan follow-up visits after discharge from hospital.

PROCEDURE–19: INTRAMUSCULAR MEDICATIONS IN NEONATES

Clinical Guidelines

- Medications are given intramuscularly (IM) for rapid absorption of drugs because muscle has rich blood supply.
- The IM route is more painful than other routes because muscle has more nerves. Medications should be administered through least traumatic and less painful route such as oral or intravenous access, when available
- In neonates, IM injections are given to administer Vitamin K and Hepatitis B vaccine, usually in the delivery room or thereafter when prescribed
- IM medications are not practiced widely for neonates to prevent nosocomial infections related to multiple needle pricks
- In neonates, IM injections are given in the anterolateral aspect of thigh in rectus femoris muscle or in vastus lateralis muscle
- Do not administer IM injections in the gluteal region in neonates. Gluteal muscles are underdeveloped leading to poor absorption of drugs. There is risk of sciatic nerve injury resulting paralysis of the limb in neonates following IM injections in gluteal region
- Follow strict asepsis and standard precautions for infection control during IM injections. Non-touch technique should be followed during handling of sterile items
- Follow "Ten Rights of Medications" and all principles of pharmacologic management. Presently 16 rights are recommended for administration of medications.

Equipment/Articles Required

- Hand hygiene supplies for hand washing and handrub
- Sterile Gloves, as per hospital/unit policy to protect from cross infections
- Sterile syringe (1 mL, 2 mL) and needle 26 G to administer medications

- Sterile cotton swabs and alcohol 70% to clean the injection site for therapeutic IM injections such as vitamin K, but for hepatitis B vaccination no skin preparation needed with alcohol swab only clean injection site should be ensured
- Sterile knife dish/small tray to carry the loaded syringe to the neonate
- Prescribed medication/vaccine (vitamin K and hepatitis B vaccine)
- Waste disposal containers, syringe hub and needle cutter, puncture proof container
- Medication record sheet/card, treatment sheet or immunization card.

Assessment and Preparation

- Assess infant's condition and mother level of understanding
- Self-preparation should be done by initial hand washing and then use of handrub
- Environment should be clean, well-lighted, and free from noise and overcrowding
- All necessary articles and items should be collected and arranged near neonate or in the procedure room for preparation of medication/immunization
- Preparation of mother: Explain to the mother about purpose of injection, precautions to be followed during IM injection and possible side effects
- Preparation of neonate: The infant should be made clean and comfortable.

Performing the Steps of Procedure with Rationale/Point of Emphasis

1. Verify the written prescription of health-care prescriber before preparation of the drug to avoid medication errors.
2. Wash hands and collect all necessary items in medication preparation area.
3. Check the label of the drug, date of expiry and amount of drug in the ampule or vial.
4. Use 1 mL syringe to ensure dose accuracy and 26 G needle to minimize muscle injury for administration of vitamin K and hepatitis B vaccine.
5. Ensure the medication is in room temperature before preparation and administration, if it was preserved in refrigerator. Cold medication causes increased discomfort when injected in the muscle.
6. Wash hand following six steps for preparation of medication to prevent infections.
7. Handle syringe and needle always in non-touch techniques or use sterile gloves.
8. Clean and break the ampule with precautions after cleaning with alcohol swab or clean the vial top with alcohol before drawing the drug, as required. For Hepatitis B vaccine vial no use of alcohol.
9. Draw up the medication in the syringe having attached needle with required dose, do not draw up additional air into the syringe, because clearing of air from the needle can affect the dose administered, as the amount is very less in neonates.
10. Change and attach a fresh needle of 26 G for administration of medication.
11. Carry the prepare drugs and sterile alcohol swabs to the neonate in sterile container for therapeutic IM injections such as vitamin K.
12. Identify the neonate and cross check the identity with mother.
13. Follow the "Ten Rights of Medications" to prevent wrong and incorrect medication.
14. Give breast milk of oral sucrose or support the infant with hand hold/containment to decrease pain sensation during IM injections. Mother can hold the neonate or can give breastfeeding before or during IM injection, if she is confident.
15. Expose and identify the injection site at thigh and hold the leg extended to make the muscle prominent and to restrict the leg movement.
16. Cleanse the injection site with 70% alcohol swab for vitamin K and allow the site to dry before giving injection.
17. Grasp the selected muscle with thumb and fingers of the left hand and introduce the needle of the syringe having the drug in it, at right angle into middle of the selected muscle. If the muscle mass is less especially in LBW infant, IM injection can be given in 60° angle.
18. Withdraw the syringe slowly for aspiration to rule out that the needle is not in the blood vessel.

19. Inject the medication slowly and observe for neonate's facial expression for pain.
20. Withdraw the needle out and press the injection site with dry swab. Do not rub the area.
21. Do not recap, bend or break the needle and disassemble syringe needle after use.
22. Comfort the neonate and allow mother to hold and care the baby, if she present.
23. Dispose the syringe, needle, swabs and gloves as per BMW rules of the hospital policy in different color coded container.
24. Wash hands and document the IM administration of medication.

Evaluation and Documentation

- Evaluate the response of the neonate and mother's reaction. Monitor the neonate for bleeding from the injection site, any side effects, discomfort, pain and vital signs
- Document the medication administered with date, time, dose, route and site of injection including presence of side effects, variations in vital signs and response of the neonate and the mother

Communication and Teaching for Homecare

- Communicate with the mother and the family about expected purpose of the medication
- Teach the parents about routine care, hygienic care, feeding, warmth and possible side effects of the injection (hard, reddened, tender), care at home and follow-up visits.

PROCEDURE–20: INSERTION OF FEEDING TUBE AND GAVAGE FEEDING IN NEONATES

Clinical Guidelines

- Gavage feeding is an alternative method of feeding to provide nutrition through a small feeding tube into the stomach passed through nose or mouth. It is given to maintain nutritional and fluid requirements of the infant to promote weight gain. It prevents malnutrition and other nutritional problems in preterm LBW and sick infants. It also prevents aspiration of feeds in preterm LBW neonates
- Gavage feeding in neonates is given as orogastric tube feeding. Nasogastric tube feeding is not recommended presently
- Tube feeding is usually given in small babies as intermittent feeding at 2 hours interval initially using EBM or formula milk. It can also be given at 3 hours interval in bigger babies and by continuous feeding as infusion using syringe pump
- Neonates less than 30 weeks of gestational age or less than 1,200 gram birth weight are unable to coordinate sucking and swallowing reflex with respiration. Initially, IV fluid therapy is given to them. These neonates require gavage feeding usually after 1–3 days. Gavage feeding can be started initially in neonates with gestational age of 30–34 weeks or birth weight in between 1,200 and 1,800 gram. Selection of mode of feeding depends upon presence or absence of sickness and individual feeding efforts of the neonates
- Indications of gavage feeding include: (a) neonates unable to take oral feed, e.g., preterm neonates, LBW infants, sick neonates and neurologically depressed neonates, (b) neonates having surgical problems, and (c) neonates with CPAP support
- Gavage feeding should not be given if there is abdominal distension with hemorrhagic or altered colored aspirate and in case of severe respiratory distress
- Early enteral feeding as minimal enteral nutrition (MEN) or trophic feeds delivered intragastric through feeding tube as gavage feeding with small volume of EBM are practiced in LBW preterm and sick infants. These feeds enhance gut growth, hormonal secretion and gut motility, thus help to prevent necrotizing enterocolitis
- Calculated amount of EBM or formula milk based on the daily fluid requirement can be given to the infants by gavage feeding
- Encourage the mother for expression of breast milk for her baby for gavage

feeding with EBM and explain about disadvantages of formula feeding.

Equipment Required

- Hand hygiene supplies for hand wash and handrub
- Unsterile clean gloves, as per unit policy
- Infant feeding tube size: 6 F used for neonates with more than 2,000 gram birth weight and size - 5 F for babies less than 2,000 gram birth weight. Feeding tube size - 8 F may also be used in neonates with some indications
- Appropriate size sterile syringe (5 mL or 10 mL) to give milk feeding
- Pediatric Stethoscope for auscultation of sound to confirm the tube position in stomach
- Adhesive tape and scissor for fixation of the feeding tube
- Tape measure to measure abdominal circumference to detect abdominal distension
- Expressed breast milk or formula milk in sterile covered container
- Diaper and diaper changing items
- Waste disposal containers
- Documentation sheet, intake-output chart and neonate case sheet.

Assessment and Preparation

- Assess the infant's vital signs, feeding behavior, sucking-swallowing reflex, and abdominal circumference. Check for presence of any abnormal movements/ seizures and respiratory difficulties and previous intake-output
  Assess parents' level of understanding and anxiety to provide necessary support
- Self-preparation should be done by hand washing
- Environment should be clean, calm and quiet, well lighted and well ventilated
- All necessary articles should be collected and arranged near neonate
- Preparation of the mother: Explain to the mother about the purpose of the procedure. Encourage to express required amount of breast milk for her infant to avoid formula feeds. Ask the mother to participate in the routine care of thebaby
- Preparation of neonate: Neonate should be stable, clean and comfortable and have no contraindications of gavage feeding. Daily morning weight must be measured for calculation of fluid and feeds.

Performing the Steps of Procedure with Rationale/Point of Emphasis

Insertion of Orogastric Feeding Tube

1. Wash hands and arrange all required articles/items near the neonate.
2. Place the neonate on supine position with head slightly elevated.
3. Select appropriate size of orogastric feeding tube.
4. Wear gloves, as per unit policy to prevent cross infection.
5. Measure the length of the feeding tube to be inserted (lip to tip). Measure from the angle of the mouth to tragus to midpoint between umbilicus and xiphisternum. There are different points of measurement for length of feeding tube (such as from the bridge of the nose to the tip of the ear lobe then down to the midpoint between umbilicus and xiphoid process). Mark at the required measured length of the feeding tube.
6. Insert the feeding tube through the infant's mouth till the pre-measured marked length has been introduced. Use infant's saliva or EBM to lubricate the feeding tube.
7. Check and confirm the position of the feeding tube in the stomach using syringe and stethoscope. Inject 1 mL of air into the stomach and hear the gurgling sound with the auscultation by stethoscope placed over the stomach area.
8. Keep the outer end of the feeding tube close.
9. Fix the feeding tube with skin friendly adhesive tape. Fix at the corner of the mouth.
10. Allow orogastric feeding tube to be left in situ for 2 or 3 days, if possible.

11. During removal of feeding tube, pinch the feeding tube and pull out gently to avoid trickling of gastric mucus into the trachea.
12. Observe the infant for any discomfort and respiratory problems. Place the infant in comfortable position and ask the mother to take care of the neonate.
13. Remove gloves, take care of the used articles and wash hands.
14. Explain to the parent about the need for gavage feeding and document the procedure.

Orogastric Tube Feeding

1. Wash hands following six steps and use handrub in between procedure.
2. Ensure infant's vital signs are stable and readiness to take feed.
3. Measure abdominal circumference just above the umbilical stump before every feed. Compare with the previous measurement of abdominal girth. When abdominal circumference increases by more than 2 cm from the baseline, it indicates abdominal distension. Then prefeed gastric aspiration is indicated.
4. Do prefeed gastric aspiration, in case of abdominal distension. Check the color and amount of gastric aspirate. Feeds may be suspended depending upon the amount and color of gastric aspirate. Analyze the amount and color of the aspirate to decide about continuing or discontinuing the feeds. Routine prefeed gastric aspirations are not recommended.
5. Confirm the position of the feeding tube in the stomach prior to give feed every time, using stethoscope to hear gurgling sound after pushing one mL air into the stomach.
6. Measure the amount of feed to be given to the infant, if abdominal distension not present and the infant is having no severe problems or illness.
7. Check the temperature of the EBM which was preserved in refrigerator. EBM should be in normal temperature before feeding to the baby.
8. Remove the plunger of the syringe (5 mL or 10 mL) and attach the barrel to the outer end of the feeding tube to give feed to the baby. Do not allow air into the tube **(Fig. 2.2)**.
9. Pour the required amount of milk in the barrel and allow the milk to flow by gravity.
10. Allow the milk to flow down slowly by adjusting the height of the barrel containing milk. Distance between the barrel and the infant's abdomen should be 8–10 cm or less in very preterm infant. Total feeding time can be 10–15 minutes. Rapid feeding may interfere with peristalsis causing cramp or abdominal distension.
11. Observe the infant during feeding for vomiting, breathing difficulty, cyanosis,

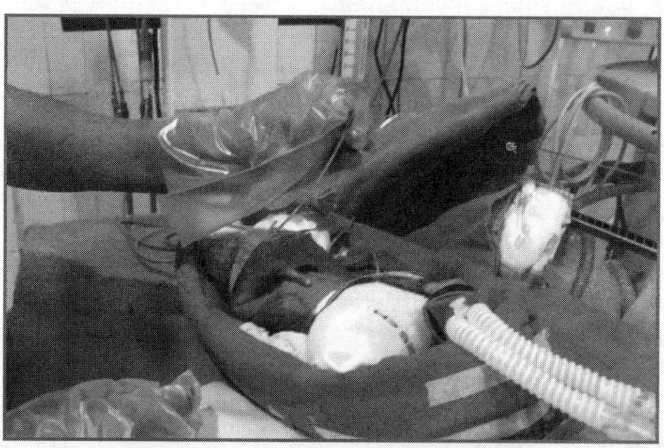

Fig. 2.2: Gavage feeding in a neonate.

choking or any other problems. There is no need of burping in gavage feeding.

12. Provide oromotor stimulation gently to the infant during feeding.
13. Close the outer end of the feeding tube with its cap after the feeding is complete. Avoid giving of water into the feeding tube to clean it.
14. Allow the infant to the mother for non-nutritive suckling on an empty breast after expression of milk, if mother present with the neonate.
15. Place the infant comfortably in lateral position for 15–20 minutes. Left lateral position reduces gastric reflux and right lateral position promotes gastric emptying.
16. Change orogastric feeding tube after 2–3 days, whenever possible.
17. Change the diaper and make the neonate comfortable.
18. Take care of the used articles and dispose the waste.
19. Wash hands and document the procedure of orogastric tube feeding.

Evaluation and Documentation

- Evaluate: Infant's vital signs, general condition, bowel sound, amount of intake and urine output, feed tolerance, stool pattern, and weight pattern. Evaluate parents concern
- Document: Amount and type of milk given, date and time of feeding, feeding tube position, measured length of tube introduced (lip to tip), abdominal girth, amount and content of aspirate (if done), infant's response during feeding, daily weight, passage of urine and meconium/ stool, any vomiting or presence of any problems.

Communication and Teaching for Homecare

- Communicate with the mother and the family members about infant's condition, improvement or deterioration of neonate's health and plan of further management. Encourage the parents to ask questions and to participate in baby care
- Teach the parents about importance of feeding with EBM, technique of expression of breast milk, disadvantages of formula feeding, hand hygiene, general cleanliness, mother's own diet and rest, continuation of care at home and plan of follow-up visits after discharge from hospital.

PROCEDURE–21: PALADAI FEEDING OR CUP/KATORI-SPOON FEEDING OF NEONATES

Clinical Guidelines

- Paladai, a modified spoon with bowl/cup or katori with household teaspoon are used as alternative methods of feeding to the infants, when infants are unable to take direct breastfeeding from mother but can swallow milk, when the milk is given in the mouth
- Preterm, LBW or sick neonates who have good swallowing reflex but poor suckling reflex, are allowed to feed by paladai or spoon. This mode of feeding is considered as bridge between gavage feeding and breastfeeding
- Neonates at about 34 (32–35) weeks of gestational age attain the ability to coordinate sucking and swallowing reflex with respiration. At 30 weeks of gestational age, neonates attain the ability to coordinate swallowing with respiration. Hence the neonates with gestation of 30–34 weeks (1,200–1,800 gram birth weight) can be fed by katori-spoon or by paladai, considering they are able to swallow the milk after 1–3 days of age. Initially on day one, these neonates are allowed for gavage feeding. Neonates more than 34 weeks of gestation or birth weight more than 1,800 gram may also require paladai or spoon feeding when they are unable to take breastfeeding directly from their mothers due to their illness or inability to coordinate suckling, swallowing and breathing actions
- Paladai or spoon feeding is given to maintain fluid and nutritional requirements and to prevent malnutrition and growth failure in preterm, LBW and sick

neonates. Feeding is given at 2 hours interval for small and sick neonates
- Calculated amount of EBM or formula milk based on the daily fluid requirement can be given to the infants by paladai or spoon feeding. It is safe for the small infants
- Remember to encourage the mother for expression of breast milk for her baby for paladai or spoon feeding with EBM and explain about disadvantages of formula feeding.

Equipment Required

- Hand washing articles and handrub
- Sterile paladai or spoon in a sterile covered container
- Expressed breast milk or formula milk in sterile covered container, i.e., cup or small bowl or katori to feed the neonate
- Small towel or bib to protect baby's dress from spillage
- Diaper and diaper changing items
- Waste disposal containers
- Documentation sheet, intake-output chart and neonatal case sheet.

Assessment and Preparation

- Assess the infant's vital signs, activity level, alertness, swallowing reflex, presence of any respiratory problems, abnormal movements and for any abnormal clinical features. Assess parents level of understanding and anxiety
- Self-preparation should be done by meticulous hand washing
- Environment should be clean, calm, quiet, well lighted and well ventilated
- All necessary articles should be collected and arranged near the neonate. Feeding utensils must be made sterile by boiling for 20–30 minutes or by autoclaving
- Preparation of mother: Explain the procedure to the mother, if she present. Allow the mother to help during feeding. Encourage her to do expression of breast milk for her baby's feeding. Ask her concern and answer accordingly
- Preparation of neonate: Make the baby clean and hold in comfortable semi-upright position. Daily morning weight must be recorded for calculation of fluid and feeds

Performing the Steps of Procedure with Rationale/Point of Emphasis

1. Wash hand and arrange all articles near the neonate.
2. Ensure the infant is clean and alert to take feed.
3. Allow the mother near the neonate and encourage to observe and participate in procedure.
4. Hold the neonate in semi-upright position comfortably with head well supported to prevent aspiration or chocking. Place the baby on lap as breastfeeding position or on the bassinet with support.
5. Check the temperature of the EBM which was preserved in refrigerator. EBM should be in normal temperature before feeding to the neonate.
6. Place the small towel or bib around the baby's neck to protect the baby's dress from spillage of milk.
7. Take the measure amount of feed from the katori or cup/small bowl into the paladai or spoon. Pour or take ½ to ¾ full amounts of milk in paladai or spoon to prevent spillage. More spillage can occur from spoon rather than paladai. Spillage interfere with required nutritional intake due to reduced amount of milk intake.
8. Hold the paladai at the side/brim **(Fig. 2.3)**. Do not put finger into the milk to prevent

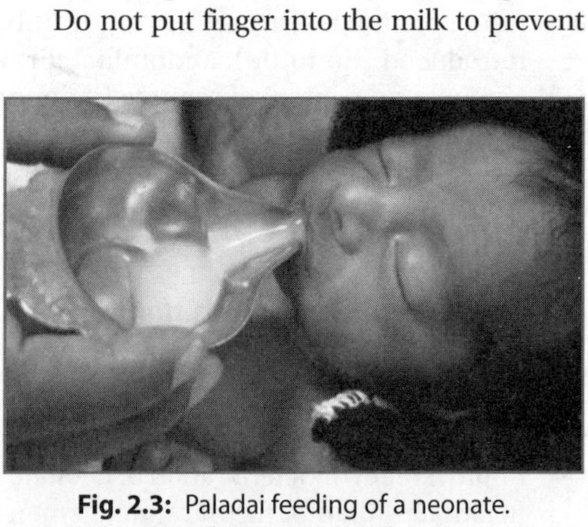

Fig. 2.3: Paladai feeding of a neonate.
(For color version, see Plate 1)

contamination. Hold spoon at the handle. Do not put finger into baby's mouth to open.

9. Place the tip of the paladai or spoon with milk at the middle of the lower lip and allow the baby to suck. The tip of the paladai or spoon can be hold at the corner of the mouth with precautions to prevent injury.
10. Pour the milk in small amount slowly into baby's mouth but not in the throat to prevent choking and aspirations. Baby will swallow the milk actively.
11. Continue the process till the calculated desired amount of milk is given to the neonate.
12. Give gentle stimulation or stroke behind the ear or on the sole of the infant, if the infant goes to sleep or does not swallow the milk actively. If the infant is still sluggish, it is better to give gavage feeding rather than paladai feeding. Force feeding must be avoided.
13. Burp the baby in between feed if air is swallowed and after completion of feed to bring out the swallowed air from the infant's stomach. Burping should be done by gentle patting or rubbing the back of the baby in partial-prone position on nurse's or mother's hand or on mother's lap by the mother.
14. Give oromotor stimulation in between two feeds and non-nutritive suckling by the mother after feeding the baby to promote sucking reflex.
15. Place the baby in lateral position with head supported a little higher than rest of the body.
16. Make the baby comfortable. Check and change the diaper, if soiled.
17. Take care articles, clean and make the utensils sterile and reset for reuse.
18. Wash hands and document the paladai or spoon feeding procedure.

Evaluation and Documentation

- Evaluate: Infant's vital signs, general condition, bowel sound, amount of intake and urine output, feed tolerance, stool pattern, and weight pattern. Evaluate parents concern
- Document: Amount and type of milk given, date and time of feeding, infant's response during feeding, daily weight, passage of urine and meconium/stool, any vomiting or presence of any problems.

Communication and Teaching for Homecare

- Communicate with the mother and the family members about infant's present condition, improvement observed and plan of further management. Encourage the parents to ask questions and to participate in baby care
- Teach the parents about importance of feeding with EBM, technique of expression of breast milk, routine care of the baby, breastfeeding technique, hand hygiene, general cleanliness, mother's diet and rest, continuation of care at home and plan of follow-up visits after discharge from hospital.

PROCEDURE–22: EXPRESSION OF BREAST MILK

Clinical Guidelines

- Expression of breast milk is indicated in some maternal and neonatal conditions when direct breastfeeding to the infant by the mother is not possible
- Breast milk expression is done to maintain milk secretion by the mother and to prevent lactation failure in case of preterm, LBW and sick infants, who are unable to suck or cannot feed from mother's breast due to some reasons
- It is practiced to relieve breast engorgement of the mother and to maintain exclusive breastfeeding to the infant by own mother's milk in case of working women
- It is better to express breast milk manually by the mother herself, rather than using breast pump. Health care providers especially the nurse and midwife should teach and demonstrate the correct technique of breast milk expression to the mother. Mother should do the expression of breast milk by herself to prevent her discomfort and pain or hurt

- When breast pump (manual or electrical) is used for expression of breast milk, be sure about use sterile breast milk bottle or container, breast shields and accessory to prevent contamination of milk and to prevent gastrointestinal infections of the baby.

Equipment/Articles Required

- Hand washing supplies
- Sterile wide mouth container or bowl with lid or cover
- A glass of drinking water for the mother

Assessment and Preparation

- Assess the mother's level of understanding and anxiety regarding infant's condition. Check the both breasts for presence of any problems
- Self-preparation should be done with hand hygiene
- Environment should be calm and quiet, clean, well-lighted and not overcrowded
- Articles should be arranged conveniently at the place of expression
- Preparation of neonate: Be sure that the infant is not very critically ill to allow the mother to visit the baby and to express near the infant. Planning to initiate early enteral feeding with minimal enteral nutrition and alternative method of feeding with EBM for the infant should be explained to the mother
- Preparation of the mother:
    - Encourage and teach the mother to do the steps of expression of breast milk
    - Allow the mother to drink a glass of water and to be relax
    - Ensure mother has maintained personal hygiene (bathing, clean dress up, hand wash)
    - Allow the mother to handle the neonate and to do expression near the infant, if possible. It will promote good let-down reflex of the mother. Touch, sound and smell of the baby increases oxytocin secretion in mother and helps in flow of breast milk
    - Maintain privacy of the mother during expression of breast milk
    - Explain about importance of early enteral feeding and exclusive breast-feeding with EBM and with mother's own milk.

Performing the Steps of Procedure with Rationale/Point of Emphasis

1. Ensure mother has done hand wash following six steps with soap and water.
2. Assist the mother to sit comfortably and to hold the container near the breast.
3. Ask the mother to drink one glass of water before expression of breast milk.
4. Help and teach the mother to massage the breast gently towards the nipples.
5. Mother will do the technique of expression of breast milk as follows:
    i. Put her thumb on the areola of the breast above the nipple and her index/first finger on the areola of the breast below the nipple. Mother should support the breast with other fingers. Thumb and index finger of mother will be placed on areola only.
    ii. Press her thumb and index finger slightly inwards, towards the chest wall.
    iii. Press her breast behind the nipple and areola between her forefingers and thumb. This will help to give pressure on lactiferous sinuses beneath the areola. Lactiferous sinuses feel like pods of peas in lactating breast. If mother can feel them, she can give pressure on them.
    iv. Repeat press and release, press and release. At first no milk will come out, but after pressing a few minutes, milk starts to drip/drop. There should not be any pain or hurt during expression. If it happens, it indicates that the technique of expression is wrong.
    v. Express from all segments of the breast following the same technique from the sides.
    vi. Avoid rubbing or sliding of fingers along the skin of the breast to prevent skin abrasions and pain. Movements of fingers should be more like rolling.

vii. Avoid squeezing the nipple only. Pressing and pulling the nipples does not help in expression of breast milk.
viii. Express from one breast for at least 3–5 minutes until the flow of milk slows. Then express from the other breast. Expression can take 20–30 minutes for both breasts.
6. Encourage the mother to express her breast milk frequently at least 8 times in 24 hours to stimulate and maintain adequate milk secretion.
7. Store the EBM with proper labeling in room temperature for 8 hours and in the household refrigerator for 24 hours or use the EBM for infant feeding immediately after expression by alternative methods as gavage feeding or paladai feeding or cup and spoon feeding.
8. Make the mother comfortable and help to complete the procedure.
9. Perform hand hygiene.
10. Document the procedure of expression of breast milk.

Evaluation and Documentation

- Evaluate the mother's level of understanding about the procedure of expression of breast milk. Re-explain and demonstrate the technique of expression of breast milk
- Document the date and time of expression, amount of milk expressed out and any pain or problems occur during expression. If the EBM is stored in refrigerator, then it should be labeled with mother's name, registration number, date and time of expression, and amount of milk.

Communication and Teaching for Homecare

- Communicate with the mother and family members about the infant's condition, plan of feeding, frequency of expression of breast milk and storing of EBM
- Teach the parents about importance and technique of expression of breast milk, storage of EBM, precautions to be followed for expression if it is practiced at home, importance of exclusive breastfeeding, maintenance of hygienic practices, maternal diet in lactational period, routine care of the infant at home, danger signs and plan of follow-up visits.

PROCEDURE–23: KANGAROO MOTHER CARE

Clinical Guidelines

- Kangaroo mother care (KMC) is a special intervention for the care of LBW infants. It is safe, simple and cost-effective method used to keep the LBW infant warm and to prevent hypothermia **(Fig. 2.4)**
- KMC is early, prolonged, continuous, and direct skin to skin contact between the neonate and mother or any other willing care giver. It has three components, i.e., skin to skin contact, exclusive breastfeeding and early discharge with follow-up care
- All stable LBW infants are eligible for KMC. More emphasis is given for the stable LBW infants having birth weight less than 2,000 gram.
- KMC can be initiated in a stable infant with intravenous (IV) fluid therapy, oxygen therapy, gavage feeding and even on CPAP and ventilator
- KMC is initiated during hospital stay in SNCU/NICU and continued at home

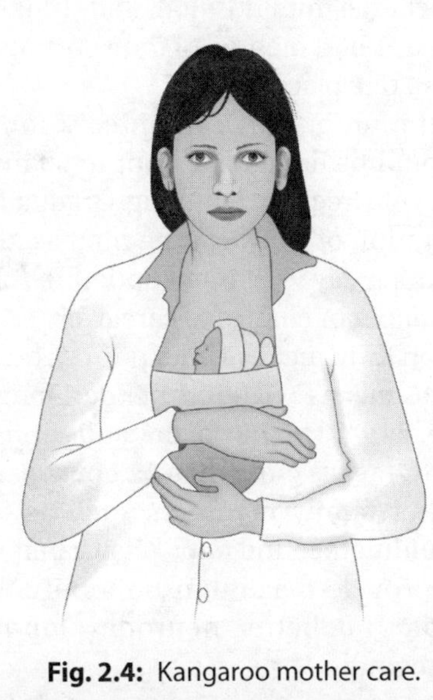

Fig. 2.4: Kangaroo mother care.

- KMC should not be confused with routine early "skin to skin care" immediate at birth in delivery room
- As per recommendation of WHO, skin to skin care immediate after birth should be practiced uninterruptedly for 1 hour for every normal healthy newborn baby irrespective of birth weight. It helps to keep the newborn baby warm in first golden hour of life and to initiate early breastfeeding
- Benefits of KMC include: (a) It provides effective thermal control and reduces risk of hypothermia, (b) It leads in increased duration and rate of breastfeeding, (c) It promotes more regular breathing and less apnea, (d) It protects from nosocomial infections and reduces incidence of pneumonia during infancy, (e) It satisfies all five senses of the infant through skin to skin contact, i.e., touch, listening to mother's voice and heartbeat, i.e., hearing, suckles from breast to feed, i.e., taste, smells mother's body odor, i.e., olfaction, and makes eye to eye contact with mother, i.e., vision, (f) It facilitates better mother and infant bonding, better neurodevelopment and makes the mother more confident to take care of LBW infant, (g) It helps in better daily weight gain, reduce hospital stay and promotes early discharge from hospital, and (h) It can be used as best method of transporting infant from one place to other
- Duration of KMC: In one session KMC should be done for 1 hour to 90 minutes to avoid frequent handling. Gradually total duration of KMC can be increased to 24 hours a day with interruption for change of diaper or change of caregiver
- Short KMC means 4 hour per day, extended KMC means 5–8 hours per day, long KMC means 9–12 hours per day and continuous KMC means more than 12 hours per day
- Other family members such as father, grandmother and aunty also can do KMC to provide maximum hours of KMC in a day for better neurodevelopmental outcome
- Continuation of KMC: It should be continued until the infant gains weight around 2,500 gram or reaches 40 weeks of postconception age. It can be continued as long as possible, if both mother and baby are comfortable, especially in winter night and after bathing
- KMC can be discontinued if the infant starts wriggling to show discomfort or pulls limbs out, cries and fusses every time in KMC position
- Evidence shows that practice of continuous KMC significantly reduced neonatal mortality and lower the rates of morbidities of neonates.

Requirements for Kangaroo Mother Care

- Hand hygiene supplies
- Mother clothing: Front open light dress as per local culture, i.e., Saree-blouse or gown
- Infant's clothing: Front open sleeveless shirt, cap, socks, mittens and nappy
- KMC bag or binder or sling to keep and support the infant in KMC position
- Sheet or shawl to wrap both mother and baby together
- KMC chair (reclining chair) or bed for mother with adjustable backrest or pillows
- Routine baby care items and diaper changing articles
- Waste disposal containers as per BMW rule
- Record sheet for documentation of KMC and neonatal case sheet
- KMC poster, KMC video in local language as IEC material to motivate the mother and family members to practice KMC for maximum duration.

Assessment and Preparation

- Assess the infant's vital signs to identify hemodynamic stability and take baby's body weight. Assess the parents' and family members level of understanding to participate in the intervention of kangaroo care
- Self-preparation should be done with hand hygiene

- Environment should be calm, quiet, clean, well ventilated and free from overcrowding
- All necessary requirements should be collected near the infant
- Preparation of mother/caregiver:
  - Ensure mother or other KMC caregiver is willing, maintain good hygiene and health, take adequate diet, have no serious illness and supported by other family members
  - Counsel the mother or other caregiver about benefits of KMC and answer to questions and clarify their doubts
  - Maintain privacy of the mother or caregiver during KMC
  - Explain about KMC position, breast-feeding during KMC, monitoring during KMC, duration and continuation of KMC, post-discharge follow-up care
- Preparation of neonate: Infant should be stable, clean and comfortable.

Performing the Steps of Procedure with Rationale/Point of Emphasis

1. Ensure mother or other KMC caregiver had taken food, had bath, used toilet, change outside dress, wear clean/sterile NICU/SNCU dress and wash hand before doing KMC.
2. Perform hand hygiene and make arrangement for KMC near the neonate.
3. Position the mother comfortably in sitting or semi-reclining posture on chair or bed with backrest or pillow in about 30–45 degree angle.
4. Maintain privacy of the mother and ask her concern.
5. Dress the neonate with cap, socks, mitten, nappy and front open sleeveless shirt.
6. Place the infant in between mother's breasts in upright position in skin to skin contact.
7. Turn the infant's head to one side in slightly extended position so that it helps to keep the baby's airway open and to allow eye to eye contact between mother and baby. This position helps to reduce the risk of apnea as mother's breathing and heartbeat stimulates the infant continuously.
8. Place the infant's hip and leg flexed in frog like position. Allow both arms of the infant to be in flexed position on mother's chest.
9. Ensure that the infant's abdomen is at the level of mother's epigastrium.
10. Provide support to keep the infant in KMC position using sling or binder or KMC bag.
11. Allow the mother to keep her one hand to hold baby's head and other hand to hold bottom of the baby to prevent dropping of the infant from KMC position.
12. Explain the mother that she can do KMC during sleep and resting.
13. Demonstrate and help the mother to give breastfeeding during KMC.
14. Cover both mother and infant together with sheet or shawl especially in winter.
15. Monitor the infant's respiration, neck position, skin color, and warmth during KMC. Teach the mother to monitor the baby in KMC position.
16. Observe for any problem of the mother during KMC session and provide support.
17. Perform hand hygiene and document KMC in details.

Evaluation and Documentation

- Evaluate infant's vital signs, feeding pattern, daily weight and improvement or deterioration of the condition. Evaluate mother's health and hygiene, level of understanding and anxiety, family support and presence of any problem
- Document the KMC, as per standard guidelines, with date, time duration per session, infant's vital signs findings, daily weight, nature of feeding, urine and stool pattern, total KMC hours per day and problems during KMC

Communication and Teaching for Homecare

- Communicate with the mother and family members about importance of KMC, family involvement, support required to the mother and need for follow-up care
- Teach the parents about continuation of KMC, special care of LBW infants, exclusive breastfeeding, assessment of infant's

temperature, maintenance of warmth by wrapping, hygienic care, environmental cleanliness, identification of danger signs, need for medical help in emergency, required screening procedures, developmental supportive care at home, immunization and plan of follow-up visits.

PROCEDURE–24: DEVELOPMENTAL SUPPORTIVE CARE OF NEONATES

Clinical Guidelines

- Developmental supportive care (DSC) is an individualized and continuous care process based on infant's cues. It improves physiological stability and protects sleep rhythms. It promotes physical growth and neurodevelopmental maturity especially in preterm, LBW and sick infants. It helps to reduce harmful environmental stimuli and stress of the infants. It provides baby-friendly womb like environment in the NICU/SNCU
- Five core components of developmental supportive care of the neonates are: (i) protected sleep, (ii) provision of healing environment, (iii) family centered care (FCC), (iv) appropriate protection from pain and (v) developmentally supportive activities of daily living (ADL)
- *Protected undisturbed sleep* for long duration promotes brain development and maturation of infants. It can be facilitated by environmental modifications, clustering of care activities, cue-based care to the individual infant, nesting, swaddling and KMC. Sleep is important to promote normal brain growth. The activity occurring during REM sleep is particularly important. Deprivation of sleep leads to neuronal death and reduced brain mass which lead to delayed or deprived neurodevelopmental outcome
- *Healing environment* for the infants, especially in NICU/SNCU, is important for optimal growth and development and reduction of pain and stress from noxious stimuli. Structured environment as similar as possible to that of intrauterine life provides support to the neonates and help them to organize their state of mind and to reduce negative impact towards better neurodevelopmental outcome. Healing environment can be provided with optimal soft noise, smoothing light, warmth with thermoneutral surroundings, sweet smell, appropriate positioning and KMC
- *Developmentally supportive ADL* for the infant should be arranged with adequate feeding with non-nutritive suckling (NNS) and oromotor stimulation, gentle massage with soft touch, dressing and undressing, skin care, sponging, diaper changing, cleanliness and hygienic measures, clustering of care activities, and participation of mother/family member during routine care and therapeutic interventions. These ADL will promote infant's growth and development, hygiene and general well-being. ADL should be carried out according to the infant's readiness and cue-based, but not based on unit protocol or healthcare professionals choice
- *Family centered care* for the neonates is the integral part of NICU/SNCU care. It promotes better parent-infant bonding and holistic wellbeing of the infant. Parents should participate in infant's care, perform KMC and take informed decisions regarding plan of management. Good communication, teaching, and encouragement helps in better parental involvement in infant care
- *Protection from pain* by assessment, anticipation, prevention and adequate management is essential for reduction of pain, stress and better neurodevelopmental outcomes. Painful procedures can result in mild or moderate or severe pain. Pain management in neonates can be done by general measures, non-pharmacological measures or using medications as pharmacological measures. Pain management is very important intervention for optimal neurological maturation
- Kangaroo mother care is the best form of developmental supportive care with

multimodal stimulation to the newborn infant for optimal comprehensive healthy outcome.

Equipment Required

- Hand hygiene supplies for hand wash and handrub
- Radiant warmer or incubator to provide rest, sleep and care to the infants
- All routine baby care articles, supplies and clothing
- Diaper and diaper changing articles
- Sterile containers with sterile sheets, gauze pieces, cotton swabs
- Waste disposal containers as per BMW rule
- Neonatal care record sheet and monitoring sheet.

Assessment and Preparation

- Assess the infant's vital signs for hemodynamically stability. Assess parents' level of anxiety and understanding related to care of newborn infant
- Self-preparation should be done by hand hygiene
- Environment should be clean, warm, calm, quiet with appropriate light and ventilation
- All care articles and equipment should be available near the neonate
- Preparation of mother/parents: Explain about the DSC, FCC to the parents and encourage them for participation
- Preparation of neonate: Make the infant clean, warm and comfortable.

Performing the Steps of Procedure with Rationale/Point of Emphasis

1. Perform hand hygiene and ensure that the neonate is warm and stable. Perform the following interventions as appropriate and whenever indicated to the infants.
2. *Nesting:* Prepare an oval thick boundary like a nest with sterile sheets around the neonate under radiant warmer on bassinet or inside incubator. Place the neonate inside the nest that holds and contains the neonate and provides intrauterine womb-like environment. Nesting promotes protected sleep and stabilizes the infant. It also helps to reduce stress and facilitate growth and development of the neonate. The infant can be placed in supine or side lying or in prone position inside the nesting. Place infant's arms and legs in flexed midline position to the trunk in supine position inside nesting.
3. *Positioning:* (a) Place the infant in *supine position* with nesting for good observation that allows flexion, midline orientation, and forward gaze. Supine position without nesting leads to retracted shoulders, delay in midline orientation and eye mouth coordination. (b) Place the infant in *lateral position* after feeding or whenever needed. Right lateral position helps in faster gastric emptying and left lateral position reduces gastroesophageal reflex. Lateral position enhances hand to mouth coordination and prevents retraction of shoulders and abduction of legs. Continuous lateral position leads to flattening of head on one side, (c) *Prone position* improves oxygenation and reduces heat loss and energy consumption. Correct and appropriate positioning of preterm neonates optimize functioning of musculoskeletal, nervous and sensory systems for better growth and development.
4. *Healing environment:* Ensure soft sound (40–45 db), soothing light (100–600 lux), thermoneutral environment as per birth weight and postnatal age, infection free environment (i.e., meticulous hand hygiene, optimum house-keeping and cleanliness, aseptic interventions, disinfection and sterilization of care items, waste management, etc.), nesting or boundaries, involvement of mother/family members during care and music therapy. Avoid overcrowding, loud noise, and bad odors. Infant should receive optimal tactile, visual, auditory, olfactory, gustatory and vestibular stimulation from the care environment to support better neurodevelopmental maturation. Healing environment supports the infants' growth and development while minimize their

pain and stress resulting from continuous exposure of unwanted and harsh stimuli.

5. *Swaddling:* Take a square baby sheet, spread diagonally and wrap the infant including head, arms, legs and abdomen fully. Swaddling makes the infant calm and regulated. It protects the infant from noxious stimuli and over-stimulating environment in NICU/SNCU or even at home. It facilitates quiet time and longer sleep of the infant. It is practiced usually during procedures exposing only the required body part of the infant thus to reduce pain sensation.
6. *Hand containment*: Place one hand firmly but gently on the infant's head and other hand on either the infant's arms or lower back, buttocks or soles of infant's feet. This technique can be performed by the mother/caregiver or health care professionals/nurse for holding and calming the preterm, LBW or sick neonates. Containment is done during sleep, during ADL and during painful medical procedures.
7. *Protected sleep:* Provide cluster care, womb-like healing environment, nesting, swaddling, containment, gentle massage and KMC to promote sleep. Modification of the care environment and cue-based care in neonatal units facilitates undisturbed sleep of the infants. Long duration of undisturbed sleep and rest are essential for the development and maturation of infant's brain.
8. *Optimal feeding:* (i) Support and swaddle the infant during feeding; (ii) Assist the mother to give breastfeeding in kangaroo position; (iii) Maintain hygienic measures and use sterile utensils or feeding articles for paladai/spoon or tube feeding; (iv) Do not give forced feeding and provide required time for the individual infant; (v) Allow NNS and give oromotor stimulation to improve sucking behavior; (vi) Initiate enteral feeding as early as possible and allow minimal enteral nutrition, and (vii) Provide dim light, reduce noise and other distractions during feeding.
9. *Non-nutritive sucking (NNS)*: Provide NNS to the neonate in the form of sucking of own fingers, mother finger, gauze lollipop dipped in mother's milk or on empty mother's breast after expression of breast milk. NNS can be started when the neonate is on gavage feeding. It helps to promote sucking behavior of the infant and to improve digestion of feeds. So, NNS helps to promote adequate feed intake, improve weight gain and reduce hospital stay by early discharge.
10. *Oromotor stimulation (OMS):* OMS along with routine care reduces the duration of gavage feeding and improves oromotor function and skills in preterm neonates. It enhances growth velocity in preterm infants with decreased time from gavage feeding to full independent feeds by mouth. There is structure OMS intervention guideline for preterm, LBW and sick neonates, that should be followed in neonatal care units.
11. *Gentle massaging:* Massage provides tactile and kinesthetic stimulations. Start gentle massaging for the neonate from head, move to the face, then to the chest, abdomen, and finally the limbs. Place fingers flat on the infant's body and massage with moderate pressure using long, firm and gentle strokes. Avoid light feathery touch. Gentle extending and flexing of limbs can be done during the massage. Apply oil for very preterm and ELBW infants instead of massaging.
12. *Skin care:* Skin is the largest organ. General cleanliness and clean cloth are essential to keep the skin healthy. Take precautions during application and removal of adhesive tape. Avoid using lotions and soap for preterm infant's skin. Change position of the neonate to prevent pressure sores. Use body oil for massage as per unit policy. Protect infant's skin from drying and injury. Minimize the needle pricks. Take care of diaper area to prevent rash or erosion.
13. *Stimulation:* Lack of stimulation and overstimulation are both harmful for the

infant. Optimal stimulation is necessary for development of sense organ.

a. Provide optimal *auditory stimulation* and protect from noise. Noise is harmful to the infant. It reduces sleep and increases stress. Noise leads to hearing loss, IVH, PVL and lower intelligence. Talk softly and discuss away from the neonate during medical round. Attend monitor alarms promptly. Reduce the volume of telephone ring and alarm sound. Avoid shouting around neonates and dragging of chairs on the floor. Allow mother speaking to the infant or singing softly or arrange music therapy.
b. Provide *tactile stimulation* by soft touch, stroking and caressing, gentle massage and by skin to skin contact in KMC. Before touching, talk to the infant to awake gently.
c. Provide *olfactory stimulation* with the mother's body smell or smell of her breast milk. Avoid bad odor and strong fragrance.
d. Provide *gustatory stimulation* by taste of own mother milk. Avoid bad taste medicine.
e. Provide *vestibular stimulation* by moving the infant gently. Mother's rhythmic breathing and chest movement is the best smoothing sensation during KMC. Avoid sudden position change and rocking or swinging movement. Do not pick the infant in a harsh manner. Adopt minimal and gentle handling of the infant.
f. Provide best *visual stimulation* with mother's face and encourage the mother for eye to eye contact in stable infant. Arrange day-night light rhythm in the NICU/SNCU. Avoid direct bright light to the neonate. Place a cover over the incubator.

14. *Pain management measures:* Assess pain in neonates by recognizing behavioral, physiological and autonomic changes and using pain evaluation scales. Provide non-pharmacological measures such as hand containment for the infant, swaddling or gently holding hands together on chest or holding legs, non-nutritive suckling, oral sucrose or breast milk drops or breast feeding, and kangaroo position. Practice minimum number of painful interventions (such as minimizing repeated needle pricks to reduce stress in neonates). Breastfeeding and breast milk drops is almost as effective as sucrose analgesia in reducing pain in neonates undergoing single painful procedure.
15. *Parent involvement*: Allow mother for dressing, undressing, diaper changing, sponging, massaging, feeding, transporting and for KMC. Assist parents to transfer or transport the infant in kangaroo position or by swaddling. Involve, encourage and teach parents to participate actively for care activities of the infant.
16. Document in details about the DSC provided to the individual infant.

Evaluation and Documentation

- Evaluate infant's condition, behavioral cues before, during and after the DSC procedures. Evaluate parents level of understanding and ability to implement developmental supportive care measures at home after discharge
- Document the findings of infant's health condition, infant's behavioral cues and measures provided to support and enhance neurodevelopmental integrity of the neonate. Keep record of parent's participation in care activities of their infant

Communication and Teaching for Homecare

- Communicate with the parents and other family members about infant's condition and importance of continuation of developmental supportive care
- Teach the parents about all aspects of developmental supportive care of the infant including its continuation at home and plan of follow-up care, as scheduled.

PROCEDURE–25: CARE OF THE NEONATES DURING RESPIRATORY SUPPORT WITH CPAP

Clinical Guidelines

- Continuous positive airway pressure (CPAP) is a method of ventilatory support applied to the spontaneously breathing patients for optimal management of respiratory distress. In CPAP, airway pressure is maintained above atmospheric pressure throughout the respiratory cycle during both inspiration and expiration. It is provided to keep the lung alveoli remain open by constant airway pressure. It splints the airways so that they do not collapse, thus improves functional residual capacity (FRC) of the lungs. It leads to better breathing and better gas exchange with less lung injury. It splints the upper airways and prevents obstructive apnea. It dilates the lower airways thus reducing airway resistance
- Delivery of CPAP to the neonate includes: (i) delivery of continuous positive airway pressure to the airway and lungs, (ii) delivery of air and oxygen mixture at the preset fractional oxygen concentration and (iii) delivery of air oxygen mixture at body temperature and at relative humidity of 100% to the neonate's nostrils
- CPAP is commonly indicated in: (a) respiratory distress syndrome (RDS), (b) apnea of prematurity, (c) transient tachypnea of newborn baby (TTNB), and (d) post-extubation from mechanical ventilation in preterm VLBW infants
- Other indications of CPAP include pneumonia, meconium aspiration syndrome, pulmonary hemorrhage, pulmonary edema, laryngomalacia, tracheomalacia, etc.
- Neonates with CPAP need three phased monitoring: (i) monitoring of neonates for adequacy of CPAP setting and to identify complications, (ii) monitoring of CPAP machine for leaks, water condensation, water level in bubble chamber and in the humidifier, and (iii) appropriateness of CPAP and interface size and fixation, presence of nasal injury and nasal block
- Adequacy of CPAP to the neonates is assessed by satisfactory cardiorespiratory status. This is confirmed by hemodynamic stable and comfortable neonate with minimal chest retractions, no grunting and normal CRT, blood pressure, oxygen saturations and normal blood gas values
- Failure of CPAP in neonates is identified by continuous chest retractions, grunting, recurrent apneas, SpO_2<90%, or PaO_2<50, PEEP >7 and FiO_2 >60%, $PaCO_2$ >55, poor respiratory effort, and when neonate is not tolerating CPAP
- Weaning of CPAP pressure and FiO_2 is done when neonate is settled and the disease process for which CPAP was started is improving. Always first reduce the FiO_2 and then the CPAP pressure in steps
- Remove the neonate from CPAP, when CPAP pressure is 4 cm and FiO_2<30% and the disease process has improved
- Continuous monitoring of the neonate's condition during CPAP and meticulous infection control practices with standard precautions are very important for optimal outcome.

Equipment Required

- Hand hygiene supplies for hand washing and handrub
- PPE for health care professionals
- CPAP Circuit, bubble chamber for Bubble-CPAP and machine
- CPAP interfaces/nasal prongs or masks and appropriate size CPAP cap
- Multiparameter monitor, pulse oximeter, stethoscope
- Oxygen source, oxygen tubing, flow meter
- Distilled water in container or bottle for CPAP water chamber
- Sterile tray containing pairs of sterile gloves, gauze pieces, cotton swabs, sheets
- Orogastric tube and suction catheter and suction machine or devices
- Articles for IV fluid therapy and syringe or infusion pump

- Tegaderm, Velcro, scissors, rubber bands, safety pins and connectors
- Neonatal resuscitation bag and masks, emergency medications, syringes
- Neonatal routine care articles, feeding articles
- Diaper and diaper changing articles
- Waste disposal containers as per BMW rule
- CPAP record sheet and neonatal monitoring sheet.

Assessment and Preparation

- Assess the neonate's respiratory status using Silverman Anderson Scoring and Downe's scoring. Assess neonate's vital signs, weight, blood gas, intake and output and presence of abnormal features. Assess parents' anxiety and level of understanding about CPAP
- Self-preparation should be done by hand hygiene and use of PPE
- Environment should be clean, calm, quiet, well lighted and well ventilated
- All necessary equipment and articles should be collected and arranged near the neonate
- Preparation of parents: Explain about need for CPAP, its therapeutic effects, possible complications and further plan of treatment. Encourage parents to ask questions and answer accordingly
- Preparation of neonate: Make the neonate clean, warm and comfortable.

Performing the Steps of Procedure with Rationale/Point of Emphasis

1. Perform hand hygiene and wear PPE.
2. Assemble the sterile CPAP circuit and fill the humidifier with distilled water.
3. Connect oxygen and air to the blender and switch on the humidifier.
4. Ensure the neonate is warm under radiant warmer or incubator.
5. Position the neonate with shoulder roll to keep the neck slightly extended in sniffing position. Clear the airway by suctioning of secretions, if present.
6. Attach pulse oximeter and multiparameter monitor to the neonate.
7. Check the patency of IV lines and ensure appropriate fluid therapy.
8. Fix the CPAP cap to the neonate, cover ears with cap and fix appropriate size prongs to the CPAP cap.
9. Ensure gap between nasal prongs and the columella to prevent nasal injury.
10. Use nasal CPAP mask around the perimeter of the neonate's nose, as per standard guidelines. Take precautions to prevent skin injury around the nose.
11. Connect nasal interface to the sterile circuit and give support to the circuit tubing.
12. Use non-pharmacological measures to reduce pain and provide comfort to the neonate.
13. Ensure temperature display on the humidifier is 37°C. There will be no condensation in the inspiratory circuit. Some condensation may be found in the expiratory limb.
14. Insert orogastric tube and fix the end of the tube to the side wall of the warmer.
15. Initiate CPAP with initial setting of CPAP pressure of 5 cm, FiO_2 of 50% and flow of 5 L/minute. It may vary depending upon the indications of CPAP.
16. Ensure desired water level in bubble chamber and humidifier. Record depth of immersion of expiratory limb.
17. Monitor and adjust FiO_2 and CPAP pressure based on the neonate's respiratory status.
18. Monitor neonate's respiratory rate, heart rate, SpO_2, CRT, blood pressure, abdominal girth, urine output, Silverman Anderson score, Downe's score, air entry, and condition of anterior fontanel. Look for apnea, tachypnea, retractions, grunting, bradycardia, tachycardia and any other problems or abnormalities.
19. Arrange for chest X-ray immediately after initiation of CPAP to the neonate to assess for lung inflation and to evaluate the etiology of respiratory distress.
20. Check the nostrils for nasal injury, secretions or any abnormalities. Do gentle

massage in each shift. Use normal saline drops, if required.

21. Assess for adequacy of CPAP or failure of CPAP and need for mechanical ventilation.
22. Wean the neonate from CPAP, when the disease process for which CPAP was started is improving gradually.
23. Remove the infant from CPAP, when FiO_2 <30%, CPAP pressure is 4 cm and disease process is improved. After removal of CPAP, frequent change of position is recommended. Oral and nasal suctioning may be needed to remove secretions. Saline nebulization may also be required.
24. Maintain standard precautions of infection control including hand hygiene and waste management for prevention of health care associated infections.
25. Document all observational findings in details in standard format for CPAP, as per institution policy.

Evaluation and Documentation

- Evaluate the neonate's improvement of respiratory status, vital signs, and disease process. Compare with baseline data. Evaluate parents' responses to the interventions
- Document date and time of initiation of CPAP, interface used, CPAP settings, respiratory status, vital signs, blood gas values, body weight, fluid intake, urine output, medications given, date and time of X-ray and its findings, problems occur during CPAP, weaning of CPAP and date and time removal of CPAP.

Communication and Teaching for Homecare

- Communicate with parents and family members about neonate's condition, effects of CPAP, plan of further management and need for involvement of mother in neonatal care for breast milk feeding, KMC and developmental supportive care
- Teach the parents about hand hygiene, cleanliness, expression of breast milk, breastfeeding, KMC, developmental supportive care, participation in care at hospital, care at home after discharge, danger signs, emergency medical help and follow-up care.

PROCEDURE–26: CARE OF THE NEONATES IN INCUBATOR/ISOLETTE

Clinical Guidelines

- Neonatal incubator is a device for the care of preterm neonates in a closed care system with controlled thermal environment. It is an enclosed crib for special care of preterm neonates, in which the temperature and humidity may be regulated. This equipment is used with specific indications. Neonatal incubator is also called as "Isolette"
- Consider use of incubator for very LBW neonates (birth weight <1,500 gram) or preterm neonates <34 weeks of gestation, as per unit/hospital policy
- Parts of the neonatal incubator include:
  - Canopy with port holes to access the neonate and wheels for locked position
  - Baby tray with mattress inside the canopy to place the neonate
  - Heat source with fan under the Baby tray
  - Skin probe to sense the neonate's body temperature
  - Air probe to measure the air temperature inside the incubator
  - Control panel for display and control knob including:
    - » Mode selectors to select air or skin mode
    - » Heater output display
    - » Temperature selection knob/key to set required temperature for the neonate
    - » Temperature display that shows neonate's skin temperature, set skin temperature and air temperature
    - » Alarm display for probe failure, power failure, heater failure, system failure, high or low skin temperature, air flow alarm, sensor alarm, etc.

- Incubator should be placed away from the wall and perpendicular to the wall for better air circulation and decreased heat loss by radiation
- Humidification may be used for neonates < 1,000 gram birth weight. Always use distilled water for humidification and change water daily. Take precautions to prevent growth of bacteria in water which can lead to neonatal sepsis. Incubator's water reservoir can be kept empty as per manufacturer recommendations. Leaving the reservoir dry may not affect the function of the incubator
- Use elbows to operate the access ports of the incubator during any procedure. Avoid banging against the sides during opening of the port. Do not keep any articles on top of the incubator
- Meticulous cleaning and disinfection of the incubator is very important for prevention of infections. All detachable parts also need cleaning and disinfection followed by reassembling. Terminal disinfection and sterilization of the incubator must be done after discharge or death or transfer of the neonate, as per manufacturer guidelines
- Regular maintenance checkup of incubator should be arranged for optimal functioning
- Consider to keep the neonate out of the incubator when the baby is stable and maintaining body temperature with heater output <25% or air temperature <30°C. This is usually occur after 2 weeks in extremely LBW neonates, when neonate's skin becomes mature and the infant started to gain daily weight with full feeds toleration.

Equipment Required

- Hand hygiene supplies for hand wash and handrub
- Neonatal incubator
- Neonatal care articles, sheets, shoulder roll
- Thermometer, cotton swabs and 70% alcohol to clean the thermometer before measuring baby's body temperature
- Bottles of alcohol and povidone-iodine, small bowl with cotton swabs
- Weighing machine and tape measure for anthropometric measurements
- Diaper, diaper changing articles and baby clothing
- Pulse oximeter and oxygen delivery system and device, if required
- Waste disposal containers
- Neonatal care sheet and monitoring sheet.

Assessment and Preparation

- Assess neonate's condition in details before placing the neonate in the incubator as baseline data. Assess parents anxiety and understanding level of neonate's condition and plan of management
- Self-preparation should be done with meticulous hand hygiene
- Environment should be clean, calm, quiet and well ventilated
- Articles preparation: All articles should be collected and arranged near the incubator. Clean the incubator using damp cloth soaked in soap solution daily, when occupied. If not occupied, then disinfect the incubator using disinfectant solution, as per unit protocol
- Preparation of parents: Explain about the need for incubator care of the neonate, plan of treatment and necessary participation in neonatal care
- Preparation of neonate: Assess the neonate's vital signs, body weight and for presence of any problem. Examine the neonate for abnormal clinical features. Make the baby clean and comfortable. Place only one neonate in one incubator

Performing the Steps of Procedure with Rationale/Point of Emphasis

1. Perform hand hygiene and ensure all necessary equipment and articles are ready.
2. Turn "ON" the incubator at least 30 minutes before receiving the neonates for rewarming the mattress, sheets and the hood.

3. Ensure adequate cleaning and disinfection of the incubator.
4. Assess neonate's vital signs for baseline data.
5. Dress up the neonate with cap, socks, and diaper. If the neonate is stable and no procedure is planned, then the neonate's body can be covered with cloths inside the incubator.
6. Place the neonate inside the incubator and monitor continuously. Keep the portholes covered.
7. Use air mode for initial stabilization, during procedure and in unstable neonate. Set the air temperature based on neutral thermal environmental temperature chart. Recommended incubator temperature for air mode should be followed based on neonate's weight and postnatal age. Record neonate's temperature every 2–4 hours and set air temperature accordingly.
8. Use skin/servo mode considering the skin maturity for better thermoregulation. Set desired temperature at 36.5°C. Attach skin probe securely with transparent adhesive as in case of radiant warmer. Ensure the neonate is not lying on the probe wires.
9. Check the probe frequently for right attachment. Assess skin condition. Change the probe site every 12–24 hours.
10. Monitor the neonate's temperature using thermometer and compare with incubator temperature initially every 30 minutes for 2 hours then 2–4 hours interval. Monitor other vital signs and clinical features to detect any abnormalities.
11. Check the temperature of the incubator every hour for first 8 hours and then every 3 hours. Compare the temperature with set temperature to assess incubator's function.
12. Handle the neonate very gently and cautiously. Take precautions for performing any procedure inside the incubator with continuous monitoring.
13. Minimize the number of entries into the incubator, because it can cause changes in the environmental temperature inside the incubator.
14. Follow the infection control practices strictly to prevent healthcare-associated infections.
15. Document all findings of assessment and procedures done for the neonate in the incubator and working condition of the incubator.

Evaluation and Documentation

- Evaluate neonate's response inside the incubator and compare temperature with previous readings. Evaluate neonate's condition for improvement or deterioration. Evaluate parent's understanding of method used to monitor and maintain neonate's temperature and treatment plan
- Document: Neonate's temperature, air temperature, mode used (air or servo) and any procedure performed such as weighing, feeding, diaper changing, medications, oxygen therapy, IV fluid therapy, etc.

Communication and Teaching for Homecare

- Communicate with the parents about the neonate's condition and plan of treatment. Encourage and motivate the parents in participation of baby care
- Teach the parents about involvement in infant's care in NICU, importance of breastfeeding, hygienic care, developmental supportive care, special care for preterm LBW infant, neonatal screening, continuation of care at home after discharge from hospital and plan of follow-up care.

PROCEDURE–27: EXCHANGE BLOOD TRANSFUSION IN NEONATES

Clinical Guidelines

- Exchange blood transfusion (EBT) involves substituting donor blood for recipient blood. During EBT small quantities of recipient's blood are alternately removed and replaced with donor blood until the desired volume of blood has been exchanged. In neonates, EBT is commonly done in case of hemolytic disease of the newborn with hyperbilirubinemia in Rh isoimmunization or ABO isoimmunization

- Early indications of EBT in neonates with hemolytic disease include: (a) cord blood bilirubin level - 5 mg/dL or more, (b) cord blood hemoglobin level - 10 g/dL or less and (c) unconjugated serum bilirubin level - 10 mg/dL within 24 hours or 15 mg/dL within 48 hours of birth or rate of rise more than 0.5 mg/dL per hour
- In case of Rh isoimmunization, the best choice of blood for exchange transfusion would be "O negative packed cells suspended in AB plasma". Other options could be "O negative whole blood" or "Rh negative blood with the neonate's ABO group"
- In case of ABO isoimmunization, the choice of blood for exchange transfusion is "O group and Rh compatible with the neonate packed cells suspended in AB plasma" or "O group whole blood and Rh compatible with the neonate"
- Fresh blood collected less than 72 hours is preferred for EBT. The quantity of blood required for "Double volume EBT" is 160 to 180 mL/kg of body weight of the neonate for one exchange transfusion to replace 80–90% of fetal blood
- The blood being used for exchange transfusion of the neonates must be cross-matched with mother's blood
- Continuous cardiopulmonary monitoring, blood pressure monitoring and pulse oximetry with intensive care are important during exchange blood transfusion
- This procedure is done in NICU/SNCU with strict aseptic techniques as surgical procedures for prevention of healthcare-associated infections
- Clinical guidelines for blood transfusion or blood product administration must be maintained during exchange blood transfusion
- During EBT at least four expert team members should perform and participate in the procedure in well-equipped set up
- The EBT process is very slow and continued for an hour or more. The completion of the procedure may require over 1–4 hours.

Equipment Required

- Hand hygiene supplies and PPE (mask, cap, plastic apron, gown)
- Sterile gowns and gloves for all care providers (doctor and assistants)
- Open care system with radiant warmer, mattress, sheets to prepare the bed for the baby
- Soft restraint to immobilize the neonate during EBT and all routine baby care articles
- Cardiopulmonary and NIBP monitor and pulse oximeter
- Freshly collected cross matched blood, as appropriate for the neonates
- Blood transfusion set and tubing with multiple connecting ports and four ways stopcock
- Exchange transfusion tray with sterile articles, such as knife, scissors, IV cannula, umbilical catheter, cotton swabs, gauze pieces, sterile specimen tubes and sterile towels/drapes to prepare sterile field
- Umbilical catheterization tray with large bore catheter
- Glucometer and test strip to assess blood glucose level in between
- Heparinized saline, calcium gluconate, 10% dextrose, as required
- Emergency medications tray with syringe, needle, fluids and resuscitation articles
- Exchange transfusion recording sheet and monitoring sheet
- Sterile bottle/bag to collect to waste/discarded blood from the neonate
- Waste disposal containers as per BMW rule.

Assessment and Preparation

- Assess the neonate's history for clinical indications to detect the need of exchange blood transfusion. Check present body weight and vital signs. Assess parents level of anxiety and understanding for the procedure

- Preparation of the exchange transfusion team members should include surgical hand washing/scrubbing and wearing of sterile PPE. At least four neonatal care providers are required. Two persons for doing exchange transfusion, one person for recording and one person for continuous monitoring and emergency treatment/management, as needed
- Environment should be clean, calm, quiet, well lighted and well ventilated
- All equipment and articles should be collected and arranged near the neonate. The procedure can be done inside the unit or in the treatment/procedure room
- Preparation of parents: Explain to the parents about the need of the procedure of EBT, side effects and precautions to be taken during the procedure. Obtain informed consent from the parent for the procedure
- Preparation of neonate:
  - Ensure the neonate is NPO for 3–4 hours before procedure to prevent aspiration
  - Make the neonate warm, stable, clean, comfortable and well restrained softly
  - Verify IV sites for patency and continuation of IV fluid therapy
  - Ensure separate IV access for exchange transfusion, fluid therapy and medications
  - Obtain pre-transfusion laboratory results for blood values (bilirubin, hemoglobin, PCV, blood glucose, etc.).

Performing the Steps of Procedure with Rationale/Point of Emphasis

1. Perform meticulous hand washing as surgical procedure to reduce transmission of microorganisms and wear cap, mask, plastic apron and sterile gown.
2. Collect and arrange all necessary supplies to promote efficient time management and organized approach to the procedure in strict aseptic technique
3. Place the neonate in supine position under radiant warmer in servo mode.
4. Attach cardiopulmonary monitor, NIBP monitor and pulse oximeter.
5. Secure arms and legs of the neonate with soft restraint for the procedure of EBT to prevent contamination of sterile field and dislodgment of catheter due to movements of neonate's limbs.
6. Check blood bag by two personnel verifying neonate's identification and cross-matching.
7. Ensure blood for exchange transfusion is in normal temperature (not exceed 37°C).
8. Set up blood tubing and prime the tubing appropriately for use.
9. Assist the doctor and assistant for gowning and donning gloves. All personnel in EBT area must wear cap, mask and sterile gown.
10. Assist during skin preparation of the cannula insertion site.
11. Assist to prepare sterile field using sterile towels to minimize contamination of area.
12. Assess neonate's vital signs and check laboratory results as baseline data.
13. Measure venous pressure before and during exchange transfusion.
14. Ensure all IV cannulation/lines are patent. Usually umbilical venous catheterization is done and use for EBT. Peripheral vein or artery can also be used for EBT.
15. Check the site of maintenance IV fluid therapy and intake-output amount.
16. Assist to connect stopcock (usually two stopcock attached) to the neonate's IV access site for EBT and connect to blood bag.
17. Connect one extension tubing with port of stopcock and place its other end in blood discard bottle/bag. The waste blood container should be below table/bassinet level to allow gravity for drainage.
18. Observe the process of exchange performed by the doctor and one assistant. Help to maintain strict aseptic technique during the procedure. The process of EBT include as:
    i. Withdrawing of desired amount of blood with gentle suction from the

neonate using sterile syringe by opening stopcock and record "blood out" amount

ii. Assess vital signs closely during the procedure to determine the neonate's tolerance to the amount and rate of blood withdrawal

iii. Rotate stopcock to waste/discard tubing and expel out the blood from the syringe

iv. Rotate stopcock to blood bag tubing and fill same increment as withdrawal amount

v. Rotate stopcock to the infant's IV access and infuse the blood slowly to the neonate and record "blood in" amount

19. Repeat the steps. This pull and push method can be repeated for 30–40 cycle with same amount of withdrawn and replacement. Aliquot can be 5–10 mL during each pull and push. Even it can be 20 mL depending upon the weight of the neonate.
20. Document the amount of "blood out and blood in" during the EBT immediately and accurately. Equal amount "blood out during aspirations of aliquots" and "blood in during injections of aliquots" helps in maintaining homeostasis. This "blood out and blood in" completes one cycle of exchange process and maintain total balance.
21. Administer calcium gluconate slowly after 50 mL of exchange, or as needed to prevent tetany, if citrate phosphate dextrose (CPD) blood is used for EBT.
22. Monitor respiration, heart rate, temperature, SpO_2, CRT, blood pressure, venous pressure, blood glucose, bilirubin, hemoglobin, PCV and other required laboratory tests (calcium, bicarbonate, etc.).
23. On completion of the procedure, clamp and disconnect tubing from the catheter. Flush IV line with normal saline or reconnect to maintenance IV fluid therapy.
24. Arrange for post-procedural laboratory tests to evaluate effectiveness of EBT.
25. Dispose blood transfusion set, tubing, discarded blood and other waste as per BMW rule.
26. Take care of all reusable articles. Decontaminate, clean, dry and arrange for sterilization of reusable items.
27. Perform hand washing and document the procedure in detail.

Evaluation and Documentation

- Evaluate the infant's vital signs after EBT for every 15 minutes or earlier to detect hemodynamic instability promptly. Continue the evaluation until the neonate returns to pre-transfusion baseline vital signs. Assess parents anxiety and level of understanding to provide necessary support
- Document the following:
  - The findings of continuous monitoring during EBT for respiration, heart rate, temperature, SpO_2, CRT, blood pressure, venous pressure, blood glucose, bilirubin, hemoglobin, PCV and values of laboratory tests
  - Keep record of EBT procedure with name of the performer and assistant of EBT, time of starting and completion of EBT, and neonate's status before, during and after the process of exchange blood transfusion
  - Document about the used blood for EBT, blood bank record, type (group and Rh) of blood used, amount of blood, time and amount of "blood in" and "blood out" along with EBT record sheet and monitoring sheet.

Communication and Teaching for Homecare

- Communicate with the parents and the family members about the procedure, neonate's condition and further plan of treatment
- Teach the parents about importance of continuation of further treatment in hospital and home along with follow-up care. Instruct the parents about possible adverse events associated with EBT and delayed transfusion reaction and need for medical help.

PROCEDURE–28: CARE OF THE NEWBORN INFANTS AT TRIAGE AREA

Clinical Guidelines

- The word "*Triage*" means sorting. "*Triaging*" or rapid screening of sick neonates with immediate attention for life-threatening conditions on arrival at hospital is very important to prevent many neonatal deaths. It is found that many neonatal deaths occur even after reaching the health care facility due to procedural delays in initiating emergency treatment and management
- Emergency Triage Assessment and Treatment (ETAT) is a sequential process of managing sick neonates as soon as they arrive in the health facility. ETAT is done based on standard guidelines to reduce facility mortality rates, particularly in first 24 hours of hospitalization
- After triaging, neonates are categories into three groups, i.e., emergency cases, priority cases and nonurgent cases
- First assess every neonate for emergency signs. If emergency signs are not present, then look for priority signs. If emergency and priority signs are not found, then the neonate should be treated as nonurgent case
- *Emergency cases* include the neonates with emergency signs such as hypothermia (temperature < 35.5°C), apnea or gasping respiration, severe respiratory distress (respiratory rate >70 bpm, severe chest retractions and grunting), central cyanosis, shock (cold extremities, CRT > 3 seconds, weak and fast pulse), coma, convulsions or encephalopathy.
  Neonates with emergency signs are at high risk. They need urgent/immediate interventions and emergency measures for stabilization followed by admission in NICU/SNCU
- *Priority cases* include neonates with birth weight less than 1,800 gram, temperature between 36.4 and 35.5°C or >37.5°C, respiratory distress (with respiration rate >60 bpm but no or minimal chest retractions), refusal to feed and lethargic, irritable, restless, jitteriness, abdominal distension, severe jaundice (appear within <24 hours of age or stains palms and soles or jaundice lasts >2 weeks), severe pallor, bleeding from any site, large neonate >3,800 grams and major congenital malformations (tracheo-esophageal fistula, esophageal atresia, anorectal malformations, meningo-myelocele, etc.)
  Neonates with priority signs are sick and seriously ill. They require immediate assessment on priority basis. These neonates also required hospitalization in NICU/SNCU
- *Nonurgent cases* include neonates with physiological jaundice, transitional stool, possetting, developmental peculiarities, minor birth trauma, minor malformations, superficial infections and all cases not categorized as emergency or priority cases.
  Neonates having no signs of emergency or priority cases are considered as nonurgent cases. They should be assessed thoroughly and treatment should be planned for out-patient department (OPD) with continuation of care at home
- There should be an earmarked "Triaging Area" at the place where a sick neonate is first brought to the health facility. All equipment and supplies should be available for emergency assessment and management of the sick neonates
- All sick neonates at triage should be given attention on management of temperature, airway, breathing, circulation, coma, convulsion and dehydration (TABCD).

Equipment Required

- Hand washing supplies and handrub to prevent cross infections
- Radiant warmer, bassinet, sheets to prepare the bed to receive the neonate
- Shoulder roll to position the neonate in slightly neck extended to keep the airway open
- Suction devices to clear the secretion from the neonate's airway or mouth wipes to clean the secretions, as needed

- Pulse oximeter to monitor neonate's heart rate and SpO_2
- Neonatal resuscitation bag, mask and other articles for resuscitation efforts
- Oxygen delivery system with nasal prongs or oxygen hood
- Glucometer, test strips, other articles for blood glucose estimation
- Articles and supplies for blood sampling for necessary laboratory investigations
- Articles and supplies for intravenous cannulation and IV fluid therapy
- Fluids and medications: Adrenaline, normal saline, 10% Dextrose, 10% Calcium gluconate, Arolyte-P or Isolyte-P solution, Phenobarbitone, Vitamin K
- Baby clothing, antiseptic solutions, syringes, needles and baby care articles
- Waste disposal containers as per BMW rule
- Treatment record sheet and emergency case sheet.

Assessment and Preparation

- Assess the infant:
  - To identify emergency signs for prompt initiation of emergency treatment and to stabilize the neonate's condition at triage area
  - After stabilization, detailed history should be taken and relevant examination should be done related to the presenting problems of the neonate
  - Then relevant laboratory investigations should be arranged and list of possible diagnosis should be made. The sick neonate may present with more than one clinical problems or with provisional diagnosis requiring treatment
- Assess parents and family members level of anxiety and understanding to provide support
- Preparation of team members should be done with prompt hand hygiene. At least two healthcare providers should be present for triage management of the neonate
- Environment should be clean, well-lighted, well ventilated and free from noise and overcrowding
- All necessary articles and equipment should be kept ready always at triage area to attend any neonate with emergency conditions. Radiant warmer should be switched "ON" before receiving the neonate to make it prewarm
- Preparation of the parents and family members: Explanation should be given softly and briefly about neonate's condition, emergency treatment and further plan of management. Medico legal aspect should be considered always in the management of all neonatal conditions and problems
- Preparation of neonate: The neonate should be promptly received in triage bed along with simultaneous assessment for emergency signs remembering the principles of "TABCD"

Performing the Steps of Procedure with Rationale/Point of Emphasis

1. Perform hand hygiene quickly and switch "ON" the radiant warmer.
2. Ensure all necessary items are ready at triage bed and take help from other team member.
3. Receive the neonate on the radiant warmer bassinet from the parent/family member.
4. Position the baby using shoulder roll with neck slightly extended.
5. Assess temperature of the neonate by "touch technique" and with thermometer. If the neonate's abdomen is cold to touch, then rewarm the hypothermic neonate by setting the radiant warmer in "Manual mode". Quick rewarming should be done up to 34°C, then gradual rewarming. Baby's temperature below 35.5°C indicates emergency signs and significant hypothermia, so that should be managed quickly.
6. Ensure the baby is dry, remove wet linen and diaper quickly, if needed.
7. Maintain normal temperature of the neonate between 36.5°C and 37.5°C. Set the warmer in "Servo mode" and attach skin probe for continuous monitoring of baby's temperature.

8. Maintain clear airway by keeping the baby's neck in slightly extended sniffing position and suctioning the secretions from mouth and nose, if required.
9. Assess SpO_2 and heart rate by attaching pulse oximeter, count respiration rate and check for presence of chest retractions, grunting, central cyanosis and apnea.
10. Initiate tactile stimulation and bag-mask ventilation, if the neonate is having apnea or gasping respiration. Follow Neonatal Resuscitation Protocol to assist the baby for breathing establishment. Continue the resuscitative measures till the neonates is having spontaneous breathing and heart rate above 100 bpm.
11. Provide oxygen therapy with nasal prongs or hood, if the neonate is having respiratory distress and monitor continuously for vital signs. Maintain SpO_2 between 90 and 94%.
12. Check CRT, whether it is normal (<3 seconds) or prolonged (>3 seconds). Check periphery for presence of cold feet and palms, for weak and fast pulse and assess for tachycardia to identify neonatal shock.
13. Insert intravenous (IV) cannula and check blood glucose by Glucometer at same time.
14. Manage hypoglycemia, if present (if capillary blood glucose less than 45 mg/dL) as per Standard Treatment Protocol (STP). In symptomatic hypoglycemia, 10% dextrose 2 mL/kg body weight over 1 minute must be administered immediately. Then plan for further treatment as per protocol. Ensure the baby is warm and not hypoxic.
15. Treat neonatal shock by fluid resuscitation, with normal saline bolus of 10 mL/kg body weight over 20–30 minutes using syringe pump to restore normal tissue perfusion (i.e., less than 3 seconds). Assess for improvement in CRT, decrease of heart rate, increase of pulse volume and urine output. Repeat normal saline bolus must be given if there is partial or no improvement of tissue perfusion after first bolus. Plan for vasopressors support on admission in NICU/SNCU to manage neonatal shock, if the signs of poor perfusion persist despite two fluid boluses with normal saline.
16. Observe for seizures, level of consciousness and features of encephalopathy.
17. Assess level of consciousness/coma using simple "AVPU" scale. In this scale, "A" indicates **A**lertness, "V" indicates responding to **V**oice that means not alert but lethargic, "P" indicates responding to **P**ain but may be unconscious and "U" indicates **U**nresponsive or unconscious. A neonate in a coma scale with "P" or "U" will consider as emergency signs and receive emergency treatment.
18. Treat neonatal seizures as per STP and arrange for admission in NICU/SNCU.
19. Assess for TABCD of the neonate (temperature, airway, breathing, circulation, convulsions, and dehydration). Manage as per emergency signs with prompt treatment.
20. Assess for dehydration and its causes such as diarrhea, hyperthermia, poor feeding, etc.
21. Provide fluid therapy as per STP and maintain intake output chart.
22. Monitor the neonate's vital signs and emergency or priority signs continuously.
23. Arrange for admission in NICU/SNCU for emergency and priority cases, but continue treatment at triage bed till everything is arranged to receive the neonate in SNCU/NICU.
24. Collect blood sample and send for emergency laboratory investigations, if possible.
25. Explain to the parents and accompanying persons about the neonate's condition, necessary investigations and plan of further treatment.
26. Follow medicolegal aspect in case of very seriously ill neonates. Obtain informed signature about the neonatal condition.
27. In case of nonurgent cases, discuss with the parent and accompanying person about plan of OPD treatment and continue care at home.
28. Maintain standard infection control precautions throughout the procedure.

29. Take care of used items and dispose waste as per BMW protocol.
30. Perform hand hygiene, report the event and document in details.

Evaluation and Documentation

- Evaluate the infant's condition continuously and treat accordingly to prevent neonatal death or long-term morbidities. Evaluate parents anxiety and level of understanding to provide necessary support
- Document: Keep record of all findings of assessment on arrival at triage and subsequent assessment, such as respiration, temperature, heart rate, SpO_2, CRT, presence of emergency signs or priority signs, blood glucose level, level of consciousness, dehydration, any other abnormal clinical features and treatment given at triage bed. Document parents reactions and response.

Communication and Teaching for Homecare

- Communicate with the parents and family members about neonate's health condition, treatment given and further plan of management
- Teach the parents about participation in neonatal care, hospital protocol for admission of the neonates, mother's accommodation, importance of breast-feeding or feeding with EBM, possible course of treatment, infection control and hygienic practices, continued home care of the infant after discharge from the facility, danger signs, need for medical assistance and plan of follow-up care.

PROCEDURE–29: ROP SCREENING OF NEWBORN INFANTS

Clinical Guidelines

- Retinopathy of prematurity (ROP) is a disorder of developing retinal blood vessels of the preterm infant which may lead to poor visual acuity and blindness
- ROP screening is recommended for all infants less than 35 weeks of gestational age and/or less than 2,000 grams birth weight. Preterm infants having 35–36 weeks of gestational age and treated with oxygen or were hemodynamically unstable also required ROP screening. It is done to examine the eye to identify any sign of ROP in the infant
- Preterm infants with risk factors such as prolonged oxygen therapy, cardio-respiratory instability, repeated attack of apnea of prematurity, sepsis, history of blood transfusion, and poor weight gain in neonatal period also need ROP screening
- First ROP screening should be performed not later than 4 weeks of age or 30 days of life in infants more than 30 weeks of gestational age. If the infants gestational age is less than 30 weeks or birth weight is less than 1,200 grams, then ROP screening should be done early by 2–3 weeks of age
- If ROP is present, then subsequent treatment and follow-up depends upon the zone of ROP, stage of ROP and presence of plus disease or AP-ROP. If no sign of ROP is present, then the infant should have visual follow-up at 4 months and 9 months of age
- ROP screening, documenting the results and communicating the findings of ROP screening to parents for further interventions are important responsibilities of all neonatal care providers for preterm infants in SNCU/NICU
- ROP screening should be done by trained ophthalmologists in NICU/SNCU by indirect ophthalmoscopy following strict infection control measures
- Preparation of neonates prior to ROP screening and explanation to the parents is very important nursing interventions. Infant should be kept NPO (nothing per oral) for 2 hours. Prescribed eye drops should be administered in correct dilution.

Equipment Required

- Hand hygiene supplies for hand wash and handrub

- Eye drops: 0.5–1% tropicamide, Phenylephrine 2.5%, topical anesthetic—Proparacaine 0.5% and antibiotic eye drops, tear drops for lubrication during procedure, clean wipes or cotton swabs, normal saline
- Ophthalmoscope and condensing lenses (20D and 28D)
- Sterile cover tray with all sterile items for ROP screening such as neonatal lid speculum, scleral depressor, sterile eye swabs/wipes, sterile gauze pieces, syringes, surgical sterile gloves, sterile gowns for ophthalmologist and assistant, small cut-sheets for draping the eyes during ROP screening
- Small sheet for swaddling the infant during the procedure of ROP screening
- Sucrose 24% or breast milk for pain management
- Pulse oximeter or monitor
- Waste disposal containers as per BMW rule
- Record sheet for documentation of ROP screening result.

Assessment and Preparation

- Assess the infant's condition, vital signs and ensure the infant is stable for the procedure. Assess level of understanding and anxiety of the parents
- Self-preparation should be done by hand hygiene
- Environment should be calm, quiet, clean, well-lighted and free from noise
- All articles and supplies should be collected and arranged near the neonate
- Preparation of the parents: Explain the importance of the ROP screening. Take informed consent for the ROP screening. Answer to the questions asked by the parents
- Preparation of the infant before ROP screening:
  - Infant should be kept nothing per oral for 2 hours
  - Instillation of eye drop 0.5–1% tropicamide one drop in both eyes every 15 minutes for 3–4 times for dilating the pupils. Instill eye drop into lower conjunctival sac
  - After that, eye drop Phenylephrine 2.5% one drop should be instilled once, 10 minutes before the screening procedure
  - Next, instill topical anesthetic eye drops Proparacaine 0.5%, just prior to the procedure
  - Pain control during the procedure should be done by giving 24% sucrose 2 mL orally 2 minutes before the procedure
  - Assess vital signs of the infant for baseline data before the procedure
  - Ensure the infant is stable, warm, clean and in comfort state.

Performing the Steps of Procedure with Rationale/Point of Emphasis

1. Perform hand hygiene and arrange all articles near the ROP screening area.
2. Make sure about inform consent and counseling for the parents.
3. Ensure the infant is stable and nothing per oral for at least 1 hour.
4. Confirm about the instillation of all eye drops.
5. Check for pupillary dilatation periodically and assess vital signs.
6. Administer sucrose 24% orally 2 mL 2 minutes before the procedure.
7. Swaddle the infant with prewarm small sheet during ROP screening procedure.
8. Assist the Ophthalmologist during the ROP screening.
9. Make the infant comfortable during the procedure. Hold the baby carefully.
10. Monitor the infant's condition for cyanosis, desaturation, bradycardia and apnea. Ask to stop the procedure immediately and call neonatologist in case any of these signs present.
11. Monitor the infant's vital signs carefully at least for 2 hours.
12. Allow feeding to the infant about 30 minutes to one hour after the procedure.
13. Instill antibiotic eye drops as prescribed for 3 days post-procedure.
14. Inform the parents about the completion of procedure and findings of ROP screening.

15. Explain to the parents about repeat screening, if required and its date, time and place.
16. Take care of the used articles and the waste.
17. Perform hand hygiene and document the findings.

Evaluation and Documentation

- Evaluate the infant's condition and parent's level of understanding for the procedure
- Document the findings of the ROP screening and plan of repeat screening or laser therapy.

Communication and Teaching for Homecare

- Communicate with the mother and the family members regarding the findings of ROP screening, indications of laser therapy, if required and need for repeat screening in simple local language. Take feedback of the discussion and ensure parents have understood the information given
- Teach the parents about need and importance of ROP screening. Discuss about continuation of exclusive breastfeeding, prevention of hypothermia, appropriate care at home, follow-up visits and immunization.

PROCEDURE–30: DISCHARGE PLANNING AND CARE OF NEONATES AT HOME

Clinical Guidelines

- Normal healthy newborn infant born by spontaneous vaginal delivery should be discharged from the hospital after 48 hours of birth once all of the following criteria are fulfilled, i.e., (i) infant is free from any illness including significant jaundice, (ii) all birth/zero dose immunizations (HBV, OPV, BCG) are administered, (iii) adequacy of breastfeeding has been established (passage of urine 6–8 times in 24 hours, onset of transitional stools and baby sleeping well for 2–3 hours after breastfeeding), (iv) mother is free from any significant illness and confident to take care of the baby at home.
- Normal healthy newborn infant born by cesarean section should be discharged from the hospital on 5–7th day of birth, as per hospital policy, once all of the above four criteria are fulfilled
- Discharge of the preterm LBW infant should be planned from the neonatal care units with consideration of the following points: (a) weight gain (1–1.5% of the body weight daily) should be consistently observed for 3 consecutive days, with minimum present/current body weight more than 1,500 grams or as per hospital policy, (b) mother should be confident to feed the neonate with breastfeeding or paladai/spoon feeding with EBM and mother learned about expression of breast milk, (c) all required nutritional supplements (multivitamin drops, vitamin D, calcium, phosphorus, and iron) are already started, (d) infant is immunized with birth/zero dose of HBV, BCG and OPV, (e) mother is confident to do KMC and temperature assessment by human touch or with thermometer, and (f) all danger signs are explained to the parents and feedback is obtained from parents regarding their level of understanding
- Body weight, head circumference and length of the infant must be always recorded at the time of discharge and should be noted in the discharge certificate
- Discharge checklist should include details of the important morbidities of the infant, treatment/therapy given (duration of oxygen therapy, phototherapy, tube feeding, KMC and use of antibiotics, inotropes, anticonvulsants, etc.), reports of laboratory and other investigations, present feeding pattern at the time of discharge, anthropometric measurements, special consultation (if done any), date and time of ROP and hearing screening, nutritional counseling, immunization given, findings of neurological examination and neuroimaging done or due date.

Requirements

- Discharge summary and discharge notes in standard format or as hospital policy
- Discharge checklist as per unit and hospital policy
- Discharge certificate of the infant
- Infant's dress, towel and clothing
- Hand hygiene supplies and hand wash and handrub
- Waste disposal containers
- Discharge Register and neonate's case sheet.

Assessment and Preparation

- Assessment of the infant for presence of discharge criteria must be done by the neonatal care team before sending the infant to home. Assessment of parents understanding level for continuation of care at home should also be done before discharge
- Nursing personnel should be well prepared to explain all points regarding care of the infant and to answer all questions of the parents
- Environment should be calm, quiet and free from excessive noise
- All papers related to discharge must be ready in hand
- Parents should be informed the exact time of discharge from the hospital and to bring necessary baby care articles and to arrange transport
- Prepare the neonate with feeding, diaper changing, appropriate dressing and wrapping before sending out of the neonatal care unit and for transport.

Performing the Steps of Procedure with Rationale/Point of Emphasis

1. Ensure mother and family members are ready to take the infant to their home.
2. Arrange all documents of the infant and send for hospital clearance, as per policy.
3. On completion of official formalities, explain the discharge advice in detail as per discharge certificate including warm, feeding, medications, immunization, due dates for screening, date of follow-up visits, etc.
4. Take signature of the parents in the hospital record and in case sheet.
5. Perform hand hygiene and prepare the infant to hand over to parents. Show the baby to the parents and explain about baby's condition.
6. Inform about current body weight, feeding pattern, sleeping pattern and output pattern.
7. Explain en-route care on the way to home during transport. Precautions should be explained for maintenance of warm, feeding, hygienic care and danger signs.
8. Instruct the mother and accompanying family members to carry the infant during transport in kangaroo position.
9. Ensure mother is confident for en-route care and home care. Explain all information further, if needed and take feedback.
10. Encourage the family members to support the mother during care of infant at home.
11. Arrange for terminal disinfection of bassinet, mattress, radiant warmer and all other care articles used for the infant.
12. Send infant's document to the record section for preservation and preserve unit record.
13. Perform hand hygiene and document the discharge procedure in hospital record.

Evaluation and Documentation

- Evaluate: Parents level of understanding about the information and teaching given
- Document: Date and time of discharge and details of discharge summary (as per standard discharge card) including relevant investigations, treatment given, course of treatment, condition of infant on discharge, final diagnosis, treatment advised on discharge for continuation of homecare and immunization given to the infant

Communication and Teaching for Homecare

- Communicate with the mother and the family members about condition of the infant on discharge, treatment to be continued, danger signs, and need of medical assistance, screening and follow-up visits. Inform about consultation with ASHA, ANM and CHO

- *Teach the parents* and explain the discharge advice in details as follows:
  - *Care at home:* Explain about exclusive breastfeeding, burping after breastfeed or paladai feeds, maintenance of warmth, hygienic measures and cleanliness, continuation of medications, bathing with lukewarm water (after umbilical cord is fallen off and birth weight is more than 2,500 grams), keeping the cord open and dry till fallen off and nothing to apply on umbilical cord, keeping the infant away from sick person and overcrowding, identifying danger signs and arrangement of neonatal screening, immunization, routine visit at Well Baby Clinic and follow-up visits. Teach about harmful traditional practices such as application of kajal in eyes, oil in nostrils and cow dung on the umbilical cord to prevent infections. Answer to the questions asked by the parents and family members
  - *Danger signs:* Explain the danger signs such as infant is cold or hot to touch, having poor feeding or refusal to feed, undue lethargic, breathing difficulty (fast breathing, chest indrawing, abnormal sound in respiration and cyanosis), convulsions or abnormal movements, excessive crying and irritability, abnormal color, bleeding from any site, abdominal distension, excessive vomiting, watery loose motion/diarrhea and superficial infections such as umbilical sepsis, skin pustules, oral thrush and conjunctivitis
  - *ROP screening* for preterm, LBW and sick neonates should be explained in detail, as per recommendation. Due date, time and place of screening must be informed
  - *Hearing screening:* Discuss about the importance and indications of hearing screening in children, especially for the preterm, LBW and sick infants.

    Early hearing test is recommended to detect congenital sensorineural deafness or severe-to-profound hearing impairment. Hearing screening helps to prevent delayed development of speech, language, and cognitive skills which may result in slow learning and difficulty in school progress.

    It is indicated in infants having prolonged ventilation more than 5 days, meningitis, severe jaundice treated with exchange blood transfusion, use of ototoxic medications (Gentamicin, Tobramycin) or diuretics, intrauterine infections (CMV, rubella, toxoplasmosis), craniofacial abnormalities and family history of childhood hearing loss.

    Hearing screening is performed using otoacoustic emissions (OAE) test or by automated Brainstem Evoked Response Audiometry (BERA), depending upon the infant's high risk conditions and problems.

    First hearing screening is recommended after 34 weeks of post-menstrual age, before discharge from hospital and before 40 weeks of corrected age. Next evaluation should be done, if first screening is abnormal, at 4–6 weeks of corrected age. Next evaluation to be done, if second screening is abnormal, before 6 months of age
  - *Developmental supportive care and early interventions with stimulations* those initiated at neonatal units should be continued at home to promote optimal neurodevelopmental outcome and to prevent developmental delay
  - *Immunizations* essential for the infant must be described as follows:
    - » It should be done as per National Immunization Schedule
    - » It can be administered at immunization clinic of subcenter, PHC, Rural hospital and at Well Baby Clinic in any hospital or from private practitioners
    - » Birth dose HBV, OPV and BCG are given before discharge in institutional delivery

- » At 6 weeks of age of the infant, recommended vaccinations include OPV, IPV, Pentavalent, PCV and Rotavirus
- » At 10 weeks of age, recommended vaccinations are OPV, Pentavalent and Rotavirus
- » At 14 weeks of age of the infant, recommended vaccinations include OPV, IPV, Pentavalent, PCV and Rotavirus
- » At 9 months of age of infants, recommended vaccinations are PCV, MR and JE
- » At 18 months of age of the child, recommended vaccinations include OPV, MR, JE and DPT
- » Explain about the immunization card, its importance, and preservation. Inform about the next due date, time and place of immunization

- *Follow-up care* for preterm, LBW and sick neonates: Inform the parents and family members about next date, time, place and schedule of follow-up visits
  - » Initially, follow-up visit is planned within 1 week of discharge from hospital. Then, follow-up visit should be done at 2 weeks interval depending upon the infant's condition and care at home. Thereafter, visits on immunization dates or at 1 month interval should be planned
  - » Visits on 3 months, 6 months, 9 months and 12 months of age are very important. Follow-up visits for high risk infant should be continued by yearly review till the child enters into school age or admit in the school
  - » Explain about the importance and continuation of follow-up care, as directed by the doctors, nurses and other team members of the follow-up clinic for the optimum growth and development of the children.

UNIT 3

Child Health Nursing Procedures for Medical Conditions

INTRODUCTION

Children are commonly hospitalized due to various medical conditions such as pneumonia and other respiratory problems, diarrheal diseases, urinary problems, blood disorders, malignant conditions, and accidental injury. Childhood diseases are not same as adult disease conditions. Pathophysiology may vary in some situations.

Nursing interventions related to medical conditions of childhood illness include basic nursing procedures, hygiene care, feeding, medications, diagnostic procedures, and therapeutic management such as oxygen therapy, fluid therapy, blood product transfusion, etc.

Care approach to the children should be different than that of adult. Young children are unable to express their problems and emotionally become more upset easily. Age-appropriate variations of level of understanding and unexpected strange situations of healthcare institutions may make the children more noncooperative and apprehensive. Individualized problem-oriented care approach should be followed for expected and optimal recovery of the sick children.

All children require comprehensive health care with prevention of health problems, health promotion, curative management of disease conditions, and rehabilitation in the family or community in case long-term sufferings with diseases or disabilities. Holistic care is essential for all children in health and illness for maintenance of physical, mental, and social well being.

PROCEDURE–1: ADMISSION OF THE CHILD IN HOSPITALS/HEALTH CARE INSTITUTIONS

Clinical Guidelines

- Hospitalization of sick children is necessary for prompt recovery from the disease conditions and for prevention of complications.
- Principles of family-centered care should be followed by all healthcare providers during the admission process and throughout the course of the child's hospitalization.
- Admission of the children in health care facilities/institutions is allowed for the purpose of observation, investigations, treatment, and for specialized skilled nursing care depending upon the sick child's clinical conditions.
- Hospital admission may be emergency or planned. Emergency hospitalization of children may require in case of any acute illness due to medical or surgical conditions, accidental injury, burns, poisoning, etc. Planned hospital admission is usually permitted in case of chronic medical and surgical illnesses of the child for therapeutic purposes or for diagnostic procedure.
- Planned admission procedure can be done systematically in sequence of required activities, but emergency admission procedure should be performed based on child's life-threatening emergency conditions or priority problems. Lengthy admission procedure may be

inappropriate, if the child's health status appears to be deteriorating rapidly.

- Each child must wear an identification band throughout the length of hospitalization. If it is not possible to place the identification band on the child's extremity, then other arrangements must be made to identify the child at all times (e.g., identification band or tag fixed on the isolette or bassinet or crib or bed).
- Children should be assigned to rooms based on gender, developmental age, diagnosis, and seriousness of the condition, communicability of illness, and projected length of hospital stay. Children are assigned a bed, crib, isolette, warmer-bassinet appropriate for their chronological age, developmental age, and/or clinical condition.
- All personal history and assessment data collected during admission process become permanent part of child's medical record.
- Stress and anxiety of the child and his or her parents/family members should be managed carefully from the time of admission in healthcare facility and also during hospital stay. Everyone's concern should be taken care for better cooperation.
- Incidental or planned health teaching should be given for optimal health outcome of the child, whenever possible to the hospitalized child with age-appropriate discussion and also to the parents and family members according to their level of understanding.

Equipment Required

For the Assigned Room and Personal Care of the Child

- Bed, crib, isolette, warmer-bassinet to provide rest and sleep to the child
- Bed linens, blanket, pillow, bath towels, washcloths, dress materials, diapers as needed
- Toiletry items, e.g., soap, body lotion, comb, toothbrush, toothpaste
- Hand washing facilities and hand rub or sanitizers
- Water pitcher, drinking glass, spoon, feeding utensils (child may wish to use own items)
- Wash basin, waste disposal containers, bedpan, urinal and weighing scale to take weight of the diaper, as required.

For Admission Process of the Child

- Hand hygiene supplies for hand wash and hand rub
- Identification band for the child, as per hospital policy or as appropriate
- Thermometer, cotton swab in a container, and 70% alcohol to clean the thermometer before measuring baby's body temperature
- Sphygmomanometer and blood pressure (BP) cuff of appropriate size for the child
- Stethoscope for auscultation of heart and lung sounds
- Pulse oximeter to assess oxygen saturation and heart rate
- Weighing scale for child 2 years of age or younger in lying position
- Standing weighing scale for older children
- Measuring tape to assess head, chest, abdomen, and mid-upper arm circumference (MUAC) and to measure recumbent length of child younger than 2 years
- Stadiometer, if available, to measure standing height of the older children. Ordinary tape measure can be used to assess standing height of the older children
- Child and family orientation brochures and identity/visitor card, as per hospital policy
- Waste disposal containers as per Biomedical Waste Management (BMW) guidelines
- Child's admission documentation forms, child's case sheet and treatment sheet.

Assessment and Preparation

- Assess the child for indication of admission in hospital. Assess the ability of the child and family members to cope the situation to plan to provide necessary support

- Self preparation should be done with practice of standard precautions to prevent transmission of microorganisms
- Environment should be clean, well-lighted, well-ventilated, and free of overcrowding
- Articles and necessary equipment should be collected and arranged for easy accessibility
- Preparation of parent and family members: Explain the need for admission and its procedure and plan of management. Allow parent to remain with the child and to take part in routine care. Answer to their questions as asked. Obtain informed written consent form for hospitalization signed from the parent or legal guardian. Explain the hospital routines, rules and regulations those need to be followed
- Preparation of child: Explain the importance and procedure of hospitalization in age-appropriate simple language. Make the child comfortable. Provide friendly and gentle approach to get cooperation. Encourage to ask questions to the older children and answer in simple age-appropriate language.

Performing the Steps of Procedure with Rationale/Point of Emphasis

Preparing the Environment for Admission of a Child in Healthcare Facility

1. Perform hand hygiene to reduce the incidence of healthcare-associated infections (HCAIs).
2. Obtain all necessary articles, special equipment, and furniture for the child. It promotes comfort for the child and family members by ensuring that required items for personal care of the child are readily available.
3. Check all equipment, lights, fan/AC, bed controls for good working order to prevent delay in admission and treatment process.
4. Inform and prepare other patients and family members about arrival of new patient/child.
5. Prepare admission bed for the child with sheets and blanket. Adjust the bed to lowest horizontal position and brakes locked. Ensure all side rails of the bed, crib, or bassinet latch in all positions to prevent accidental fall and injury. Lower height of bed makes it easier and safer for child to get in and out of bed. Brakes should be in locked position to prevent hazardous movement of the bed or crib or bassinet.
6. Ensure everything is ready to receive the child in admission bed and for prompt initiation of need-based problem-oriented treatment.

Assessing the Child on Admission

1. Greet the child by name and the family member. Introduce yourself to promote friendly welcome. Anticipate questions and anxiety level to provide support as required
2. Escort the child and parent/family member to the child's room and bed. Introduce them with other patients of that room
3. Assist the older child to sit or lie down in the bed or crib. Allow the family members to stay with the child. Allow the child to sit on parent's lap during assessment, if feasible, or in the bed or in the crib. Make sure side rails are up for safety. Note the child's condition on admission when receiving at bed
4. Apply identification band or tag to the child and to parents (if applicable)
5. Determine reliable person who will be able to provide necessary information related to child's past medical history or complete history of the events that led to child's admission. Person accompanying the child may not know details history of child's illness
6. Collect detailed history of illness and related information for hospitalization as per standard format of the health facility
7. Ascertain the history of previous hospitalization of the child. Determine child's perception and temperament in relation to

previous experiences with hospitalization and healthcare personnel. This helps to consider appropriate and individualized approach to nursing care and treatment for the hospitalized child
8. Perform hand hygiene before physical assessment of the child
9. Assess vital signs including respiration, heart rate, temperature, BP, oxygen saturation by pulse oximetry, and pain level. This provide baseline parameters to compare with future monitoring findings
10. Assess the signs and symptoms of illness, present on admission in the hospital
11. Obtain the following information, as child's health condition permits:
    - Body weight measurement is essential for calculating medication dosage for the child
    - Length or height measurement is required for calculation of body surface area and body mass index (BMI)
    - Head circumference measurement helps to detect cranial problems and abnormalities
    - Mid upper arm circumference is important to identify level and grade of malnutrition
    - Abdominal girth measurement is needed to identify abdominal distention
12. Examine the child from head to toe for presence of abnormal clinical features
13. Record history of child's health and illness and all examination findings as baseline data
14. Discuss health care topics with the child and family members related to the participatory care that are relevant to the age and development of the child
15. Involve the parent/family member during routine care of the child and allow the child as per his or her own ability to perform self care
16. Ensure and validate the mechanism to contact family members when they are not present in the hospital with the child
17. Notify the attending physician or healthcare prescriber of the child about the admission and arrival of the child at the unit. Inform the presence of any emergency or unusual findings of the child immediately
18. Obtain treatment order on admission from the physician/healthcare prescriber.
19. Initiate prescribed treatment/management of the child promptly avoiding any delay
20. Discard the waste generated during the admission procedure as per BMW rules
21. Take care of reusable items by decontamination, cleaning, and disinfection or sterilization. Perform hand hygiene
22. Document the child's admission in hospital record system and register.

Orienting the Child and Family Members to the Hospital Unit/Ward

1. Orient the child (if condition permits), and family members to the physical setup of the unit (source of drinking water, wash basin, toilet, urinal).
2. Demonstrate the use of lights, bedside table, bed control, side rails and bathroom facility.
3. Explain unit/ward routine, meal schedule, hand washing guidelines, waste disposal and other hygienic practices, visiting rules, available services in the health facility, support systems, smoking policy, play facilities, and communication pattern.
4. Encourage parents/family members to notify the staff for their needs and problems.
5. Inform the parent and child about healthcare providers and attending physician who will meet and see the child during hospitalization. This will prevent family's confusion.
6. Determine whether or not family has brought any medications, supplies or devices from home for child's use. Discuss with physician, if any of these can be used. Otherwise send them back to home with the family. This prevents child's property from getting lost.
7. Label the child's personal devices with child's name and medical record number

8. Answer to the questions asked by parents or family members to clarify their doubts.
9. Discuss about the financial aspects and expenditure for child's hospitalization, as per institutional policy especially in private sectors.

Securing the Valuable Items of the Child

1. Place child's clothes and toiletries in assigned locker or closet. This prevents child's clothing and other care items from getting mixed with others.
2. Encourage child's family to take all valuables, costly items, and money to their home, whenever possible. If family member is unavailable to take the valuable items to home, then list all items and preserve safely in presence of another employee and keep record.
3. Obtain parent's or family member's signature when handing over and returning the valuable items. Keep one copy of receipt as hospital document.
4. Allow personal dolls, toys, story books, musical tapes, and play materials to help the child to cope in the hospital environment.

Special Points to Remember for Newly Hospitalized Child

- Follow evidence-based scientific principles of therapeutic and nursing interventions for the disease process of the sick child
- Provide individualized need-based support to the child and family members to reduce stress and anxiety in friendly approach along with family involvement
- Make the child and family member comfortable. Ensure for best treatment and care
- Attempt to gain confidence of the child and parents during the period of hospital stay
- Hospitalization of the child is the break in the unity of the family. So, emotional support should be considered first for the child and family, then management of the physical problems should be provided to the sick child
- Special approach must be followed for terminally ill or dying children and their family.

Evaluation and Documentation

- Evaluate child's and family's understanding of admission process and orientation to the unit. Determine the area of concern of the family and the child to plan for necessary support accordingly
- Document the admission process in hospital record and assessment data in child case sheet including history of illness, examination findings and investigation reports, if any.

Communication and Teaching for Homecare

- Communicate with child and parents about the child's health status, plan of management, discharge planning, financial aspects, importance of family participation and about hospital rules and regulations
- Teach the child (as appropriate) and parents about the followings:
  - Rest, sleep, activity limitation, dietary restrictions, personal hygiene including hand wash
  - Environmental hygiene and cleanliness with appropriate waste disposal
  - Emergency conditions or danger signs requiring immediate medical attention
  - Use of medications, adverse effects of drugs and necessary precautions
  - Use of recreational and diversional measures for the child to cope with hospitalization
  - Care at home after discharge from hospital for continuation of treatment
  - Plan for follow-up visits, its date, time and place
  - Need for contact with community healthcare workers (ASHA, ANM, CHO), if needed
  - Importance of regular health check up and practice of health promotion activities.

PROCEDURE-2: ASSESSMENT OF VITAL SIGNS OF INFANTS/OLDER CHILDREN

Clinical Guidelines

- Vital signs are physical signs concerning functions essentials to life and include respiratory rate, heart rate, body temperature, and BP. Alteration of these signs helps to detect abnormal physiological functioning of the body system. Vital signs are objectively measurable and verifiable
- Some healthcare professionals consider patient's level of pain to be a "fifth" vital sign, although this is not accepted by all. While all healthcare professionals agree that experience of pain by the individual is a critical feature of his or her adaptation to illness. Level of pain is considered as subjective
- Other important signs of illness, such as SpO_2, CRT, skin color, activity pattern and level of consciousness, should be assessed to identify the health status of the child and to diagnosis the disease process
- Various electronic automated devices are available to measure heart rate, SpO_2, respiration, temperature, and BP including ECG (e.g., pulse oximeter, BP monitor, multiparameter monitor, cardiorespiratory monitor, etc).
  Manufacturers' instructions must be followed to use all these devices. Comparison should always be done between electronic devices findings with routine examination findings by healthcare providers
- Purposes of vital signs measurement include to assess general health status of the child, to assist in diagnosis of illness and to observe the therapeutic effects of medications or medical interventions or surgical procedures
- Vital signs should be measured to assess the baseline health condition of the child on admission at triage bed or after receiving in the assigned bed inside the unit. In case of critically ill child, reassess vital signs at every 30 minutes interval till the child's condition is stabilized. Routine assessment of vital signs should be done at 4–6 hours intervals are as per unit policy. In emergency conditions, assess vital signs promptly
- BP is measured in neonates if clinical signs of hypotension are present or in case of renal disease or in congenital heart disease such as coarctation of aorta is suspected. Universal screening of neonates is not recommended
  BP should be measured in a child younger than 3 years of age with history of neonatal condition requiring intensive care, symptoms of hypertension or hypotension, elevated intracranial pressure, recurrent urinary tract infections, renal or cardiac disease, in case of malignancy or transplant (solid, bone marrow), and treatment with medications known side effects to affect BP. When child older than 3 years of age is seen in medical setting BP should be measured. A decrease in BP is a late sign of shock in children.
- Use of mercury thermometer and mercury BP instrument to assess body temperature and BP is not recommended at present to prevent mercury hazards.
- Standard precautions of infection control measures should be followed to prevent cross infections during the procedure.
- Recording and reporting of vital parameters should be done promptly and accurately as it is one of the most important legal documents regarding the improvement and deterioration of the health condition of the sick hospitalized child.

Equipment Required

- Hand hygiene supplies for hand wash and hand rub
- A clean tray containing digital thermometer, pediatric stethoscope, pediatric size sphygmomanometer (aneroid) with appropriate size BP cuff, a bowl with dry cotton swabs, a bottle of 70% alcohol or alcohol wipes (if available)
- Watch or clock with second hand or digital readout to count respiration and heart rate

- Electronic automated devices (pulse oximeter, multiparameter monitor, BP monitor), if available and as per child's condition
- Chart having normal ranges of age-appropriate vital signs of the children
- Waste disposal containers as per BMW rules
- Vital signs documentation sheet/monitoring chart and child's case sheet.

Assessment and Preparation

- Assess the associated factors and signs of alteration of vital signs (e.g., tachypnea, bradypnea, tachycardia, bradycardia, hypothermia, hyperthermia/fever, hypotension, hypertension and other abnormalities). Review the child's record for medical diagnosis, history of illness, and current medications used. Assess the child and family members for anxiety, level of understanding, and ability to participate during the procedure
- Self-preparation: Review the age-appropriate range of vital signs of children, those should be readily available in hand during the procedure for quick reference
- Environment clean, calm, quiet, well lighted, free from noises and overcrowding
- All necessary articles and items should be collected and arranged near the child's bed
- Preparation of parents: Explain the steps of the procedure and equipment to be used for the procedure briefly. Discuss about importance of vital signs measurement of the child
- Preparation of child:
  - Explain the procedure to the child, if condition allows, in age-appropriate language
  - Allow the child to handle the equipment, if he or she is able to do that
  - Review child's medical record for previous vital signs, when available to get the baseline data for comparison. Check record for desired parameters
  - Note the child's medical diagnosis and history of respiratory problems, cardiac problems, infections or any other disease conditions or difficulties which may alter the vital signs
  - Make the child clean, comfortable, calm and quiet in supine position, whenever possible.

Performing the Steps of Procedure with Rationale/Point of Emphasis

Assessing Respiratory Rate

1. Perform hand hygiene and assemble all necessary items near the child bed.
2. Determine whether child is taking any medications that may affect respiratory rate and depth, e.g., salicylates can increase rate and depth of respiration.
3. Assess the child's respiratory rate first, before disturbing the child for other procedures that may affect the respiratory rate. Count respiration when the child is calm and quiet. Don't touch the infant and young child before counting respiration, if possible, because touch can stimulate the child and alter respiratory rate.
4. Count rate and rhythm of respirations of the child:
   i. Observe the abdomen for movement during respiration in infant and young child. As young children are primarily diaphragmatic breathers
   ii. Observe thoracic movements in older child. As older children depend more on their intercostal muscles for respiratory activity
   iii. Count respirations in infant for 1 minute. Infants are episodic breathers, it is normal for them to vary their respiratory rate and pattern. So count for full 1 minute to obtain more accurate measure of respiration
   iv. If respirations are irregular in older children, then count the number of respirations for one full minute
   v. If the older child is having regular respirations, then count respirations for 30 seconds and multiply by two (2) to get breathing rate per minute.
5. Note depth and pattern of respirations and presence of chest retractions, abnormal

sounds in respirations, grunting, nasal flaring, cyanosis (central or peripheral), pallor, restlessness, anxiety, fussiness, irritability, level of activity and position of comfort (e.g., sitting up or leaning forward)

- This helps to identify respiratory distress and signs of hypoxia. If respiratory distress is noted, then immediately auscultate breath sounds and report to appropriate healthcare professional/physician for prompt initiation medical management. Immediate medical attention is required to evaluate possible causes of respiratory distress and to prevent respiratory failure.

6. Make the child comfortable. Perform hand hygiene.
7. Communicate with team members about the abnormal respiration immediately.
8. Record respiratory rate in breaths per minute and all other observational findings.

Measuring Apical Heart Rate by Auscultation and Measuring Peripheral Pulse by Palpation

1. Determine the site for counting apical heart rate and peripheral pulse.
2. Ensure the child is not crying, not agitating and having no pain and anxiety. These conditions usually increase the heart rate. A quiet, cooperative or sleeping child will contribute to more success when auscultating the heart rate. Noisy respirations, crying infant and environmental noises detract from the ability to detect heart sounds and possible murmurs or presence of any other abnormalities.
3. Perform hand hygiene to prevent transmission of microorganisms.
4. Cleanse the stethoscope chest piece and ear pieces with alcohol wipes/swabs before and after examination to prevent cross infections. Discard the used alcohol swab/wipes in the waste disposal container
5. Insert ear pieces with tips bent forward toward face, considering normal anatomy of ear
6. Palpate the chest wall and identify the site of auscultation at point of maximal impulse:
   i. In children younger than 7 years age, auscult heart rate at just left of the midclavicular line and in fourth intercostal space
   ii. In children older than 7 years of age, auscult heart rate at left midclavicular line and in fifth intercostal space.
7. Warm the chest piece of the stethoscope by rubbing it in your palm. Cold stethoscope can cause discomfort or startle the child
8. Place diaphragm of stethoscope over the point of maximal impulse and count heart rate. Counting for full 1 minute gives more accurate heart rate, particularly when sinus arrhythmia or other irregularity is present. Always count heart rate for full 1 minute, if the heart rate is irregular. If the child is having regular heart rate, then count for 30 seconds and multiply by two (2) to get heart rate beats per minute.
9. Note rhythm and quality of heart sound of the child.
10. Report the presence of murmur or any other abnormality to the physician. Murmurs are not uncommon in infants, but must be evaluated for potential pathology.
11. Measure peripheral pulse by palpation as follows **(Fig. 3.1)**:
    i. Identify the site; radial and brachial pulses are most frequently used for easy accessibility in upper limbs. The dorsalis pedis pulse can be palpable on the dorsum of the foot or posterior tibial pulse can be felt in lower extremities
    ii. Locate the child's pulse and palpate with your first two or three fingers. Do not use excessive pressure, it may occlude the pulsation. Don't use thumb to check pulse because the thumb has

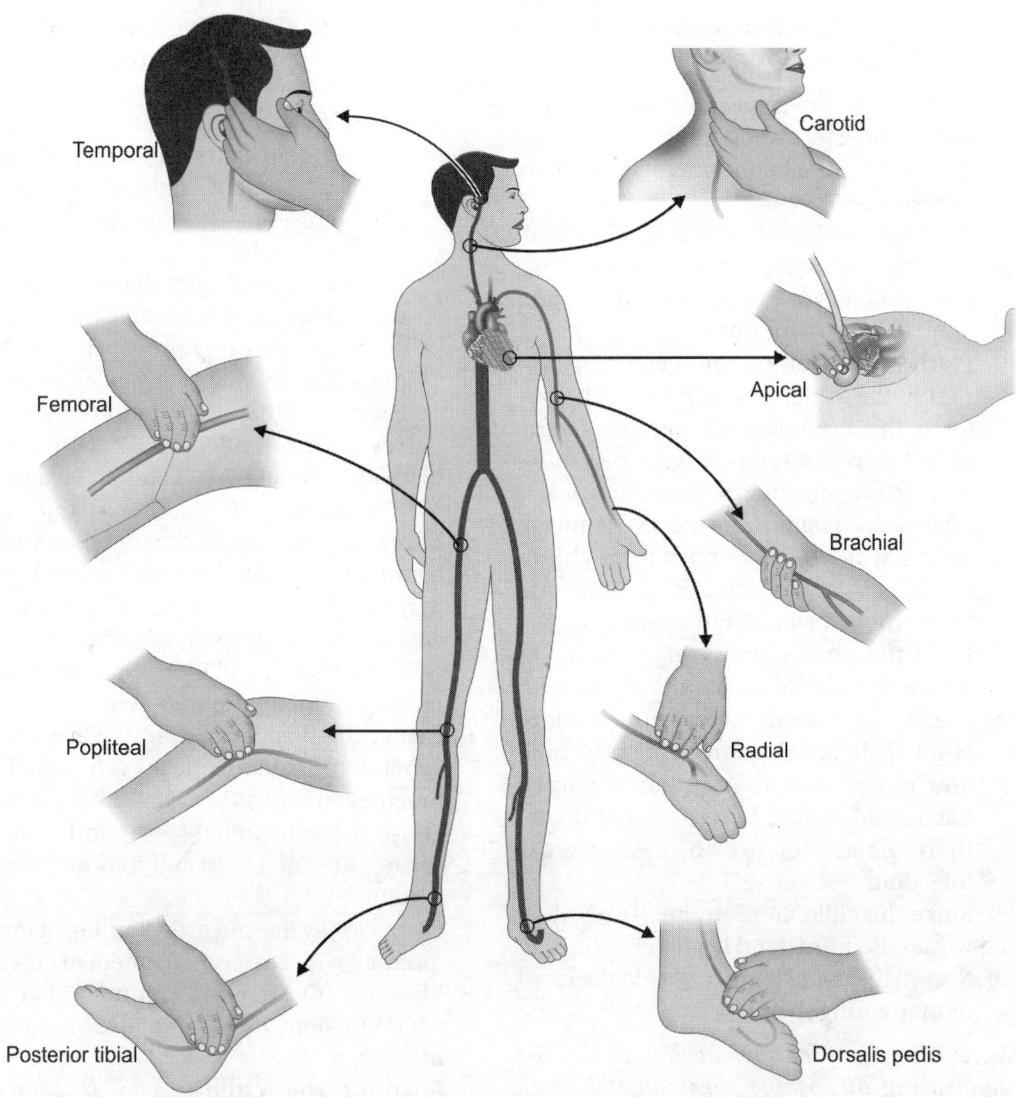

Fig. 3.1: Different sites of assessment of pulse of older children.

a pulse and may be confused with the child's pulse

iii. Note rhythm of pulse. If the pulse is irregular, then count for full 1 minute. If the child is having regular pulse, then count for 30 seconds and multiply by two (2) to get pulse beats per minute

iv. Check and count peripheral pulse in all four limbs, whenever indicated.

12. Compare heart rate and pulse rate. Find any difference in pulse rate in limbs.
13. Compare the heart rate with the display of it in the monitor or pulse oximeter.
14. Perform hand hygiene to reduce transmission of microorganisms.
15. Record heart rate, pulse rate, and other abnormal findings. Note the site used to obtain heart rate and pulse rate and child's present activity level (e.g., asleep, quiet, crying, fussing, restlessness). Documentation of assessment findings in child's record provides basis for comparison and considers as part of legal record. Report the abnormal findings.

Measuring Axillary Temperature using Digital Thermometer

1. Perform hand hygiene and make the child comfortable for temperature assessment.
2. Take out the digital thermometer from its container.
3. Wipe the thermometer with alcohol swab from bulb to stem in circular motion.
4. Dry the child's one axillae with dry cotton swab to remove moisture.
5. Place the tip of the thermometer at apex or roof of the axillae and support with arm. Keep the thermometer parallel to the child's arm and hold close to the child's body to keep the thermometer in place.
6. Wait for beep sound from the thermometer. Take out the thermometer from child's axillae gently to note the temperature and to interpret the temperature reading.
7. Read the child's body temperature to record it in the child's monitoring sheet.
8. Clean the thermometer with alcohol swab again after use from stem to bulb and preserve in the container gently. Each child should have personal digital thermometer for use to prevent cross infections.
9. Make the child comfortable. Discard all wastes. Perform hand hygiene.
10. Record the noted temperature in the chart or monitoring sheet.

Note: Temperature measurement can be done using disposable thermometer (e.g., chemical dot thermometer), as per availability. Electronic thermometer can be used to measure oral or rectal or tympanic temperature, whenever indicated in some special childhood conditions. Use of electronic devices should be done as per manufacturer's guidelines following basic anatomy of the body parts and contraindications for use of the devices.

Measuring Blood Pressure (BP) by Auscultation Method

1. Review child's previous BP readings, if available.
2. Analyze child's clinical diagnosis and current medications that can affect on BP.
3. Perform hand hygiene. Clean the diaphragm of stethoscope with alcohol wipes
4. Select the site of BP measurement. Use right arm whenever possible
   - Use same site and position of previous BP measurement, if already taken. If child refuses to use same site, then use another extremity
   - Do not use extremity that has injury, wound or foreign devices (e.g., IV cannula, arteriovenous fistula or renal dialysis shunt) or having altered circulation (e.g., Coarctation).
5. Select appropriate size BP cuff. The bladder width of BP cuff should be about 40% of the arm circumference midway between the olecranon (elbow) and the acromion (shoulder). Using too small cuff may falsely elevate the BP measurement and too large cuff may give falsely low reading. Use manufacturer's guidelines on the cuff for appropriate selection
6. Center the bladder of the BP cuff on the extremity proximal to the pulse (e.g., at the brachial site, position about 1–2 inches above the antecubital fossa) and snugly secure the cuff. Loose cuff may give false reading
7. Do not apply the cuff over clothing. It may interfere with correct placement of cuff
8. Measure BP after 3–5 minutes of rest, when possible, to prevent false elevation of BP
9. Position the child's arm (selected extremity) at heart level to get accurate reading
10. Locate the pulse at the site. Place the bell of the stethoscope where the pulse is felt, below the bottom edge of the cuff
11. Close the sphygmomanometer valve and inflate the BP cuff to a pressure above the point at which artery pulsation is obliterated. Stabilize the extremity during BP measurement. Movement may cause extra sounds and interfere with ability to hear pulsations
12. Deflate the BP cuff at a rate of 2–3 mm Hg per second to ensure accurate measurement

13. Note Korotkoff sounds, beginning with onset of tapping sound. This correlates with phase I, which represents systolic pressure
14. Note muffling of the sound, if applicable. This represents phase IV and may occur more commonly in preadolescents
15. Note disappearance of sound. Silence correlates with phase V, which corresponds with diastolic pressure
16. Do not reinflate BP cuff during deflation. If it is necessary to repeat BP measurement, then allow few minutes in between another measurements
17. Fully deflate the BP cuff on completion of measurement and remove the cuff from arm
18. Make the child comfortable. Remove the instrument. Take care of all articles used
19. Perform hand hygiene. Record and inform the BP findings, extremity used and cuff size
20. Interpret the BP as high or low. Compare with previous BP findings, if taken already and with the BP value measured by the automated device method.

Evaluation and Documentation

- Evaluate the findings of child's vital signs (respiration, heart rate, body temperature, and BP) measurement for presence of any abnormalities and compare with previous findings, if already assessed
- Document the findings of vital signs assessment with date and time. Keep record of the presence of abnormal clinical features and child's response. Record about the sites of measurements and equipment used.

Communication and Teaching for Homecare

- Communicate with child and parents about the health status of the child, plan of management, tentative duration of hospital stay and anticipated prognosis of illness
- Teach the parents about use of thermometer, counting of respiration, recognition of abnormal vital signs (e.g., respiratory distress, fever) and need for contact of the healthcare provider for medical help. Instruct about participation in routine care of the child in hospital and continued care at home after discharge. Discuss about use of medications with necessary precautions and plan of follow-up care.

PROCEDURE–3: ANTHROPOMETRY OR ASSESSMENT OF GROWTH PARAMETERS OF CHILDREN

Clinical Guidelines

- Anthropometry is the science of measuring the human body. Usually body weight, length or height and head circumference are measured to assess the physical growth of the children and to detect any abnormal deviations as failure to thrive or growth retardation. Chest circumference and MUAC measurements also help in detection of abnormal growth and nutritional status of the children
- Growth parameters assessments are obtained at each visit to the healthcare facilities or at each home visit by the healthcare provider to detect growth failure. It is essential for all children on admission to healthcare institutions, as baseline data for planning of treatment
- Daily weight recording at same time, ideally in the morning before breakfast, using same weighing machine of hospitalized children is essential and important for calculation of IV fluid therapy and dose of medications. It should be measured in all hospitalized children, especially for children with abnormal cardiac and renal functions with evidence of accumulation of fluid as edema, fluid and electrolyte imbalances, excessive loss of body fluids in diseases conditions and to assess nutritional status
- Recumbent length is measured usually up to 2 years of age of the child in lying down position using infantometer or simple tape measure. After 2 years of age, standing height is measured using

stadiometer, a measuring device affixed to a wall or height assessment rod attached to weighing scale or electronic length/ height measurement device or wall tape measure (prepared by using ordinary tape measure on a wall).
  - Length or height is an important growth parameter. Measurement of this parameter is essential to detect stunting (low height for age) and wasting (low weight for height). It is also required to calculate BMI, which indicates and helps to estimate obesity, overweight or underweight. BMI is calculated by dividing body weight in kilograms by height in meter squared.
- Head circumference is related to brain growth and development of intracranial volume in children. Head circumference measurement helps to detect abnormal increase in size and shape of the child (e.g., hydrocephalus, microcephaly, oxycephaly, etc.). It is measured as occipitofrontal circumference (OFC) over the most prominent points of head
- Chest circumference and MUAC measurements help to assess growth and nutritional status of the children. Abnormal shape of chest in children is found in malnutrition, rickets and congenital heart diseases. Measurement of MUAC is required to identify severe acute malnutrition (SAM) among children, which is a significant contributing factor of childhood illnesses and deaths.
- Assessment of growth parameter can be done on child's bed or in the procedure room in presence of the parent for safety and privacy of the child and to gain their cooperation.

Equipment Required

- Hand hygiene supplies for hand washing and hand rubbing to prevent cross infections
- Weighing scale (as appropriate): Lying-in weighing scale for younger child (infant/ toddler) or stand-up scale for older child or bed scale for bed ridden child
- Measuring tape or infantometer for assessment of recumbent length for younger child and Stadiometer or measuring tape for assessment of standing height of the older child
- Drapes or sheet or paper to place on weighing scale pan/tray and on infantometer
- Disinfectant solution for cleaning the weighing scale tray/pan
- A bottle of 70% alcohol and cotton swabs in a container to clean the tape measure, if used
- Standard Growth Chart to identify normal or abnormality of growth parameters
- Calculator to assess BMI of the child
- Waste disposal containers as per BMW rules
- Documentation sheet or child's case sheet.

Assessment and Preparation

- Assess child's previous growth pattern and most recent findings of weight, length/height, head circumference, chest circumference, and MUAC. Assess child's and family members understanding level about the importance of assessment of growth parameters
- Self preparation: Follow standard precautions of infection control and gentle approach
- Environment should be warm, clean, well ventilated and well lighted
- Articles preparation: All necessary articles and equipment should be arranged near the child at bedside or at procedure room, as convenient. Cleanliness must be maintained
- Preparation of parents: Explain the procedure of anthropometry and its importance to the parents. Encourage them to participate during the measurement to reduce stress of the child and to get cooperation. Answer to their questions in simple words.
- Preparation of child: Explain the procedure of anthropometry in age appropriate language. Make the child clean and comfortable. Answer to his or her concern

related to the measurement procedure, whenever needed.

Performing the Steps of Procedure with Rationale/Point of Emphasis

Measuring Body Weight

1. Note the previous body weight of the child, if available. It serves as baseline data to detect any weight changes.
2. Perform hand hygiene and assemble all required items near the child.
3. Use digital weighing scale with a pan/tray to place the child during weight measurement for the children aged below 24 months of age.
4. Ensure the weighing scale is cleaned/disinfected and placed on firm flat surface.
5. Ensure the room is warm and no fan is running. Weight can be measured at bed side or in the treatment room or procedure room.
6. Place a light drape/sheet or paper on the scale pan and calibrate the scale to "0" position.
7. Completely undress the infant/toddler and safely place on the pan at the middle of the weighing scale. Children aged below 24 months should be weighed nude without any cloths for accurate body weight determination. Remove the dress and diaper of the child. One small sheet can be used to cover the child on the tray/pan of the scale, if complete undressing is not allowed. Child can have diaper in place. Remember to deduct the weight of sheet and diaper from the total weight recorded.
8. Keep your one hand slightly above the child while on weighing scale to prevent accidental fall and injury
   i. If the child is extremely fearful or active, then weight measurement may be done by having the parent hold the child in his or her arm and stand on adult weighing machine. Weigh parent holding the child first and then weigh the parent alone. To assess child's weight, subtract weight of parent alone from the weight of parent and child together.
9. Use stand-up weighing scale for ambulatory children older than 24 months of age. Determine whether the child is able to stand and balance on the weighing scale. Ensure the scale is in "0" position. Place a piece of paper or drape on the scale
   i. Ask the child to remove shoes and heavy clothing. Light clothing is allowed unless otherwise specified. Privacy must be maintained. Do not make the older child nude
   ii. Assist the child to stand on the weighing scale safely with arms hanging at his or her sides of body
   iii. Ask the child to be still on the weighing machine. Ensure the scale is not shaking.
10. Note the child's weight in gram for young infant and in kilograms for older child. Weight in kilograms is used for calculation of medication doses and IV fluid therapy.
11. Carefully remove the infant/toddler from the weighing scale. Redress the child and put on diaper. Return the child to parent's arm or crib securely. Assist the older child to step down from stand-up weighing scale, if needed.
12. Dispose the drape or paper from the weighing scale. Disinfect the weighing scale (as per institutional policy) each time after use to prevent transmission of microorganisms.
13. Dispose all waste. Rearrange reusable articles and equipment for next use.
14. Ensure the child is comfortable. Perform hand hygiene.
15. Document the child's weight on child's hospital record and on growth chart.

Measuring Recumbent Length and Standing Height

1. Note the child's age and previous length or height measurement value, if available. It helps to detect changes in child's length or height

2. Perform hand hygiene. Make the child comfortable for measurement of length or height.
3. Ensure infantometer or measuring tape is clean for assessing recumbent length of the young child up to 2 years of age.
4. Place light drape or paper on flat surface or on flat measuring board or on infantometer to provide comfort and to protect from cross contamination.
5. For use of infantometer, lay the infant/toddler in supine position, placing the vertex of the child's head at the top of the board and soles of the feet firmly against the footboard of infantometer. This allows full extension of body for accurate length measurement.
   Hold the child's head at midline point and extend legs fully. Having parent hold the child's head provides emotional comfort for the child and helps with full extension of child's body. Hold the child's legs gently. Then note the child's length.
6. For use of measuring tape, stretch a tape measure on a flat surface and measure from crown of the child's head to heel of the child's foot, alongside child's body boundaries. Ensure child's body and legs are in full extension.
   Use of tape measure is less accurate method than use of infantometer for length measurement. Tape measure should only be used when infantometer or other devices are not available.
7. After recording the child's length, carefully remove the infant/toddler from the flat surface or infantometer and return to the parent's arm or crib or bed.
8. For measuring the standing height of older children use stadiometer or prepare a stand-up height scale on the wall using ordinary tape measure (wall tape measure)
   i. Determine whether the child is able to stand and balance on height scale
   ii. Move the child to the area where stadiometer or wall tape measure is attached
   iii. Ask the child to remove shoes. Child should not wear hat or hair ornaments
   iv. Assist the child to stand with back to the height scale/wall/stadiometer. Child's heels, buttocks and shoulders should be in contact with the wall or height bar of the scale. Child should look straight ahead without tilting the head
   v. Raise height rod and extend height assessment bar high over child's head to prevent injury. Lower the height rod to top of child's head to note the height. Ensure that height assessment bar is perpendicular to height rod
   vi. Keep eye to eye contact with the child and apply gentle traction to the jaw, if required and note the height measurement
   vii. Place a bar or rod on child's head to mark the height, when "wall tape measure" is used
   viii. Mark the child's height on the scale/stadiometer/wall tape measure.
9. For electronic length measurement devices, follow manufacturer's instructions.
10. Note and record child's length or height in centimeters, not in inches.
11. Make the child comfortable. Answer for any questions.
12. Take care of the reusable articles. Dispose all waste. Perform hand hygiene.
13. Document the length or height on child's growth chart and/or related record, specific for the child's care and treatment.

Measuring Head Circumference, Chest Circumference. and Mid-upper Arm Circumference

1. Note the child's last recorded head circumference, chest circumference and MUAC, if available. It ensure baseline data and helps to identify changes in child's head circumference, chest circumference, and MUAC.
2. Perform hand hygiene. Clean the tape measure with alcohol swabs or alcohol wipes.
3. Place the child in supine position or in sitting position on bed or parent's lap

or on examination table with support to prevent accidental fall and injury.
4. Ensure proper tension of the tape measure during measurement, not too tight or too loose.
5. For measuring head circumference, place the tape measure over the most prominent point of the occiput at the back, around the head just above the eyebrows (i.e., over supra-orbital ridges) in front and above the pinna on the sides. These are points of largest circumference of child's head.
6. Measure chest circumference by placing the tape measure around the chest at the level of breast nipples in between inspiration and expiration.
7. Take MUAC measurement at midpoint of left upper arm, between the tip of acromion process of scapula and olecranon process of ulna. Use simple tape measure or special MUAC measurement tape. Measure MUAC firmly and gently without compressing the arm. Allow the arm to hang freely. There should be no cloths on the arms.
8. Carefully return the child to the parent's arms or crib or bed and provide comfort.
9. Clean the tape measure. Discard the used swabs or wipes. Perform hand hygiene.
10. Note and record child's head circumference, chest circumference, and MUAC in centimeters.
11. Document all findings of measurements on the child's on growth chart and in hospital record in case hospitalized child. Report the abnormal findings.

Evaluation and Documentation

- Evaluate child's growth parameters on standardized growth charts and detect the presence of any abnormalities for prompt initiation of management. Compare child's growth parameters with baseline data to identify any changes and to teach the parents about optimal care of the child for favorable growth and development. Evaluate the parent's knowledge regarding child's growth progress and its deviations
- Document child's exact chronological age (e.g., 4 years 5 months or $4^{5}/_{12}$), weight, length or height, head circumference, chest circumference, MUAC, and BMI on child's growth chart and treatment specific hospital/clinic records.

Communication and Teaching for Homecare

- Communicate with child and parents about health status of the child, findings of all growth parameters, measurements and plan of management in simple language and as asked by family members
- Teach the parents about child's rest, sleep, activity pattern, dietary recommendations, water intake, hygienic practices, play, recreations, and diversional measures. Discuss about the medications to be used, nutritional supplements, and discharge planning from hospital with emergency health conditions requiring medical attention, continued care at home and plan of follow-up visits. Instruct the parents about importance of preservation of growth chart and other health records.

PROCEDURE–4: OXYGEN THERAPY TO INFANT AND OLDER CHILDREN

Clinical Guidelines

- Oxygen is a drug used to improve its concentration in inspired air when there is deficiency of tissue oxygenation. It is administered as temporary measures to treat hypoxemia and hypoxia but does not replace the definite treatment of underlying cause of those conditions. Oxygen should always be given based on oxygen saturation level and child's clinical presentations. Usually oxygen is given in 40–60% concentration, but in some conditions 100% oxygen need to be delivered
- Oxygen therapy is indicated when the oxygen saturation level is below normal level or in the conditions where the demand of tissue oxygenation is increased. The need for oxygen, the type of oxygen

delivery system, and the amount of oxygen to be delivered depends upon child's respiratory status and comorbid health conditions

- Common indications of oxygen therapy include breathlessness (due to respiratory infections, asthma, pulmonary embolism, emphysema, cardiac diseases, etc.), cyanosis, accidental injury, bleeding, shock, anemia, circulatory failure, critically ill child, convulsions, unconsciousness, during anesthesia, and in postanesthesia period, etc.
- Oxygen supplementations is administered to the children by use of nasal prongs/nasal cannula, nasopharyngeal catheter, mask (simple face mask, venturi mask, partial rebreathing mask, nonrebreathing mask, and bag-valve mask), hood or endotracheal tube. Nasal cannula and nasopharyngeal catheter are contraindicated in children with nasal obstructions (e.g., nasal polyp and choanal atresia). Nasopharyngeal catheter is contraindicated in case of maxillofacial trauma, basal skull fracture, coagulations problems and in neonatal population. Commonly used devices for oxygen therapy are nasal prongs, oxygen mask, and oxygen hoods or head boxes
- Pulse oximetry monitoring is recommended during oxygen administration to assess the expected saturation level. Normal saturation levels in healthy children are considered to be in the range between 97 and 99%
  - Attach the sensor probe of pulse oximeter to the selected site. For optimal performance, keep the sensor site at the level of heart. This allows measurement of the light transmitted through a pulsating arterial vascular bed to calculate the percentage of hemoglobin saturated with oxygen. Rotate the sensor site as unit specific criteria to reduce the risk of tissue breakdown at probe site
  - Avoid placing the sensor probe over thick skin, nail polish and false nails and in the extremities that are moved excessively by the child and at areas where perfusion is known to be poor
  - Suggested probe sites for infants are great toe with the cable extending toward the heel, ball of foot below the toes, palm of the hand, wrist, and forehead
  - Suggested probe sites for older children are index finger with light source centered on the fingertip and forehead
  - Alarm limits should be determined considering the child's age, underlying condition and past history of normal parameters for that particular child
- Restrict use of ignition sources where oxygen therapy is administered (e.g., cigarettes, candles, sparking toys) to prevent fire hazards. Place fire precautions display.

Equipment Required

- Hand hygiene supplies for hand wash and antiseptic hand rub
- Disposable clean or unsterile gloves, mask, and face shield or goggles
- Oxygen source, as available (piped-in-system or oxygen cylinder or oxygen concentrator or liquid oxygen reservoir)
- Oxygen regulator, oxygen flow-meter, and oxygen tubing
- Humidifier and sterile water for humidification chamber
- Oxygen hood, nasal prongs/cannula, oxygen mask, as directed
- Gauze pieces and mouth wipes in a container/bowl to remove secretions
- Pulse oximeter, as indicated to measure oxygen saturation and heart rate
- Paper tape for fixation of nasal prongs and scissors
- Water soluble lubricant for catheter insertion, if used
- Extra blanket or sheet
- "No smoking" sign
- Waste disposal containers as per BMW guidelines
- Documentation sheet, treatment sheet and child's case sheet.

Assessment and Preparation

- Assess child's history of illness and examine the child to identify the rationale for oxygen administration. Assess vital signs and presence of respiratory difficulties
- Self preparation should be done with hand hygiene and use of gloves
- Environment should be clean, calm, well lighted and well ventilated
- Equipment and necessary articles should be arranged at child's bedside. Oxygen cylinder, if used, should be secured within metal cage in an upright position. Fire safety should be followed. All electrical equipment and oxygen equipment should be checked for proper working order. Extension cords should not be used
- Preparation of parents: Explain the need of oxygen therapy and fire safety. Demonstrate how the equipment is placed on the child's face. Allow one parent at child's bedside and to use diversional measures for the child to cope with the situation
- Preparation of child: Explain according to the level of understanding about need for oxygen therapy and discomfort that may occur during therapy. The child should not wear synthetic clothing. Ensure nostrils are clean and no discharge present. Make the child comfortable. Answer to the questions as asked by the older child in simple language.

Performing the Steps of Procedure with Rationale/Point of Emphasis

1. Perform hand hygiene and assemble all necessary items near the child for organized approach and efficient time management especially during emergency condition.
2. Select appropriate size of nasal cannula/ prong or oxygen mask to prevent nasal injury, skin abrasion, leakage of oxygen and obstruction.
3. Remove all ignition sources and display "No Smoking" sign near the child's bed.
4. Connect the regulator and flow-meter to the oxygen source at wall unit of central supply or freestanding oxygen cylinder/ tank.
5. Connect humidifier and oxygen tubing to the oxygen setup to provide moisture in the system. Humidified air is less drying to the nares and to the lungs.
6. Fill the humidifier with sterile water between the minimum and maximum marks. Use sterile water to decrease the incidence of bacterial growth and to prevent mineral buildup within the system.
7. Connect the distal end of the oxygen tubing to the oxygen delivery device (prong/ mask). It completes the cycle of supplying oxygen from the source to the child.
8. Turn on the flow meter to the prescribed amount of oxygen flow. Check to assess whether you feel oxygen flowing through the system to ensure the child actually receives the required amount of oxygen. Always follow the oxygen flow rate as directed by physician.
   By nasal cannula/prongs, flow of oxygen may be maintained in infants and young child up to 3–4 L/minute and up to 6 L/ minute for older children and adolescents. For oxygen masks, flow rates can vary from 5 to 10 L/minute.
9. Perform hand hygiene and don gloves. If the child is coughing or has copious secretions, mask and goggles may also be worn for safety and protection from pathogens.
10. Attach pulse oximeter to the child's limb to measure oxygen saturation, as directed. Attach pulse oximeter sensor to the selected site with the light source on one side of the tissue pad and the sensor on the other side, facing each other.
11. Place the child in supine or semi-fowler's position. Raising the head of the bed helps to protect the airway from the vomitus and secretions. Infant should be placed in midline in "sniffing position" to maintain proper alignment of the mouth, pharynx, and trachea.

12. *For use of nasal prongs/cannula,* place the cannula/prongs just inside the external meatus of the nares. Loop the head attachment around the child's ears and tighten it under the chin or loop it around and behind the child's head and tighten. Instruct the child to breathe through nose in age-appropriate and simple language.
    Paper tape or other adhesive materials may be used to secure the tubing to the child's face. Care should be taken to keep the cannula tubing and straps away from the neck to prevent airway obstruction in infants. Avoid undue pressure on the nasal tissue from tightening the attachment too much. Watch for redness, erosion, irritation, discomfort, and for tissue breakdown at nares at any pressure points
13. *For use of oxygen mask,* place oxygen mask over mouth and nose. Oxygen tubing travels downward and away from the child's head. Tighten the straps attached to the mask until you can easily fit one finger between the strap and the face of the child. Avoid too tight application of strap. Appropriately secure mask allows the prescribed amount of oxygen to flow into the respiratory system
14. *For use of nasopharyngeal catheter,* lubricate the tip of catheter with water soluble lubricant. Gently insert the appropriate size catheter to a depth equal to the distance from the side of the nose to the front of the ear. So that tip of the catheter is just visible in the pharynx below the soft palate when mouth of the infant is open. Do not use force to place the catheter. If resistance in placement is met, do not proceed with nasal catheter and choose other device. Secure the catheter to the child's face using paper tape or other adhesive material to prevent dislodgement of the catheter when the child moves.
    Improper insertion of nasal catheter can cause gagging and nasal or pharyngeal trauma. Improper size of catheter can lead to nasal obstruction and irritation. Catheter sizes less than 8F are less effective in oxygen delivery and may easily obstruct with mucus. Use of nasopharyngeal catheter may be limited with excessive mucus drainage, mucosal edema, or presence of deviated septum.
15. *For use of oxygen hood,* place the hood on the crib or bed so that the child's head is inside the unit. Hood should not rest on the child's neck. Child should be able to turn her or his head side to side easily. Child's entire head should be inside the oxygen hood with enough free space
16. Ensure that the target oxygen concentration level is achieved and available. Monitor SpO_2 and assess the child's respiratory status and general condition for signs of improvement or deterioration
17. Change the humidifier, oxygen tube and water daily after use of 24 hours. Reuse all these articles after cleaning and sterilization. Take care of all wastes
18. Perform hand hygiene. Report all findings and document the procedure of oxygen therapy.

Evaluation and Documentation

- Evaluate the respiratory status, SpO_2, temperature, heart rate, and features of improvement or deterioration of the child. Evaluate the level of understanding of the child and parent to provide necessary support regarding use of oxygen
- Document—type of oxygen delivery system used (prong, mask, hood, catheter), setting of the oxygen flow meter, time of initiation of oxygen therapy, SpO_2 level, temperature, heart, respiratory status (rate, retractions, grunting, cyanosis, nasal flaring), skin condition of the nares with presence of any redness or irritation due to pressure of the prongs.

Communication and Teaching for Homecare

- Communicate with child and parents about need for oxygen supplementation, safety concerns with special attention to avoid smoking, electric toys, and open flames. Inform about child's respiratory

condition and about plan of continuation of treatment
- Teach the parents about participation in child's routine care, signs of worsening and continuation of care at home after discharge and plan of follow-up visits.

Refer: Oxygen Therapy for Neonates, in Procedure - 13 in the Unit - 2 of this Manual.

PROCEDURE–5: NEBULIZATION THERAPY OR AEROSOL TREATMENTS TO THE CHILDREN

Clinical Guidelines

- Nebulization is the process of producing a fine spray or mist from liquid, using a machine called as nebulizer. Nebulizer is available as electric or battery-run device for the treatment of breathing problems. Nebulizers may be easier to use for the children than metered-dose inhalers. Nebulization may be done by rapidly passing air through the liquid or by vibrating a liquid at high frequency, so that the particles produced are extremely small
- The use of medicated mists such as bronchodilators, antivirals, corticosteroids, or mucolytic agents to treat lung or bronchial diseases is termed as aerosol therapy. Aerosol is solution dispensed as a mist or any suspension of particles in air or gas
- Healthcare professional and nursing personnel should be confident and skilled about the use of aerosol delivery devices and the medications being delivered as aerosol therapy, including their contraindications, potential side effects, and desired outcomes of children
- Indications for aerosol treatment include the need to deliver aerosolized medications to patients in acute respiratory distress or with reduced respiratory flow and the need to deliver a topical medication in aerosol form to the lung parenchyma
- Types of aerosol devices for pediatric populations include small volume nebulizers, large volume nebulizers, metered dose inhaler, and dry powder inhaler. Selection of an aerosol device depends on child's age, clinical conditions, and single-patient use or multiple-patient uses. A face mask, rather than a mouthpiece, should be used for infants and children younger than 3 years of age.
- Delivery of aerosol treatments requires knowledge and skills related to aerosol delivery devices and their limitations for use including assembly, care, safety precautions, and reuse of those devices (as per manufacturer's instructions). Family members and older children need demonstration and return demonstration of the procedure for long-term use of this aerosol treatment
- Aerosol treatments can be administered in a number of settings, including hospital, clinic, extended care facility, school, home and during medical transportation
- Standard precautions of infection control measures must be followed during nebulization therapy. Continuous monitoring of the child's health status must be done during aerosol treatment. Anxiety and stress of the child and parents should be managed carefully.

Equipment Required

- Hand hygiene supplies for hand wash and use of antiseptic hand rub
- Disposable gloves, protective mask or face shield and apron/gown for care provider
- Age-appropriate aerosol delivery device including aerosol generator (small volume nebulizers, large volume nebulizers, metered dose inhaler or dry powder inhaler) and interface (mouthpiece, face mask) and power source
- Prescribed medications, isotonic diluents and syringes (2 mL, 5 mL)
- A container with mouth wipes or gauze pieces and sputum mug with disinfectant
- Oxygen delivery system, as ordered and pulse oximeter
- Resuscitation articles and emergency medication tray with necessary items
- Articles for monitoring of vital signs and stethoscope

- Extra clothing, sheet, blanket, pillow to make the child comfortable
- Waste disposal containers as per BMW guidelines
- Documentation sheet, treatment sheet and child's case sheet.

Assessment and Preparation

- Assess child's respiratory rate, work of breathing, oxygen saturation, breath sounds, features of respiratory distress, heart rate, and presence of any other abnormal clinical features before initiating nebulization.
  Determine the type of age-appropriate equipment to be used for the child and ability of child to manage mouthpiece or face mask. Identify the anxiety and knowledge level of the child and family members regarding medical reason for the aerosol treatment, use of device, ability to perform of aerosol therapy and care of the equipment at home, if needed
- Self preparation should be done with hand hygiene and use of appropriate personal protective equipment (PPE)
- Environment should be clean, well-ventilated, well-lighted and free from overcrowding
- Articles should be assembled near the child. Infection control measures must be followed
- Preparation of parents/family members: Explain the procedure according to level of understanding. Allow the parent for holding the child and for use of diversional measures. Encourage to ask questions and reply
- Preparation of child: Explain the procedure to the child in age-appropriate language. Make the child clean and place in comfortable position. Answer to the questions as asked.

Performing the Steps of Procedure with Rationale/Point of Emphasis

1. Perform hand hygiene and assemble all required articles and supplies near the child.
2. Select appropriate aerosol device. Effectiveness of aerosolized medication depends on position of child to the equipment, particle size, ventilatory pattern, airway clearance, and dose of medication used.
3. Check the prescribed dose of the medication to be administered.
4. Ensure the child is prepared and positioned for nebulization. Place the child in semi-Fowler's or upright or sitting position comfortably with the help of the parent.
5. Perform hand hygiene. Wear gloves and protective mask. Protective measures from exposure to aerosols, medications and patient generated droplets must be strictly followed.
6. Assemble the aerosol delivery device, power source and the interface (mouthpiece, face mask). Follow the specific manufacturer's directions for the equipment that is being used. Each manufacturer has unique directions for connecting the various disposable parts of the aerosol equipment.
7. Fill the nebulizer chamber with prescribed liquid using a syringe to measure the precise amount of isotonic diluent or medication ordered. Close the chamber. Use only sterile fluids for aerosol solutions and dispense them aseptically. Diluents that are not isotonic may increase reactivity. Delivering aerosolized medications or mist may vary, because the actual amount of aerosolized material delivered into the lungs varies with the tidal volume of the child.
8. Position the child comfortably and place the interface (mouthpiece, face mask). When using a mouthpiece, it is important that the child seals the lips around the mouthpiece and breaths only through the mouth. Children younger than 3 years of age are usually not able to cooperate well enough to use a mouthpiece and to achieve the desired seal around the device. Use of face mask is recommended for the children younger than 3 years of age. Using

a mask attached to the nebulizer cup, which is held over the nose and mouth, enables the treatment to be dispersed as a mist, thus eliminating the need to keep a mouthpiece in place. Parent can hold the mask in position, but necessary precautions should be explained.

9. For infant, hold the baby in comforting upright position and support the head and neck, and place the face mask over the mouth and nose. Increasing the comfort level of the infant will enhance the ability to finish the treatment without the infant crying. Crying reduces particles deposition in the lungs.
10. For older children, elevate the head of the bed or place him or her in sitting position. Place the mask over his or her mouth, forming a tight seal to prevent escaping of medication without being delivered to the lungs.
11. Turn on the compressor and use for the prescribed time. With aerosol treatment, the duration may vary slightly, but an extended treatment may lead to an increase in noncompliance.
12. Monitor the child's vital signs and signs of any adverse reactions to the treatment. Adverse reactions commonly include tachycardia, cardiac arrhythmias and palpitations. Continue to assess the child for improvement of respiratory status. Delivering aerosol treatment directly to the lungs results in stabilization of respiratory status. Continuous monitoring is recommended during nebulization.
13. On completion of the treatment, remove the mask from the child's face and turn off the compressor. Help to remove mouthpiece in case of older child. Maintain safety of the child and the equipment during the therapy.
14. Assist the child to rinse the mouth with water after each administration of inhaled steroids. This prevents oral irritation or overgrowth of opportunistic organisms.
15. Make the child comfortable in safe position in bed with side rails up to protect the child from falling out of bed.
16. Remove equipment from child's bedside. Arrange for cleaning and disinfection according to institutional policy and manufacturer's instructions. Clean equipment decreases the risk of cross infections and increase nebulizer output.
17. Dispose all waste in appropriate containers. Remove gloves. Perform hand hygiene
18. Document the aerosol treatment and observational findings in child's record sheet.

Evaluation and Documentation

- Evaluate child's response to the treatment, comparing the findings with the pretreatment assessment of work of breathing and breath sounds.
  Evaluate child, family and caregiver's ability to perform the procedure, e.g., delivery technique, administration of medication, calculation of medicine dose, cleaning of the equipment, assessment of respiratory problems and need for the treatment at home
- Document the following:
  - Date, time and frequency of aerosol treatment administered to the child
  - Respiratory status of the child before and after the treatment
  - Name and amount of medications and diluents given
  - Type of aerosol delivery device and interface used
  - Presence of any adverse reactions to the treatment
  - Training given to child or parents or caregivers who will perform the procedure at home.

Communication and Teaching for Homecare

- Communicate with child and parents about the need of aerosol treatment at hospital and/or at home, health status of the child and plan of future management
- Teach the parents or caregivers about the followings:
  - Routine care of the child at hospital and at home after discharge from hospital

- Demonstrate safe use of aerosol delivery device, use of oxygen, and technique of aerosol treatment. Show the cleaning technique and assembly of the aerosol delivery device
- Explain the purpose of medications, preparation, dosage, indications and their side effects
- Inform about the signs and symptoms of respiratory distress requiring aerosol treatment and when to report to physician or healthcare prescriber or to hospital
- Instruct about hand hygiene, cleanliness, asepsis, diet, rest, sleep and activity at home
- Discuss details of discharge advice, continued care at home, and follow-up visit plan.

PROCEDURE–6: INTRAVENOUS FLUID THERAPY USING PERIPHERAL CATHETERS TO THE SICK CHILD

Clinical Guidelines

- Peripheral IV catheters are placed by cannulating superficial veins. Potential sites of peripheral IV access in children include the back of the hand, the arm (including the antecubital fossa), the foot, the leg and the scalp. Commonly used veins of upper limbs are fifth interdigital vein, cephalic vein, median antebrachial vein, median basilic vein and basilic vein. Commonly used lower limbs veins for IV cannulation are median marginal vein, lateral marginal vein, and small saphenous vein **(Fig. 3.2)**
- The choice of access of peripheral IV site depends on the hemodynamic status of the child, general condition of the vasculature, expertise of the nurse/physician/technician, availability and quality of supplies and nature of the IV fluid being infused
- Peripheral IV catheters are used for direct administration of primed IV fluid, intermittent use for medications and for blood product transfusion. These also can be used for venous blood sampling for laboratory analysis and parenteral nutritional supplementations.
- Disposable IV cannula/catheters of various lengths and sizes are available from several manufacturers. Infants and children with small veins may tolerate large-volume IV rates with small-bore (20 G to 24 G) catheters. Peripheral IV catheters in children may remain in place as long as there are no signs of extravasations or any other complications. They do not need to be changed on a routine basis.
- Placement of IV catheters must be done in strict aseptic technique with practice of standard precautions of infection control measures. Normal anatomy of the veins must be considered. Skilled approach should be done to prevent complications.
- When placing IV lines in extremities, then access the most distal site first and use non-dominant hand. Do not use the antecubital veins until other sites have been exhausted, because catheters in the antecubital region, or any joint, can be easily disturbed by joint flexion. If immobilization is done at the joint, that may cause joint stiffness and pain.
- Monitoring of IV site is very important for early identification of complications and for the prompt interventions. Complications of intravascular therapy with peripheral access include bleeding, hematoma, infiltration, phlebitis, bacteremia, septicemia, nerve damage, and mechanical problems like breaks in the catheter, migration of catheter, accidental catheter removal, etc. Precautions should be followed to prevent these complications.

Equipment Required

- Hand hygiene supplies for hand wash and hand rub to reduce cross infections
- A sterile tray containing all sterile articles such as gloves, cotton swabs, gauze dressing, small bowls for use of antiseptic solutions, small dressing forceps for skin preparation

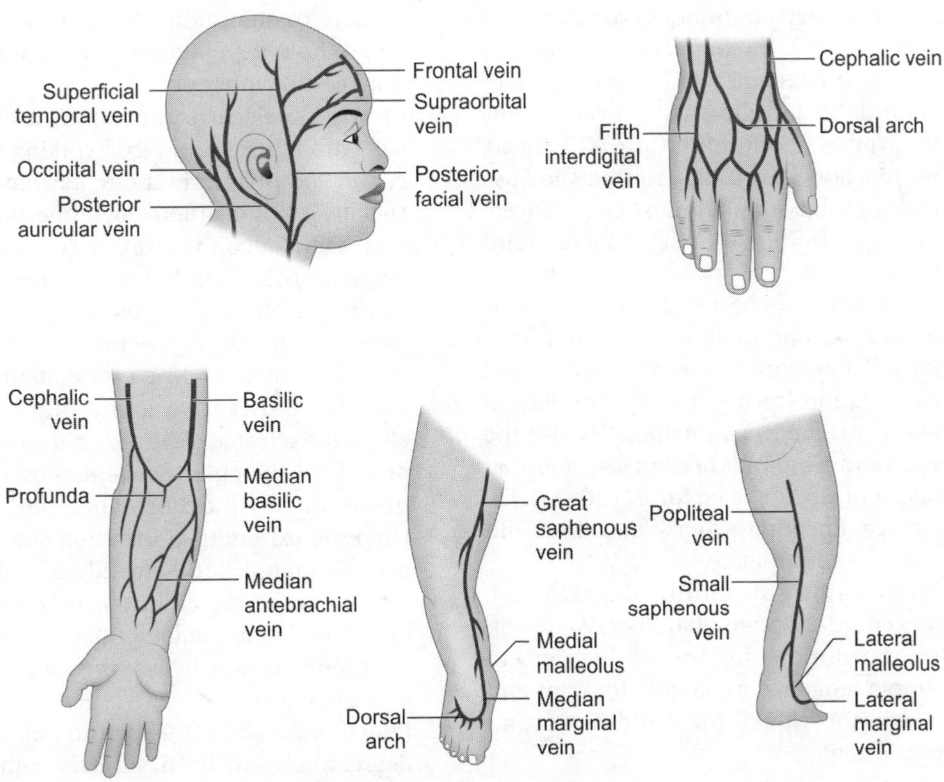

Fig. 3.2: Sites for peripheral intravascular access.

- A clean tray containing a bottle of 70% alcohol, a bottle of povidone-iodine, or a bottle of 2% chlorhexidine-base preparation, a bottle/ampule of normal saline, vial of injection heparin (if heparin lock is used), local anesthetic topical agents/cream, appropriate size IV cannula/catheter packet, syringe packs (3 mL, 5 mL, and 10 mL), IV fluid bottle/bag as prescribed, IV fluid administration tube set, or micro-drip set, 3-way/multiple connector or adaptor, tourniquet (if needed), skin friendly adhesive tape, transparent dressing, clean cotton swab, soft piece of cloth to remove anesthetic cream, and scissors
- Transfer forceps or lifter to handle sterile articles
- Syringe pump or infusion pump and pressure monitoring (PMO) line, IV fluid stand
- Waste disposal containers as per BMW rules
- Intake-output chart, documentation sheet, treatment sheet, and child case sheet.

Assessment and Preparation

- Assess child's health status, skin condition, previous intake and output, history of fluid loss and severity of disease process. Assess the level of anxiety and understanding, ability and readiness for process information of both the child and family members
- Self preparation should be done with hand hygiene and practice of aseptic technique. Help of one assistant usually required to maintain asepsis, especially during placement of IV cannulation
- Environment should be clean, calm, well-lighted and free from overcrowding

- All necessary equipment, supplies and necessary articles should be collected and arranged near the child. Sterile articles should be handled with precautions to prevent contamination. Cleaning, disinfection, sterilization routines and use of disposable supplies must be practiced, as per institutional policy and standard guidelines
- Preparation of parents: Explain the purpose, risks and benefits of IV fluid therapy. Allow parent's involvement to get cooperation during the IV cannulation and continued IV infusion. Discuss the signs and symptoms of extravasations that may indicate the need for IV catheter site change. Encourage to ask questions and answer appropriately
- Preparation of child: Explain the procedure of IV cannulation or IV infusion as appropriate for the child's age in simple language especially for pain and discomfort. Make the child clean and comfortable.

Performing the Steps of Procedure with Rationale/Point of Emphasis

Insertion of Peripheral IV Catheter and Initiation of IV Fluid Therapy in a Child

1. Perform hand hygiene and assemble all necessary items near the child.
2. Identify the site and the vein for insertion of peripheral IV catheter/cannula.
3. Apply topical anesthetic agent on the selected IV cannulation site and allow that to remain on the skin for appropriate length of time (e.g., 1 hour for EMLA cream, 15 minutes for lidocaine iontophoresis over intact skin, 1 minute for injectable lidocaine). This helps to reduce pain during IV cannula insertion.
4. Remove topical anesthetic cream with soft cloth before beginning the IV cannulation
5. Select catheter size, open the outer pack and prepare all supplies without contamination.
6. Perform hand hygiene and don gloves. Obtain the assistance of an additional person to maintain sterile technique and to hold the child securely to prevent unnecessary attempts.
7. Cleanse the skin over the chosen insertion site with antiseptic swabs, working from center to outward in a circular motion. Usually alcohol, then povidone-iodine and again alcohol swabs are used to prepare the skin before IV cannula insertion. Allow the area to dry for 30 seconds. This decreases the numbers of organisms on the skin at cannulation site.
8. Ask the assistant to apply tourniquet above the selected cleaned site, if required or to hold the child's extremity to apply pressure above the cannulation site.
9. Hold the extremity of insertion site with non-dominant hand steadily to reduce discomfort of the child during cannula insertion. Using dominant hand, remove the protective sheath over the catheter or take assistance.
10. Puncture the skin of the insertion site at 45 degree angle with the bevel of the catheter needle up and parallel to the vein.
11. Reduce the angle of the catheter needle and insert $^1/_8$ to ¼ inch into the vein until retrograde blood flow appears in the catheter. This allows insertion of catheter into the vein lumen without puncturing the posterior wall of the vein.
12. Release the tourniquet or applied pressure by the assistant. It prevents rupture of vein as needle is advanced into vein lumen.
13. Advance catheter into the vein while gently removing inner needle from the catheter, leaving only catheter sheath in place to establish the catheter in vein.
14. Stabilize the catheter in place with nondominant hand and cover the hub with a cap.
15. Fix the catheter in place securely with gauze dressing and tape or cover with transparent dressing to the site. This prevents catheter movement and accidental dislodgement. Transparent dressings provide greater visualization of the site. If there is any blood at insertion site, clean

the blood with sterile swab before fixing the IV catheter.

16. Connect primed IV infusion set to the catheter hub to provide direct entrance of IV fluid to flow through the catheter. It also helps to assess the patency of the catheter.
17. Initiate the flow of prescribed IV fluid or normal saline through the catheter and assess for signs of infiltration. If the needle of catheter has punctured the posterior wall of the vein, then fluid will fill into the surrounding tissue causing localized edema or hematoma.
18. Start prescribed IV fluid infusion and regulate the rate of infusion. Use syringe infusion pump for small amount of fluid and medications. Set the syringe pump with PMO line and the syringe filled with prescribed fluid in aseptic technique. Micro-drip infusion set is usually used for the young child having 60 drops equal to 1 mL. Set the drop rate carefully to maintain infusion of fluid within prescribed time limit.
19. Check the rate of infusion and the remaining amount in the syringe or fluid bag or bottle after few minutes. Check the IV site for infiltration of fluid at regular interval.
20. Use and place "saline lock or heparin lock" for intermittent infusions, as prescribed.
21. Secure the IV line and tubing with additional tape and arm-board and surgical netting, as needed to prevent accidental removal. Secure connection is required to prevent air embolizations or migration of the catheter.
22. Maintain strict intake and output chart. Adjust IV fluid requirement with the amount of intake of enteral feed and any other fluid intake. Monitor for any complications.
23. Make the child comfortable and relax. Allow to parent to support the child.
24. Discard all used supplies and disposable items. Take care of reusable articles.
25. Perform hand hygiene. Document the IV fluid therapy in child's treatment sheet.

Maintenance of IV Infusion

1. Perform hand hygiene and gather the necessary supplies, as needed.
2. Assess the IV site every hour for presence of any complications and for prompt initiation of interventions. Discontinue the IV infusion as indicated (e.g., infiltration of fluid or hematoma formation).
3. Infuse IV fluid via controlled infusion device. Hang IV fluid not more than 4 hours at any one time during fluid infusion, if feasible. This prevents accidental fluid overload and reduces complications from IV infiltration.
4. Infuse calculated amount of prescribed IV fluid for the child. Take into consideration of other fluid intake (e.g., any oral intake or IV medications or blood products) to provide total fluid requirements as per age, body weight and disease condition of the child.
5. Follow aseptic technique during preparation and administration of fluid therapy.
6. Countercheck prescribed IV fluid, as directed by physician or healthcare prescriber to maintain appropriate fluid and electrolyte balance.
7. Look for any signs and symptoms of fluid and electrolyte imbalance in the child.
8. Maintain intake and output chart strictly in each nursing shift and for total in 24 hours.
9. Change the IV tubing using aseptic technique, as per unit/institutional policy, or no more frequently than every 24–72 hours or when contamination occurs or suspected.
10. Label the IV tubing with date, time and initials of person who hung tubing to identify exact change date and time.
11. Change the IV access site dressing in aseptic technique when the site appears soiled, damp or loose. This reduces bacterial contamination. Follow wound site care guidelines.
12. Label the dressing with date, time and initials of the person who reapplied the dressing.

13. Make the child comfortable and allow to parent to support the child.
14. Discard all used supplies. Take care of reusable articles.
15. Perform hand hygiene. Document the IV fluid infusion details in child's treatment sheet.

Removal of Peripheral IV Catheter

1. Perform hand hygiene and arranged all required articles near the child.
2. Explain about the need for removal of IV cannula to the child in age appropriate simple language and to the parent.
3. Don gloves to maintain asepsis and to reduce transmission of microorganisms.
4. Close the clamp on IV administration set. Turn off the IV controlled infusion device. Ensure all connections are clamped or closed. These stops the flow of fluids and prevents potential infiltration while removing peripheral catheter.
5. Remove old adhesive tape and dressing from and around the insertion site gently.
6. Apply slight pressure over catheter insertion site using gauze pad or cotton ball, while withdrawing peripheral IV catheter. It facilitates easy removal of catheter.
7. Continue holding pressure at insertion site for 1-2 minutes after removal of IV catheter to prevent bleeding from the site.
8. Remove gauze and cotton swab. Assess insertion site for signs of bleeding, infiltration, infections or phlebitis. Intervene promptly to manage the complications.
9. Apply small sterile gauze dressing over the insertion site and fix with adhesive tape.
10. Dispose all used items and waste as per BMW rules. Take care of reusable articles.
11. Perform hand hygiene. Document the procedure of removal of IV catheter, its reason and all related findings in child's record.

Evaluation and Documentation

- Evaluate child's IV site every hour for appearance of the site and signs of complications. Note presence or absence of redness, swelling, drainage, tenderness and discoloration
- Document date and time of IV insertion or removal of IV cannula, insertion site, type and size/gauge of the catheter, numbers of attempts during insertion, child's response during insertion, and date, time, type and amount of flush solution, if used. Maintain intake and output chart with details of fluid infusion. Record the presence of any complications in child's case sheet.

Communication and Teaching for Homecare

- Communicate with child, if condition permits, and with parents about the child's health status, disease process and plan of management. Answer to their questions, as asked
- Teach the parents about hand washing, general cleanliness, precautions for prevention of dislodgement of catheter and extravasation, dietary restrictions (if any), oral fluid intake, and signs of complications of IV therapy. Discuss with the parents about duration of hospital stay, plan of discharge, continued care at home, medication use, need for medical help in emergency and plan of follow-up visits.

Refer: Intravenous Fluid Therapy for Neonates, in Procedure - 17 in the Unit - 2 of this Manual.

PROCEDURE–7: PLACEMENT OF GASTRIC FEEDING TUBE AND GAVAGE FEEDING TO OLDER CHILDREN

Clinical Guidelines

- Gavage feeding is given with introduction of feeding tube placed into the stomach through nose or mouth. Gavage means forced feeding through a tube passed into the stomach. It is a form of enteral feeding as orogastric or nasogastric routes. Other routes of enteral feeding include gastrostomy tube feeding and jejunostomy tube feeding
- Nasogastric or orogastric enteral tube placement is done by passing a small bore

feeding tube through the nostril or mouth into the oropharynx and then through the esophagus to the stomach. These tubes are used for both diagnostic and therapeutic purposes

- Gavage feeding may be given as intermittent feeds, also called a bolus feeds or as continuous drip of feed or combination of these methods, which is best for the child. Most common practice is intermittent feeds. Continuous drip enteral feeding is given using enteral feeding pump, which controls delivery of feeds. Enteral feeding bag with administration set/tubing and/or pump (as indicated), and fluid stand or pole are extra requirements for the continuous drip feeding
- Nutritional and calorie requirement of the children in relation to disease states should be considered during selection and preparation of feeds and fluids. The food should be in liquid or semi-liquid form at room temperature
- Total fluid requirements must be maintained to prevent dehydration and fluid overload. Calculation of fluid requirement usually done based on body weight of the children, which needs adjustment of IV fluid intake with that of intake by oral route, if any
- Gavage feedings are indicated for children who are unable to ingest an adequate amount of nutrition orally. These may include children who are unconscious, unable to swallow, ventilated, or transitioning from parenteral nutrition
- The child receiving gavage feeding must have a functioning gastrointestinal tract (e.g., audible bowel sounds and occurring peristalsis) for digestion and absorption of nutrition
- Feedings provided by the way of gastrointestinal tract as gavage promote gut barrier structure and function. These are most cost effective than parenteral nutrition. These provide the child with a much lower risk for complications (e.g., catheter sepsis, thrombophlebitis) and prevent poor nutritional status or worsening of malnutrition
- Enteral tube position and function are evaluated before each use. Assess patency of the tube without leaks, kinks or occlusion. Intake and output through the enteral tube must be monitored at frequent interval, as per child's condition and unit policy
- Placement of enteral tube should be changed every 3–7 days or as per unit or policy. Place the enteral tube in other nostril when reinserted. This prevents necrosis of the nares tissue and ensures patency of the tube. The enteral tube may need to be flushed or irrigated with sterile water to maintain its patency.

Equipment Required

For Placement of Nasogastric or Orogastric Enteral Tube

- Hand hygiene supplies for hand wash and hand rub
- Clean or nonsterile gloves, eye protection and mask, as per unit policy
- Enteral feeding tube of appropriate size, generally 5F or 6F or 8F
- Water soluble lubricant to lubricate the tube
- Syringe 5 mL and stethoscope to check the tube position in the stomach
- Adhesive tape and scissors to fix the feeding tube
- A cup of water, tissue paper, small towel
- Extra pillow for positioning the child and sheet for restraint, if needed
- Emesis basis and waste disposal container as per BMW rules
- Documentation sheet and child's case sheet.

For Intermittent or Bolus Enteral Feeding

- Hand hygiene supplies for hand wash and had rub
- Clean or non-sterile gloves, as per unit policy
- Enteral tube in situ—nasogastric or orogastric

- Syringe - 5 mL and stethoscope to check the tube position in the stomach
- Syringe -10 mL or 20 mL or 50 mL to give the feed, depending upon total amount of feed
- Prescribed amount of feed in a covered container and measuring cup
- Small towel, wash cloth, extra pillow
- Waste disposal containers as per BMW guidelines
- Documentation sheet and treatment sheet.

Assessment and Preparation

- Assess child for the followings:
  - History of nasal deformity, surgery or trauma to assess the patency of nares and easy passage of nasogastric tube
  - History of esophageal or gastric surgery, which may complicate placement of enteral tube
  - History of cardiac, renal, pulmonary and hepatic diseases. These may limit the intake of fluid volume and type of feeds or formulas to be administered
  - Measure child's daily weight for calculation of amount of feeds and medications
  - Auscultate for presence of bowel sounds and palpate the abdomen to ensure that it is soft, non-distended and non-tender to identify any problems of gastrointestinal tract
  - Examine for signs and symptoms of gastric distention or irritation, potential risk for aspiration, clinical features of respiratory distress and malnutrition, edema and for conditions that increase metabolic demand and therefore increase calorie requirements
  - Check for orthodontic appliances, if the tube is inserted through the mouth. It can be dislodged during the procedure and possible aspiration may occur
  - Identify the child's and family's cognitive level, anxiety, stress, readiness, and ability to process information related to gavage feeding
- Self preparation should be done with practice of standard precautions of infection control
- Environment should be clean, calm, quiet, well lighted and well ventilated
- All necessary supplies and equipment should be collected and arranged near the child. Precautions should be taken to prevent cross contaminations. Cleaning, disinfection and/or sterilization must be done as per institutional policy and standard guidelines
- Preparation of parents: Explain the procedure of enteral feeding, its importance and precautions to be followed to prevent complications. Allow participation of parent/family member for gaining cooperation and to reduce stress of the child during the procedure
- Preparation of child: Explain the procedure gavage feeding, its risk and benefits to the child, as age and developmentally appropriate language. Discuss the child's role in assisting with passage of the orogastric or nasogastric tube and during gavage feeding.

Performing the Steps of Procedure with Rationale/Point of Emphasis

Placement of Nasogastric or Orogastric Enteral Tube

1. Perform hand hygiene to prevent cross infections and assemble all necessary items near the child for efficient time management and organized approach to the procedure.
2. Ensure smallest size small-bore feeding tube is used. The small diameter of the tube causes less gagging on insertion of the tube and is more comfortable once placed in situ. The small diameter of the tube may also allow the child to continue oral intake and ingest food around the tube, when indicated.
3. Position the child comfortably:
   i. Infant and toddler may need to be restrained in supine position before the procedure begins. It should be

done either with swaddle-type restraint or a second person securely holding the child. When the child is in supine position, arrange towels or pillows under the shoulders to slightly extend and elevate the head

ii. The older child may be placed in sitting position for placement of feeding tube if the child can cooperate. Otherwise a second care provider can effectively support and keep the child calm during the procedure. Help to child to bend the head slightly extended

iii. Extending the nasopharynx during initial tube insertion may help to decrease the gag reflex of the child. Once the feeding tube tip is passed distal to the pharynx, the head may be slightly flexed to anatomically to direct the tube insertion into the esophagus, that enhance swallowing and prevent passage of the tube into the trachea

iv. Keeping the child's hands away from the feeding tube helps to prevent the child from pulling out the tube. Restraint may not be needed if diversional measures are used effectively to distract the child during the procedure.

4. Determine the length of enteral tube to be inserted. Using the enteral tube, measure distance from the tip of nose to the earlobe and from the earlobe to the midpoint between xiphoid sternum and umbilicus. Note mark on the tube. Note the measured tube length that will remain external which will help to assess exact tube position in stomach.
5. Place emesis basis and tissue papers within easy access of the child.
6. Place towel over child's dress/gown to protect clothing from emesis or secretions.
7. Perform hand hygiene and wear gloves. Wear eye protection and mask to provide protection from potentials droplets or secretions. The child may cough and splash secretions. These help to reduce transmission of microorganisms.
8. Lubricate the distal tip of the feeding tube with water soluble lubricant. It reduces friction and prevents trauma to the area during insertion. Water soluble lubricant will not lead to pneumonia.
9. Insert the feeding tube gently into nostril or mouth, aiming down and back to follow the anatomical path.
10. When enteral tube reaches the pharynx and the child gags, ask the child to swallow. Swallowing promotes esophageal peristalsis, which facilitates passage of the enteral tube.
11. Continue to pass enteral tube until measured segment of the tube is at the nares or mouth. Don't pass the enteral tube beyond the mark. Tube should reach the stomach
    i. Inserting enteral tube too far may result in looping the tube in the stomach, causing kinking, ineffective drainage, or advancing the tube into the duodenum
    ii. Signs of respiratory distress, coughing or cyanosis indicate that the tube is in respiratory tract. Remove the tube at once if there are signs of respiratory distress.
12. Secure the enteral tube temporarily to avoid accidental dislodgement and verify the tube placement in the stomach.
13. Check the enteral tube placement by aspirating stomach contents using a syringe, if aspiration is not contraindicated. Assess the characteristics of aspirate. Gastric aspirate is thin, clear and off white in color. Test acidity level of the aspirate by pH strip/tape. Level of pH - 5 or less suggests gastric placement. If pH level is > 5, it indicates respiratory, esophageal or intestinal placement or may be due to intake of acid suppression medications by the child
    i. Tube position in the stomach can be checked using syringe and stethoscope to auscultate the gush of air pushed by the syringe in the stomach
    ii. Failure to obtain aspirate from the tube does not indicate that the tube is placed improperly. There may be less stomach content or the enteral tube

may not be in contact with the gastric fluid.

14. After confirmation of proper tube placement, secure the tube with adhesive tape or transparent dressing to the child's face (usually at cheek), avoiding interference with the child's visual field. Avoid causing pressure and irritation to nasal mucosa.
15. Close the outer end of the feeding tube with the cap, unless directed to keep open.
16. Dispose all waste in appropriate containers. Take care of reusable items.
17. Remove gloves and other protective gears. Perform hand hygiene.
18. Document the procedure of insertion of feeding tube and related findings.

Intermittent or Bolus Enteral Feeding Through Nasogastric or Orogastric Tube

1. Perform hand hygiene and gather all necessary supplies near the child
2. Place the child in supine position, before the procedure begins, with the head of the bed up 30 degrees (if not otherwise contraindicated). Older children may be placed in sitting position or in a position of comfort. These help to prevent aspiration of gastric content and to promote flow of feed by gravity during feeding. A semi-Fowler's position or head of bed up or right side-lying position promotes gastric emptying and peristalsis
3. Measure prescribed amount of enteral feed to be given into sterile graduated measuring cup or catheter-tip syringe to promote safety for the delivery of feeds
4. Place a towel or washcloth under child's indwelling enteral tube or below child's chin and chest. It protects clothing and linen from emesis or secretions or spillage of feeds
5. Verify the placement of feeding tube in the stomach to prevent complications
6. Use sterile syringe to administer bolus feeding. Select appropriate size syringe (50 mL/20 mL/10 mL) according to the amount of total feed to be given and age of the child
7. Assess for residual gastric fluid, if indicated. Use syringe to aspirate for residual fluid. Monitoring residual fluids helps to prevent overfeeding and to detect early signs of feeding intolerance. Gastric residuals may be elevated because of formula intolerance, delayed gastric emptying, sepsis or underlying gastrointestinal disease process
8. Note the color and consistency of the aspirate. If more than one half of the previous feeds volume is obtained as aspirate or if there is change in color of the aspirate, hold the present feeding and notify the physician/healthcare prescriber
   - Follow the standard guidelines for continuation of feeding. If there is small amount of aspirate, then continue the enteral feeding procedure. Some authority suggests returning the aspirate to the stomach, if not contraindicated. Gastric aspirates contain enzymes, electrolytes and secretions essential for digestion, so discarding aspirates repeatedly could lead to electrolyte imbalances
9. Administer feed by attaching the syringe without plunger to the outer end of the feeding tube. Pour the measured feed volume in the attached barrel of the syringe. Allow the feed to flow slowly by gravity. Gradually add the total volume of feed into the syringe. Don't allow air entry into the syringe and feeding tube. Raising or lowering the syringe can adjust the rate of flow of feeding
   - The flow of feeding may need to be initiated by giving little pressure. Avoid forceful pressure during feeding. Enteral feeding delivered too rapidly may interfere with peristalsis, causing abdominal distention, possible cramping, regurgitation and/or diarrhea. Enteral feeding should flow freely by gravity to administer the feeding over about 15 minutes, which is a typical time frame for feeding
10. Observe the child during the feeding for intolerance and complications such

as elevated gastric residuals, emesis, abdominal distention, bradycardia or apnea

- Stimulation of the vagal nerve by the enteral tube can cause bradycardia or apnea. Feeding intolerance can occur with decreased gastric peristalsis secondary to underlying disease process, leading to inability to digest formula feeds

11. After feeding is complete, gently clear the feeding tube and catheter-tip syringe with measured amount lukewarm water flush. This prevents the feeding tube from clogging. Depending on child's age and diagnosis, free water adding is required to avoid potential dehydration that can result from high osmolality formulas
    - Excess free water may lead to fluid overload. Free water may not be indicated for many children with specific diagnosis, e.g., pulmonary, renal and/or cardiac conditions. Assess and monitor total volume of free water including flush volumes
12. If feeding tube is discontinued after each feeding, remove adhesive tape first, then pinch or clamp the enteral tube and withdraw/pull the tube out of the nares or mouth with slow, smooth and steady movement. This avoids leakage of contents from the tube, preventing possible aspiration of contents during removal of tube
    - Cleanse the feeding tube and syringe thoroughly with warm water and rinse well, if they are reused. Repeated use of feeding tube and syringe can be done up to 24 hours. Changing disposable supplies every 24 hours prevents bacterial growth
13. Change the placement of enteral tube every 3–7 days or as per unit policy
14. Administer oral care frequently, if the feeding tube is in place, unless contraindicated
15. Provide comfort measures to the child. Change adhesive tape as required and consider use of skin barrier to protect skin surface from the irritating effects of adhesive tape
16. Gradually, initiate oral feeding when the child's condition permits and decrease the duration of tube feeding to reduce complications and discomfort of the child related to placement of nasogastric or orogastric tube
17. Dispose all waste in appropriate containers and take care of reusable supplies
18. Remove gloves. Perform hand hygiene. Document the procedure of enteral feeding in details in intake and output chart and related findings.

Evaluation and Documentation

- Evaluate the placement and patency of the tube, integrity of skin around nares and at the adhesive tape area. Monitor intake, output and signs of respiratory distress, and compare with baseline data
- Document: Date and time of insertion of feeding tube, tube size and length inserted, child's tolerance of the procedure, method of confirmation of tube position and function, intake in feeds and amount of flushing water per feeding, any vomiting, any changes in tube placement and condition of skin around nares, mouth and under adhesive tape.

Communication and Teaching for Homecare

- Communicate with child and parents about the child's health condition, need for gavage feeding, response to this treatment and plan of further management
- Teach the parents about hand hygiene, general cleanliness, oral care, comfort measures and participation during routine care of the child in hospital. Instruct about care at home after discharge and follow-up visits for continuation of treatment.

Refer: Gavage Feeding for Neonates, in Procedure - 20 in the Unit - 2 of this Manual.

PROCEDURE–8: ORAL CARE OF INFANT AND YOUNG CHILD

Clinical Guidelines

- Oral hygiene and care of oral cavity is an important aspect of personal hygiene

to maintain cleanliness of mouth and to enhance sense of well being. Clean mouth improves appetite and digestion. This prevents bad taste, bad odor, oral infections, and tooth decay
- During illness, the children may have high body temperature, mouth breathing, inadequate nutrition and poor salivary secretions including dryness of mouth and mucous membrane and cracking of lips which lead to oral infections. So, it is important to provide appropriate care of the oral cavity to prevent further complications
- Oral care can be given as general mouth care for the children whose general health status is good and they are able to do it as self care. Independence should be encouraged to promote good habits of oral hygiene among children. Older children can take own oral care, if they not very sick and unable to maintain self care of this hygienic need
- Special mouth care is required for sick child who is unconscious, very ill, cannot able to swallow or not allowed any oral feed. Special oral care is also needed for the child having hyperpyrexia, any surgical interventions, oral infections or malignancy and in any sickness. Mentally retarded children also need help of oral hygiene or special mouth care
- Preventive dental care and regular dental check up is necessary as a part of oral hygiene
- Bottle feeding should always be discouraged to prevent baby-bottle tooth decay and its potential adverse sequelae as otitis media and diarrhea. Use of feeding bottle always leads to poor oral hygiene and dental problems
- During chemotherapy, assessment of oral cavity and maintenance of oral hygiene on daily basis must be emphasized. Pediatric oncology patients should be referred to pediatric dentist for evaluation, before initiation of chemotherapy or radiation therapy. Special emphasis should be provided to maintain oral hygiene of the children receiving chemotherapy with standard guidelines for oncology nursing
- Professional care provider should wear gloves before performing oral care to prevent contact with body fluids as standard precautions.

Equipment Required

- Hand hygiene supplies for hand wash and hand rub
- For oral care of infants—soft washcloth or gauze pads, clear warm water, clean gloves
- For oral care of toddlers and young children—soft bristle brush, toothpaste, dental floss, clear water, nonsterile gloves (use personal toothbrush and toothpaste of the child)
- For oncology patients (for self care or with assistance) - soft bristle brush, a bowl with gauze pieces/pads, toothpaste, dental floss, clear water, antiseptic mouth wash (as prescribed), sterile water, normal saline, medications (if prescribed), nonsterile gloves
- For special mouth care for unconscious or very sick children:

  A tray containing the following items:
  - A bowl with gauze pieces/mouth wipes to cleanse the oral cavity and teeth
  - Swab sticks, toothettes (disposable single use oral care sponge swabs attached to a stick)
  - A container with one pair of small dressing forceps to hold mouth wipes/ gauze pieces, one pair of dissecting forceps to remove mouth wipes, a padded tongue depressor for unconscious child to open the oral cavity and swab sticks to apply medications
  - Baby toothpaste or cleansing agents (sodium bicarbonate) to cleanse the mouth
  - Antiseptic mouthwash, as prescribed
  - Feeding cup with clean water to rinse child's mouth, depending upon child's condition

- A kidney tray to receive the waste water
- Glycerin or Vaseline to apply on lips to prevent cracked lips or medications for mouth
- Waterproof sheet or mackintosh and treatment towel to protect child's clothing
- Waste disposal containers as per BMW guidelines
- Procedure documentation sheet to record the oral care given to the child.

Assessment and Preparation

- Assess child's health condition, condition of oral cavity and ability to do age-appropriate self care activity for oral care
  - Assess oral cavity for integrity and color of tongue, gums, teeth, mucous membrane and lips. Check for presence of any irritations, potential infections, trauma and other abnormal conditions. Observe for tooth eruptions and placement. Assess child's ability to salivate, swallow and eat food. Assess for presence of any pain in oral cavity
  - Assess parent/caregiver's knowledge and ability regarding oral care, tooth eruptions and oral problems and tooth decay
- Self preparation should be done by practice of standard precautions of infection control
- Environment should be clean, calm, and well lighted
- Articles preparation should be done according to the type of oral care. Cleaning, disinfection and sterilization of care items should be done as required. All necessary supplies should be collected and arranged near the child
- Preparation of parents: Explain the importance and procedure of oral care. Encourage them to participate and learn the technique of oral care to perform or to assist the child
- Preparation of child: Explain the procedure in age-appropriate language. Make the child comfortable to perform the oral care. Assist the child during self oral care activity.

Performing the Steps of Procedure with Rationale/Point of Emphasis

1. Perform hand hygiene to reduce transmission of microorganisms.
2. Gather all necessary supplies near the child's bed for organized approach.
3. Wear gloves before performing special oral care to prevent contact with body fluids as standard precautions, especially in case of infected child and unconscious child.
4. *Provide oral care to the infants* with following steps:
   i. Position the infant on parent's lap or infant seat. Support infant's head and access to his or her mouth. If required, take help of second person to support or restraint the infant
   ii. Make a gentle and non-aggressive approach to prevent the infant crying and fear
   iii. Clean infant's gums and teeth (if teeth are erupting) after each feeding. Wrap a soft cloth or gauze piece soaked with warm water around your finger and wipe or massage the gums. Regular cleaning of gums provides comfort during eruptions of new teeth and soothes the irritated gums. It helps to remove excess plaque and bacteria. Teach this step to the mother, if she is present with the child
   iv. Add a small amount of baby toothpaste (the size of a rice grain) to the soft cloth or mouth wipes and wipe the erupted teeth. Take precautions to avoid swallowing of toothpaste by pasting it properly on the soft cloth. Adult brand toothpaste should not be used for the infants. Fluoridated toothpaste can be used for young children
   v. Remove the toothpaste using water soaked soft cloth or gauze pieces or toothettes. Infants are unable to spit out the excess toothpaste.

5. *Perform oral care for toddlers or young children* as follows:
   i. Engage the toddler and young child in the self care activity of tooth brushing, if developmentally appropriate and the child is medically stable. Allow the child to brush his or her teeth, followed by the mother/caregiver brushing the child's teeth until the child can achieve the ability to complete the task successfully. Be cautious of the amount of toothpaste for younger children, as they may swallow it. Too much fluoride can lead to enamel fluorosis or discoloration of teeth
   ii. Clean teeth and gums using "very soft" or "soft" toothbrush with thin bristles and small enough head to fit within child-sized oral cavity. This prevents plaque buildup and dental caries. Brush the child's teeth and gums gently
   iii. Use pea-sized amount of toothpaste and check that child is not swallowing it. If the child is unable to spit out the toothpaste, use water soaked gauze piece to cleanse the teeth. Small dressing forceps can be used to hold the gauze piece to cleanse the child's mouth
   iv. Floss the child's teeth once a day, if needed, to prevent plaque forming
   v. Brush child's teeth at least twice per day. If the child eats highly sweetened foods, then an extra brushing should be performed
   vi. Supervise the child during oral care and brushing up to at least 8 years of age.
6. *Provide special mouth care to very sick or unconscious children* as follow:
   i. Turn the child's head to one side to facilitate drainage of water from mouth and to prevent aspiration of water and cleansing agents
   ii. Protect child's clothing and bed with waterproof sheet and towel
   iii. Use tongue depressor to open child's mouth, whenever needed
   iv. Cleanse oral cavity gently with mouth wipes or gauze pieces soaked in cleansing solution and wrapped around a dressing forceps. Remove mouth wipes from the dressing forceps using a dissecting forceps only, to prevent cross contaminations
   v. Cleanse child's mouth with sterile water and remove cleansing agent
   vi. Ensure mouth is cleaned properly, before applying any medications
   vii. Apply glycerin or petroleum jelly to the lips to prevent drying and cracking
   viii. Provide special mouth care as indicated at 4–6 hours intervals
   ix. Take precautions to prevent any injury during special mouth care to very sick or unconscious child. Take help from other person/parent as required.
7. *Perform oral care for oncology patients* as follows:
   i. Review health records and discuss with family members about medical interventions that may be affecting oral mucosa (e.g., chemotherapy, radiation)
   ii. Assess child oral cavity for presence of oral infections or other problems
   iii. Assist the child, as needed, to perform oral hygiene. Brush with soft toothettes (it is disposable single use oral care sponge swabs attached to a stick). Toothbrush may cause bleeding of the gums
   iv. Use floss when there are no mouth sores or bleeding. This prevents food particles to remain in between teeth that can lead to cavity formation
   v. Ask the child to rinse and spit with mouthwash (chlorhexidine 0.1%), sterile water, sodium bicarbonate or Nystatin in presence of fungal infection, as prescribed. These solutions or medication help to keep the oral mucosa clean and free of debris. These solutions or medication should not be swallowed by the child
   vi. Apply oral analgesic agents, as prescribed, if the child is having pain due to stomatitis. Continue meticulous oral hygiene

vii. Restrict any oral intake of food for 30 minutes afterward to promote absorption of medication into the oral mucosa. Assess child's ability to eat food and swallow. Avoid hard and acidic foods to prevent irritation, abrasions and sore in oral cavity
viii. Apply lip balm or petroleum jelly on the lips to prevent cracking
ix. Take care to maintain oral hygiene three or four times a day for oncology patients
x. Encourage the child to sufficient amount of water to prevent drying of oral mucosa.

8. Make the child comfortable. Ask for presence of any discomfort or problems.
9. Dispose waste in appropriate containers. Take care of reusable supplies.
10. Remove gloves. Perform hand hygiene. Document the procedure of oral care and use of any medication or solution in child's record.

Evaluation and Documentation

- Evaluate child's oral cavity for presence of any problems and improvement found from previous state. Evaluate child's and caregiver's ability with understanding to perform appropriate oral care and dietary habits that support good oral health
- Document the time of oral care given, status of oral cavity and lips, cleansing agents/medication used and teaching provided to the child and parent/family member.

Communication and Teaching for Homecare

- Communicate with child and parents about the importance and procedure of oral hygiene and inform about the presence of any problems
- Teach the parents and child about age-appropriate oral care at hospital and home with precautions, need for adequate diet and water intake, identifications of clinical features of oral infections or other oral problems, need for dental check up and treatment, prompt management of any health problems with follow-up care.

PROCEDURE–9: BATHING INFANT OR YOUNG CHILD

Clinical Guidelines

- Bathing is a hygienic practice that provides sense of cleanliness and comfort to all individuals. Bath can be given as sponge bath and tub bath. Older ambulatory children can use bathroom for thorough bath, under supervision. Daily morning bath should be provided, unless it is contraindicated. Bath is given to the sick children on bed at hospital or home and known as bed-bath. Avoid unnecessary handling of sick child during bathing
- Tub bath is the common method of bathing the infant and young children. Dip tub bathing of the children by immersing in lukewarm water helps to observe child's behavior in water and gives the child a chance to do exercise. It makes the child happy and stimulates his or her blood circulation
- Child's age, medical condition and hemodynamic stability helps to determine the type of bath to be given. Review the child's treatment chart to determine the type of bath, when last bath given and child's last recorded body temperature
- Find out the special needs of the children before starting the dip tub bath. Some restrictions for bathing may apply to the child with surgical incisions, traction, IV catheter, casts, urinary catheters and artificial airways
- Weight recording and vital signs measurement can be done during daily morning bath for hospitalized children. Fingers and toe nails should be checked during bathing. Arrange to cut the nails using nail cutting scissors or nail cutter, whenever needed. Skin conditions (especially skin folds, perianal region), conditions of eyes, mouth, genitalia and general behavior of the child should be assessed during bathing and prompt management should

be initiated for any abnormal conditions. Prevention of cross infections should be emphasized by use of individual or personal bathing items like separate soap, wash cloth, towel, bath tub, comb or hair brush, etc.

Equipment Required for Tub Bath

- Hand washing supplies for hand wash and hand rub
- Waterproof apron for care provider to protect the dress
- Clean non-sterile gloves to prevent cross infections, as per hospital policy
- Baby dress/clothing - frock, shirt, cap, socks, and diapers
- Baby sheet, linen, and dry blanket especially in winter season to remake the baby's bed
- Two Bath towels - for wrapping and drying the baby
- Two wash cloths - to give bath to the infant
- Sterile cotton balls/swabs in a covered sterile bowl, if required
- Basin with lukewarm water to be used for bathing the child. Water temperature for bathing should be 100°F or 37.8°C
- Two water jugs - one with hot water and another with water having normal temperature
- Bath thermometer to measure the water temperature
- Baby Soap to clean the baby's skin, as recommended
- Baby Oil to apply on baby's dry and rough skin, if needed
- Baby Powder, as recommended. Usually baby powder is used for axillae or perianal area or groin to prevent bad odor. It should not be irritating to the baby's skin
- Soft bristle hair brush or fine toothed comb
- Diaper changing supplies and disposable cleaning wipes, as available
- Waterproof sheet or mackintosh and towel to protect the bed/crib
- Waste disposal containers as per BMW rules for clothing and linen
- Procedure documentation sheet for bathing the child and related observational findings.

Assessment and Preparation

- Assess the child's health status, body temperature, skin conditions and presence of any abnormal features or special medical or surgical conditions with specific instructions. Identify the feasibility and type of bathing to the child
- Self preparation should be done with hand washing and following standard precautions of infection control measures. Take help of the parent to make the child cooperative during bathing and observation
- Environment should be clean, calm, quiet, well lighted, well ventilated, warm and free from draughts. No fan should be running near the procedure area. Close the nearby window
- Articles preparation: All supplies should be collected and arranged near the child's bed/crib or in the procedure room. Prepare bath table in the procedure room. Table should be attached to the wall. All required supplies should be arranged on the table for easy access. Child should be protected from falling from the table. Table or bed should be protected with waterproof sheet or mackintosh. Cleanliness of all required equipment must be maintained to prevent nosocomial infections
- Preparation of parents: Explain the importance of procedure of bathing and allow the parent to participate during the bathing. Instruct about special precautions
- Preparation of child: Explain the importance and technique of bathing in age-appropriate language and ask for cooperation during the procedure. Provide comfort and safety to the child. Check the diaper of the infant and young child. Change if it is soiled before initiating bathing to ensure cleanliness.

Performing the Steps of Procedure with Rationale/Point of Emphasis

Giving a Sponge Bath

Refer: Bathing (Sponge Bath) and Diapering the Neonates, in Procedure - 9 in the Unit - 2 of this Manual.

Giving a Tub Bath

1. Perform hand hygiene to prevent transmission of microorganisms.
2. Collect and gather all necessary supplies near the child or in procedure room for time management and organized approach to the procedure.
3. Ensure that the opposite side rail of the crib is raised, if the tub bath is given on crib.
4. Ensure the child is not having any problem that is contraindicated for tub bath.
5. Fill the bath tub with lukewarm water (two to three inches). Water temperature should be about 100°F or 37.8°C to prevent scalding of child's skin. If water thermometer is not available, then test the water temperature using the inside of your wrist or elbow.
6. Perform hand hygiene again and don gloves as standard precautions, whenever needed.
7. Undress the child to prepare for bath. Ensure diaper area is clean, before placing the child in the bath tub with water.
8. Gradually slip the infant/young child into the water in bathtub while supporting the neck and head. Take precautions to prevent water to enter into the ears. Close both external ear orifice of the child with the thumb and one finger, if possible or use cotton plug.
9. Wash child's face with wet wash cloth and dry with towel.
10. Wash the child's body with soapy cloth, beginning at the shoulder and arms continuing to the lower extremities. Cleanse the skin folds thoroughly. Take special attention to buttocks, groins, genital area and perianal region. Starting with the cleanest area progressing to the area that is most soiled helps to keep the bath water cleaner.
11. Change the bathing water before rinsing. Then rinse the child thoroughly with a clean, damp washcloth to remove the soap completely. This helps to prevent skin irritation of the child.
12. Dry the child's body using dry towel thoroughly with special attention to skin folds. Avoid chilling.
13. Wrap the child with sheet or blanket and ready for hair wash.
14. Discard the used water and take fresh lukewarm water for hair wash.
15. Wash child's hair to maintain cleanliness, to prevent drying of scalp and formation of cradle cap, with the following steps:
    - Ensure wrapping of the child in a warm sheet or blanket to stabilize his or her body temperature during hair wash and securing the child's arms close to the body
    - Place the child or infant in football hold position in one hand (e.g., left hand) and washing hair with other hand (e.g., right hand)
    - Position the child's head over the wash basin or bath tub for hair washing. Support the child's back and neck, while allowing the head to drop slightly backward at an angle that prevents water and soap from running into the child's eye
    - Close the external ear orifice of the child with cotton plug or with thumb and finger
    - Lather the child's hair and scalp with mild soap or shampoo to cleanse the hair and scalp and prevent seborrhea
    - Wash the child's hair using damp soapy cloth and rinse thoroughly. Residue of soap or shampoo on hair may irritate the child's scalp
    - Dry the child's hair and scalp with dry towel thoroughly
    - Comb the child's hair with fine toothed comb or soft-bristle brush. It helps to remove crusts from infant's scalp, if there is cradle cap on infant's head
    - Remove the blanket or sheet used for wrapping on completion of hair wash.
16. Dress the child adequately with dry clothing to prevent loss of body heat.
17. Apply body powder or body oil to the child, whenever necessary.
18. Position the child for comfort and with safety in crib/bed. Ensure bedside rails are up.
19. Cleanse and rinse the wash basin or bath tub and other reusable items. Dry and

store in the storage area for reuse. Follow standard precautions of infection control.

20. Dispose the waste in appropriate containers to prevent transmission of microorganisms.
21. Remove gloves. Perform hand hygiene. Document the procedure of bathing.

Evaluation and Documentation

- Evaluate child's health status and presence of abnormal clinical features during bath. Compare with baseline data to detect improvement or deteriorations of health condition. Evaluate child's ability to perform self care for bathing and response to hygienic practices. Evaluate parents ability to give bath to sick and small child with precautions
- Document the time and type of bath given to the child, child's response to bath, observational findings, presence of any abnormalities and parent-child interaction (when parents are giving bath or participating during bathing procedure).

Communication and Teaching for Homecare

- Communicate with child and parents about child's health condition and presence of any abnormal conditions
- Teach the parents about importance of personal hygiene and regular bath, precautions during daily bath and bathing of sick young child. Instruct the parent to inform healthcare providers, if any abnormal skin lesions or any other abnormalities are found
  - Inform the parent that at home mother or caregiver can give bath to the infant and young child on stretched legs or on lap, if they like to avoid tub bath. Make the parent aware that infant and young child should never be left alone when bathing whether in the tub of water or in bathroom
    - » Demonstrate the bathing procedure to the parents, especially for sick child, and take return demonstrations to assess their ability and competency to perform the basic bathing procedure with precautions for the child.

Refer: Bathing (Sponge Bath) and Diapering the Neonates, in Procedure - 9 in the Unit - 2 of this Manual

PROCEDURE–10: CARE OF INFECTED EYES AND ADMINISTRATION OF OPHTHALMIC MEDICATIONS

Clinical Guidelines

- Clean eyes are important aspect of personal hygiene. Regular eye cleaning is done during bathing along with face cleaning using clean washcloth. Special care and cleaning of eyes required when it is infected and any injury occurred or any surgical interventions are performed for any disease conditions
- Always ensure clean eyes before administration of any ophthalmic medications for its optimal therapeutic effects. Eye cleaning should be done using sterile cotton swabs soaked in sterile water or normal saline for better removal of secretions and crusts. Clean the eyes from inner canthus to outer canthus, using separate swabs each time for complete removal of eye discharges. This helps to prevent blocking of nasolacrimal duct
- Eye infections are common in infants and older children. Conjunctivitis is the most common inflammatory condition.
- It occurs due to viral and bacterial infections and may be a highly contagious disease condition. Strict maintenance of hand hygiene helps to prevent spread of infection from one eye to the other and transfer of infection from the affected person to others
- Care of the infected eyes should be done following aseptic technique to treat the infections, to administer prescribed medications, to maintain cleanliness of the eyes and to prevent complications. Routine eye care is not recommended, unless indicated
- Eye drops and ointments are prescribed for treatment of infected or diseased eyes.

Principles of pharmacologic management must be followed during administration of medications to the eyes

- Follow the Principles of Pharmacologic Management. *Refer Unit - 1 of this Manual for the Principles*
- Follow at least "Ten Rights" for administration of medications to the children.

Equipment Required

- Hand hygiene supplies for hand wash and hand rub to prevent cross infections
- A sterile tray containing all sterile items including gloves, a small bowl with cotton swabs, a small bowl with normal saline or sterile water (as prescribed), and sterile gauze pieces or tissue papers
- A clean tray containing prescribed eye drops or ointment and a small towel
- Waste disposal containers
- Documentation sheet, child case sheet and treatment sheet.

Assessment and Preparation

- Assess the child for presence of signs and symptoms of eye infections and its complications. Identify child's previous experiences with receiving ophthalmic medications. Assess child's and parent's understanding of need for care of infected eyes and importance of administration of ophthalmic medications
- Self preparation should be done with appropriate hand hygiene
- Environment should be clean, calm, and well lighted
- Articles required for the procedure should be collected and arranged near the child. Aseptic technique must be followed using sterile items for eye care
- Preparation of parents: Explain the importance of care of infected eyes and need for medications. Allow the parents to observe the procedure, so that they can do it at home, whenever necessary
- Preparation of child: Explain the procedure of eye care, its purpose and possible discomfort during the administration of medications in age-appropriate language. Encourage the child to cooperate during the eye care and medications to promote safety.

Performing the Steps of Procedure with Rationale/Point of Emphasis

1. Ensure about child's eye condition and verify child's identity.
2. Verify the treatment from medical record. Confirm whether the medication is to be administered into both eyes or in only one eye and into which eye, if in only one. It will reduce medication error.
3. Perform hand hygiene. Assemble all care items near the child. Check the expiry date of the drugs. Medications should be at room temperature. If it is not warm, hold the eye drop vial between hands to make it warm. Cold medication increases discomfort.
4. Perform hand hygiene again and don gloves to reduce transmission of microorganisms.
5. Position the child supine in bed or other flat surface, and ask to look up.
6. Restraint the child, if only required in case of noncooperation. Obtain other person to hold the child and to make the child to lie still, if needed.
7. Cleanse the eye with sterile cotton ball or gauze soaked with normal saline to remove sticky discharge and crust. Cleanse from inner canthus of the eyelid to the outer canthus. Use a new sterile cotton ball each time for sweeping the eye. Previous medications or eye discharge may remain sticky around the eye. Using a new cotton ball or gauze for each sweeping of the eye helps to cleanse the area easily and to prevent contaminations.
8. Assess the child's eye condition during cleansing.
9. Administer medication into the eye as follows **(Figs. 3.3A and B)**:
   - Place your dominant hand (holding the medication vial or tube) against the child's forehead. With the other hand, pull down the lower eyelid to expose

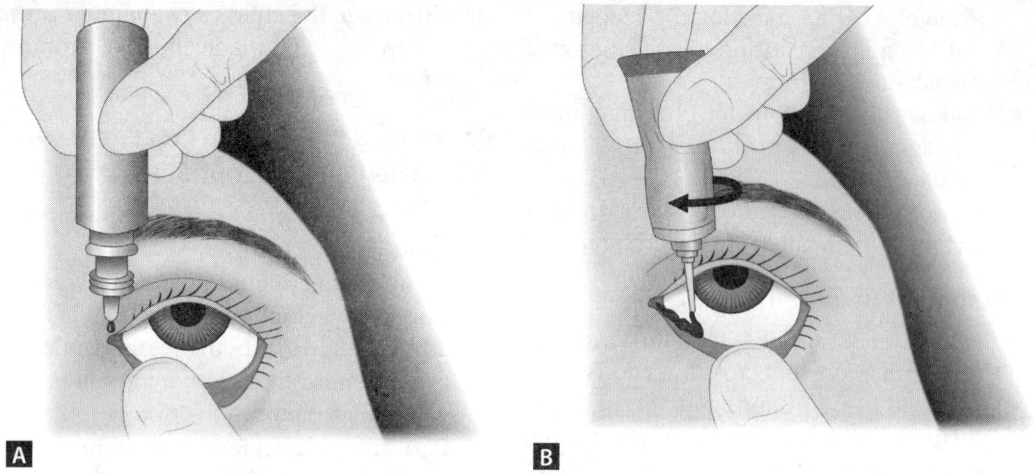

Figs. 3.3A and B: Administration of ophthalmic medications. A. Installation of eye drops. B. Administration of eye ointment.

the conjunctival sac for placement of medication

- Instill correct amount of prescribed eye drops, using dropper, into the conjunctival sac. Be careful not to touch the dropper to the eye to prevent contamination. Ask the child to keep the eye open for few seconds, otherwise eye drops may expel out
- Apply ointment by twisting the ointment tube at the end to dislodge the ointment from the tube and place a thin ribbon of ointment along the entire conjunctival sac from the inner canthus to the outer canthus. Instruct the child to keep his or her eyes closed for up to 1 minute after administration of ointment.

10. Wipe off the excess medication with a cotton ball or tissue paper. It prevents irritation of the skin surrounding the eyes due to medication.
11. Place the child comfortably. Arrange for safe storage of medications. Each child should have his or her own medication to prevent cross-contamination. Ophthalmic medications (eye drops or ointment) should not be shared with others.
12. Dispose the waste. Take care of reusable items. Remove gloves. Perform hand hygiene.
13. Document the procedure of care of infected, eye condition, medications administered to the child, and any teaching given to the parent and child.

Evaluation and Documentation

- Evaluate the child for therapeutic effects and side effects of ophthalmic medications. Evaluate child's response and understanding level related to this procedure. Determine whether the child and family members have additional areas of concern and discuss accordingly
- Document the condition of the child's eyes, date and time of procedure done, type and dose of medication administered, site of medication (right eye, left eye or both), presence and absence of adverse effects of medication used and child's tolerance of procedure.

Communication and Teaching for Homecare

- Communicate with child and parents about child's eye condition and plan of further management. Encourage to ask questions and answer in simple language
- Teach the parents about hand hygiene, other hygienic practices, general cleanliness and causes of eye infections. Dis-

cuss about signs of complications of eye infections, adverse reactions and safe storage of medications. Demonstrate and take return demonstration of technique of administering ophthalmic medications with precautions, for both eye drops and ointment. Instruct the parents about continuation of treatment at home whenever required, need for medical assistance in case of complications and plan of follow-up visits.

PROCEDURE–11: MEDICATIONS TO THE CHILDREN—ORAL, SUBLINGUAL AND BUCCAL

Clinical Guidelines

- Follow the Principles of Pharmacologic Management. *Refer Unit - 1 of this Manual for the Principles.*
- Follow at least "Ten Rights" for administration of medications to the children
- Purposes of oral medications are mainly for therapeutic effects to cure diseases or to treat deficiency conditions. Oral medications/drugs is given before some diagnostic procedures and also to prevent some disease conditions
- Use *oral route* for administration of medications to the children because it is least invasive method and less traumatic than intramuscular (IM) and IV routes. The gastrointestinal (GI) tract provides a vast absorptive area for medications. This absorption from GI tract, as well as distribution, metabolism, and elimination differs with maturation of the GI tract. Factors such as gastric pH, gastric emptying time, motility, absorptive area, enzyme activity, and dietary factors affect absorption

  Oral medications are used for the infants and young children as syrup and drops. Tablets and capsules are administered to the older children. Accurate measurements of liquid medicine is prime importance to prevent dosing error of medications
  - Administer oral medications in a manner consistent with the child's age and developmental abilities. The following guidelines for the specific age group should be highlighted during administering oral medications:
    » *For the infant:* Up to 3–4 months of age, liquid medication should be given using oral syringe. The rooting and sucking reflex stimulates the infant to suck the medication from the syringe and swallow it. For 5–12 months of age, put liquid medication in an oral syringe and administer in small amounts toward the side of mouth, not toward the throat and lightly stimulate the infant to swallow. Oral medicine can be placed on a spoon in a small amount of sweet-tasting food or breast milk and fed to infant. Never give honey to an infant because of risk for botulism
    » *For toddler:* Explain in simple terms and language about the reasons of medications. Use same technique as followed in infant. Involve parents during medications and permit expression of their feelings
    » *For preschooler, school-aged children, and adolescent:* Explain the purpose of procedure in simple language. Offer choices on technique to gain child's cooperation
- *Sublingual* (under the tongue) and *buccal* (between the cheek and gum) routes are transmucosal administration of medications to the children used for particular drugs. Medications from these routes are absorbed by the oral mucosa, which has rich vascular supply and lacks a stratum corneum epidermidis; therefore absorption by this route is rapid. Medications given through these routes can be detected in the blood within 1 minute and peak levels are generally achieved within 10–15 minutes.
- Expiration date of the medication must be checked always, if the date is expired do not administered that drugs
- History of drug allergy should be obtained. Allergic medications must be avoided to

prevent life-threatening allergic reactions

- Adverse or side effects of administered medications must be monitored frequently and need to explain to the parent
- Recording of medication administration is an important legal documents of treatment given to the sick individual and it must be maintained accurately to prevent medication errors especially for sick child.

Equipment Required

- Hand hygiene supplies for hand wash and hand rub to reduce cross infections
- Nonsterile gloves for standard precautions, as per hospital/unit policy
- A tray containing - correct prescribed medications (drops/syrup/tablets/capsules), oral syringe or medicine cup, covered container with drinking water, spoon, small towel, mouth wipes, gauze pieces
- A small tray to carry the prepared medicine to the child for administration
- Treatment sheet or medication card, child case sheet
- Waste disposal containers
- Medication documentation/record sheet.

Assessment and Preparation

- Assess child's present health status, history of drug allergy and previous experience with oral medications. Assess child's and parents level of understanding and ability to perform the procedure of oral medications
- Self preparation should be done with hand hygiene
- Environment should be clean, calm, and well lighted
- All necessary supplies should be collected and arranged in the procedure room for preparation and then near the child for administration of medications. Prepare medicine should be carried to the child safely
- Preparation of parents: Explain the therapeutic effects and side effects of the medicine and technique of administration of oral medications. Allow the parent to participate during administration of medication. Teach this procedure and its precautions
- Preparation of child: Explain the procedure of oral medication in age-appropriate language. Make the child comfortable. Allow the expression of anger and feelings.

Performing the Steps of Procedure with Rationale/Point of Emphasis

1. Verify the treatment order with the child's medical record. Check correct drug, dose, route, frequency, time and patient's name. Check record for history of any drug allergy.
2. Collect all supplies for administration of medications in the procedure room.
3. Perform hand hygiene. Don gloves, as per hospital policy, for standard precautions.
4. Obtain the medication and read the label to verify with the treatment order.
5. Check expiration date and any change in color of the medication to be administered.
6. Ensure that the form of medication to be administered orally to the child is appropriate for age and health condition.
   - Many children are unable to swallow tablets/pills or capsules, so they may need in the form of syrup or drops. Solid medications that are not sustained-release preparations may be crushed and mixed with small amount of liquid or food.
7. Prepare medication for administration to the child. Measure all liquid medications using oral syringe for accurate measurement or using medicine cup. Use tuberculin or 1 mL syringe for medications less than 1 mL.
   - Household spoons are inaccurate for measurement and there may be spillage of medications during oral administration. Accurate measurement is very important because small error in amount of medications could be dangerous for the child.
8. Take the prepared medications and medication record to the child for administration
9. Verify the child's identity by comparing name of the child from identifier, such

as parent or caregiver or child with identification band and from medication record to prevent error

10. *For administration of oral medications:* Position the child upright with head elevated (if not contraindicated), or pick up and hold the small child or infant to give medication in the mouth. Upright position helps in swallowing and prevent choking and aspiration
11. Administer the medication into the child's mouth slowly. Deliver liquid medications in small amounts, placing the syringe to the side of the child's mouth and allow swallowing the medicine in between. Administration of 0.2–0.5 mL medication at a time prevents choking. Placing the syringe to the side of mouth prevent gagging
12. *For administration of medications in sublingual or buccal route:* Place the medication under child's tongue (sublingual) or between the cheek and the gum (buccal). Alternate side of the mouth should be used for subsequent doses in these routes
    - The child should not be allowed to take any food or to drink any liquid or to do smoking while the medication is in his or her mouth. Eating, drinking and smoking interfere with absorption of medications
13. Stay with the child until the medication is swallowed. Older children can take tablets or capsules by themselves. Never leave any medication at bedside of the child, it could be forgotten or can be taken by another child. Allow parents to administer the oral medications, if they are willing, but that should be under nursing supervision
14. Make the child comfortable and observe for any abnormalities or side effects
15. Dispose syringe and all other disposable items in appropriate BMW containers
16. Remove gloves. Perform hand hygiene. Document the medications administered.

Evaluation and Documentation

- Evaluate the child's reactions to the procedure and presence of therapeutic and adverse effects of administered medication. Evaluate child's and family's understanding of medication effects
- Document date, time, type, dose, route and name of medication. Record the presence or absence of adverse effects and tolerance of procedure of oral medication. Keep record of the teaching and demonstration given to parents and older children for self care.

Communication and Teaching for Homecare

- Communicate with child and parents about child's present health status, improvement or presence of any problems, plan of future management and additional areas of concern
- Teach the parents about technique of oral medications and necessary precautions that should be continued at home. Instruct about prevention of illness by hygienic practices, and good dietary habit. Discuss about daily routine care of the child, need for emergency medical help after discharge from hospital and plan of follow-up visits.

PROCEDURE –12: PARENTERAL MEDICATIONS TO CHILDREN—INTRAMUSCULAR AND SUBCUTANEOUS

Clinical Guidelines

- Follow the Principles of Pharmacologic Management. *Refer Unit - 1 of this Manual for the Principles*
- Follow at least "Ten Rights" for administration of medications to the children
- Medications are given intramuscularly for rapid drug absorption because muscle has rich blood supply. The IM route is more painful than other routes because muscle has more nerves. Alternative less painful routes should be considered when available as oral or IV access.
    - Common and easy site for IM injections is vastus lateralis for the age group of infant, toddler, preschool-aged and

school-aged. The vastus lateralis is relatively large muscle in infants and free from major blood vessels and nerves.
  - Needle length for IM should be for infant - ½ inches, for toddler-½ inches–1 inches and preschooler and school-aged -1 inches. Volume of IM medication should be for infant - 0.5 mL, for toddler - 0.5–1 mL, for preschooler - 1 mL, and for school-aged - 1.5–2 mL. Needle insertion angle should be 70–90 degrees for IM injections and volume of medication should not be more than 2 mL
  - Other sites (i.e., ventrogluteal, dorsogluteal, and deltoid) for IM injections are usually not used for the young children. For grown up adolescent age group with good muscle mass, the adult guidelines can be followed for IM injections
  - Avoid IM injections in the area of impaired tissue integrity which will further damage or have potential risk for spread of infection or abscess formation
- Medications are given subcutaneously (SC) when a slower rate of absorption is desired, because fatty tissue has fewer blood vessels. This site can only be used for medications that do not cause tissue irritation. Needle length for SC injections for infant or child should be - 3/8 inches, for adolescent - ½ inches to 5/8 inches. Needle gauge for SC injection should be 25–27 G. The amount of medication for SC injection should be no more than 0.5 mL to small child and 1 mL for preschooler or school-aged child or adolescent to prevent complications of injection site.

Equipment Required

- Hand hygiene supplies for hand wash and hand rub to prevent cross infections
- A tray containing prescribed medications, sterile syringe pack of appropriate size, sterile needle of age-appropriate gauge size and length, sterile cotton swabs or wipes in covered bowl, bottle of 70% alcohol or alcohol swabs, single use gloves for administration of medications, knife dish or a small container to carry the prepared syringe with medication to the child, and adhesive band-aid/bandage for covering injection site (as per unit policy)
- Transfer forceps or lifter to handle to sterile items
- Treatment sheet or medication card, child case sheet
- Waste disposal containers as per BMW guidelines
- Medication documentation or treatment record sheet.

Assessment and Preparation

- Assess for child's vital signs, general health status, age, muscle mass, skin conditions and presence of any physical limitations which will impact for choice of site for IM or SC injections
  - Assess child for previous experience with receiving injections and history of drug allergy
  - Assess parents' level of understanding about the medications and ability to participate during medications and to learn the SC injections whenever required
- Self preparation should be done with hand washing and practice of other precautions
- Environment should be clean, calm, well lighted and well ventilated
- Necessary supplies should be collected and arranged in medication room for preparation of medication. Prepared medication and medication card/treatment sheet only to be taken at child's bedside to administer medication. Aseptic technique and handling of sterile items should be done carefully to prevent contamination and infection at injection site
- Preparation of parents: Explain the need for medication, its action and side effects. Allow parent to support the child during injections to promote child's coping
- Preparation of child: Explain the procedure of injections, its purpose and about pain during injection in age-appropriate

simple local language. Tell the child to stay as still as possible and not to move during injection to prevent further trauma. Never give false information. Provide therapeutic play (toys, play materials) and distract the child by storytelling or other measures. Use topical anesthetic when time allows for reducing pain and trauma of injections (as per hospital policy). Make the child clean and comfortable.

Performing the Steps of Procedure with Rationale/Point of Emphasis

Administering Intramuscular Injections to the Child

1. Verify the medication order with the medical record to detect possible transcription errors.
2. Perform hand hygiene to reduce transmission of microorganisms.
3. Assemble all necessary supplies in the medication room for time management.
4. Obtain prescribed medication and read the label to verify with the order. Check the expiration date, if expired, do not administered. This helps to decrease the chance of medication error by ensuring "right drugs".
5. Bring the medication to room temperature before administration, if storage was in refrigerator. Cold medication causes increased discomfort when injected.
6. Check the amount of medication to be administered to determine syringe size and appropriateness for the child. Limit the volume of medication according to the age of the child and the size of the muscle to be used (Refer clinical guidelines for IM injection of this procedure). Use 1 mL syringe to administer medication volume of 0.5 mL or less for dose accuracy. Large volumes of medication injected into small muscle can result in leakage of medication out of the muscle and lead to muscle atrophy.
7. Choose appropriate needle length for the site and muscle size (Refer clinical guidelines of this procedure). The needle must be long enough to enter the muscle mass and minimizes injury to the tissue and leakage into subcutaneous tissue.
8. Select needle gauge based on what is available for the appropriate needle length for the child and medication viscosity. Usually 22- or 23- or 24- or 26 gauge needle is appropriate for the children depending on age and muscle mass. Large gauge needles have narrower bore and thus produce a jet under high pressure, which causes more damage to the tissue.
9. Don gloves to maintain standard precautions to reduce transmission of microorganisms.
10. Draw up the medication with aseptic and non-touch technique in the medication room. As sight of needle can increase the child's fear and anxiety. Draw up correct amount of medication into the syringe with exact dose. Medication must be measured accurately because a small error in amount of drug could result in dangerous dosage variation
    Do not draw up additional air into the syringe, because clearing the needle of air can affect the dose to be administered.
11. Use a separate filter needle to draw medication up from an ampule or rubber-topped vial and then change to appropriate-sized needle before giving injection. This prevents small particles such as glass or other substances from entering the syringe.
12. Verify the medication for second time again from treatment sheet/record. Carry the syringe with medication in a sterile knife dish/kidney dish to the child for administration along with medication card/record.
13. Verify the child's identity by comparing name on medication record with child's identification band and any other patient identifier or parent to ensure right patient thus to prevent medication error.
14. Position comfortably and restrain the child securely for giving injection. Position may help the muscle to relax thus causing less pain. Restraint decreases chance of injury

from child's movement. Assistance from other person may require for securing the child. Parents may remain with the child to give support but they should not be responsible for securing the child.

15. Distract the child by storytelling or blowing bubbles. To decrease the perception of pain sensation at IM injection site, manual pressure can be applied on the injection site by the thumb of nondominant hand for 10 seconds before giving injection to the child. Other non-pharmacological measures can be used for pain reduction.
16. Cleanse the IM injection site with alcohol swab or alcohol wipe and allow drying before injection. This decreases entry of microorganisms and minimizes pain at the injection site. For therapeutic IM injection, skin preparation should be done with alcohol swab. But for vaccination by IM injection, use of alcohol is not recommended (Refer **Figs. 3.4A to D**).
17. Insert the needle quickly at 70–90 degree angle. Aspirate to check for blood, if blood found during aspiration, remove the needle. Then replace that needle with another sterile one and start over. This facilitates needle entry into the muscle. Aspiration prevents IV or intra-arterial administration of drug.
18. Inject the medication slowly. Slow injection may reduce local damage and pain.
19. Withdraw the needle after injecting total volume of medication. Apply pressure over the site with a dry sterile cotton ball

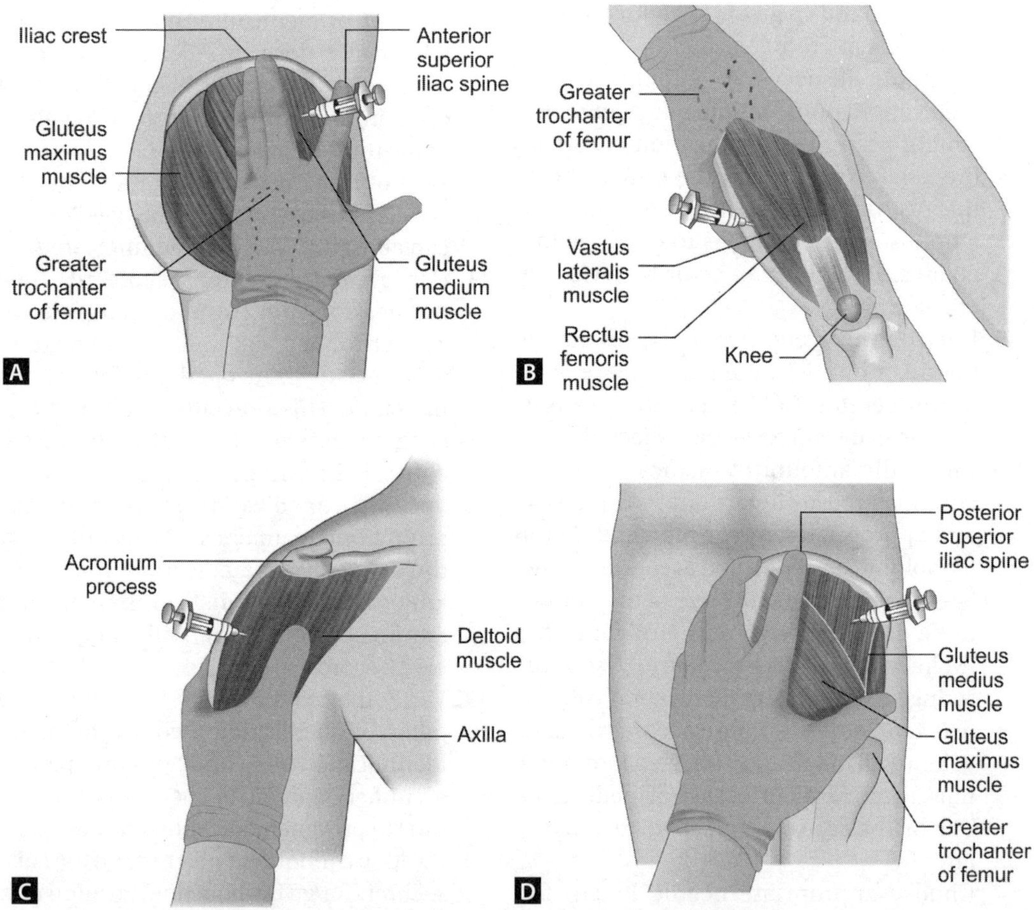

Figs. 3.4A to D: Sites for the Intramuscular injections. A. Ventrogluteal; B. Vastus lateralis; C. Deltoid for older children; D. Dorsogluteal for older children.

or gauze to prevent bleeding. Alcohol should not be applied over injection site as it may sting and prolong bleeding.

20. Follow the "Z-tract method" for caustic medications, such as iron. This helps to prevent leakage of medications into subcutaneous tissue, decreasing pain and other complications
    - To inject medication using Z-tract method, use a new sterile needle. Using new needle avoids medication being on the outside of the needle and coming in contact with tissue as the needle is inserted
    - Pull the skin with nondominant hand laterally or downward away about ½ inch (1.25 cm) from the injection site. Insert the needle into the muscle at 90-degree angle at the injection site where you initially placed your finger to displace the skin. Pulling the skin and subcutaneous layers displaces them out of alignment with the underlying muscle to trap the drug in the muscle after the structures return to their normal position
    - Aspirate for blood return, if blood is aspirated discontinue the procedure. If no blood appears, inject the drug slowly. Wait for 10 seconds, if possible, before withdrawing the needle. Withdraw the needle slowly and release the displaced skin and subcutaneous tissue to seal the needle track. Waiting before withdrawing the needle after injection helps to ensure dispersion of medication.
21. Do not recap the needle after administration of medication. Destroy the needle and syringe before disposal using hub cutter. Dispose the syringe and needle in puncture-proof sharp container to reduce chance of needlestick injuries.
22. Place adhesive bandage/band-aid over the injection site, as per unit policy. Young children will like it and feel that there will be no leak out from the injection site, if bandage/band-aid is used.
23. Make the child comfortable during injection and praise for cooperation. Clear all supplies from child's bed. Allow the parent to comfort the child. This promotes positive nurse-patient relationship and decreases long-term negative effects of painful procedure.
24. Discard all waste. Take care of all reusable supplies as standard precautions.
25. Remove gloves and perform hand hygiene to prevent cross infections.
26. Return to the child a short time later for positive interaction. Assess signs of adverse reactions to medications and bleeding from the injection site. This provides opportunity to further evaluate the child's physical and emotional response to the procedure.
27. Document the procedure of administration of IM injections and related findings.

Administering Subcutaneous Injections to the Child

1. Follow the **step 1 to step 5 same as IM injections.**
2. Check the amount of medication in SC route to be administered. It helps to determine syringe size and appropriateness for the child. Limit the volume of medication according to the age of the child and the size of the adipose tissue (Refer clinical guidelines for SC injection of this procedure). Large volumes of medication injected into the SC tissue can result in tissue injury.
3. Choose appropriate needle size in gauge and length for SC medication considering child's size and SC injection site. Viscous medication requires a larger gauge needle. Use the needle with smallest bore. Usually 25–27 gauge needle is used for SC injection to children. Do not use a needle longer than 5/8 inches. Longer needle may result in intramuscular instead of subcutaneous administration.
4. Follow next steps as **step 9 to step 14, as for IM injections.**
5. Distract the child by storytelling or blowing bubbles to decrease perception of pain sensation.
6. Evaluate the child's amount of subcutaneous tissue. Choose the most

appropriate site considering the adequacy and condition of subcutaneous tissue and duration of therapy. Subcutaneous injections sites include abdomen, lateral upper arm and thighs. There is wide variation in the amount of subcutaneous fat in the children. This may necessitate choosing an alternative site in the child. Give choice to the child (Refer **Fig. 3.5** for Sites of subcutaneous injections).

7. Restrain the child securely. Assess the need for additional help for holding the child during SC injection and obtain help as indicated. Parent should not be responsible for securing the child but may remain with the child to give support, such as holding the child's hand. This decreases chance of injury from movement of limbs or body parts, because even cooperative children have a tendency to move during injections.
8. Cleanse the injection site with antiseptics soaked cotton swab and allow drying. Allowing the antiseptic solution to dry promotes antimicrobial action of antiseptics and minimizes pain at injection site
   - Insulin injections in SC route do not require skin preparation with antiseptics but skin cleanliness at the injection site must be ensured.
9. Grasp the SC injection site and elevate the tissue. Insert the needle quickly at 45-degree angle, if there is little tissue or at 60–90-degree, if subcutaneous tissue is abundant. Elevating the site helps to separate the subcutaneous tissue from the underlying muscle.
10. Aspirate to check for blood, if blood is seen in the syringe, remove the needle. If blood is not present, slowly inject the medication. Slow injection reduces local damage and pain.
11. Do not aspirate when administering injections of insulin or heparin.
12. Withdraw the needle quickly at the same angle at which it was inserted and apply pressure over the injection site with a dry sterile cotton ball to prevent bleeding.
13. Follow next steps as **step 21 to step 27, as for IM injections.**

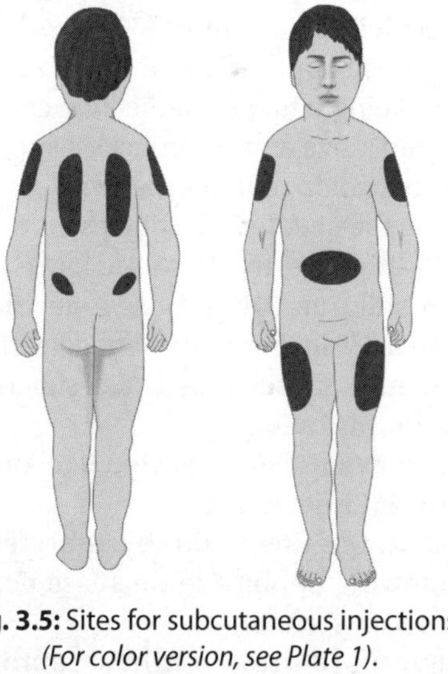

Fig. 3.5: Sites for subcutaneous injections *(For color version, see Plate 1).*

Evaluation and Documentation

- Evaluate the child for changes in vital signs, hemodynamic status and other signs as appropriate after medication to identify therapeutic effects and adverse effects of medications. Evaluate for signs of complications like infections and abscess formation at injection site. Monitor the child for 15 minutes after SC injections of drugs that may potentially cause allergic reactions or side effects
  - Evaluate child's response to the injection and understanding level of both child and family members to determine the areas of concern
- Document date and time of injection, type and dose of medication, route and site of injection, adverse effects (if any), child's response and tolerance of injection. Keep record of the teaching and demonstration, if any given to parents for SC injection.

Communication and Teaching for Homecare

- Communicate with the child and parents about child's health status, duration of injections, potential side effects and plan of further management

- Teach the parents about hygienic measures and routine care of the child at hospital and home, continuation of required medications after discharge from hospital, signs of complications, need for medical help and follow-up schedule. Teach the child in age appropriate simple language about self care, promotion of health and prevention of illness
  - If subcutaneous medications (e.g., Insulin) are to be given at home, demonstrate the SC injection technique to the competent family members and older child (if he or she can do it) and take return demonstrations. Instruct in details about site for SC injections, method of draw up medications, techniques to administer medication, signs of adverse effects, safe storage of medications and supplies (syringe, needles), safe disposal of syringes and needles, and about medical supply vendors. Provide written instructions for injection technique and necessary precautions to be followed at home.

PROCEDURE–13: ADMINISTRATION OF INTRAVENOUS MEDICATIONS TO CHILDREN

Clinical Guidelines

- Follow the Principles of Pharmacologic Management. *Refer Unit -1 of this Manual for the Principles*
- Follow at least "Ten Rights" for administration of medications to the children
- Medications are given by IV route for rapid absorption when an IV line is in place. The IV route of administration of medications is less traumatic than other routes when an IV line is already inserted
- Methods of administration of IV medications include-(a) IV push, used with small volumes that are injected over short period of time, usually 1–5 minutes, (b) Syringe pump, used to administer medication over a specific period of time using smaller volume infusion tubing and PMO line, (c) Volume control chamber (Buretrol, Burette, Volutrol), used when the medication can be diluted in the established IV fluid; volume is usually restricted to 150 mL or less, and (d) Small volume container (IV fluid bag/bottle containing small volumes)
- Rate of infusion of IV medication is determined by the nature of the particular medication. Always verify with reference source. This minimizes adverse effects associated with high serum levels. Medications must be administered within one hour of prescribed time
- Emergency medicine tray with all necessary supplies should be readily available to manage any drug reactions, adverse effects and complications after IV medications.

Equipment Required

- Hand hygiene supplies for hand wash and hand rub to prevent cross infections
- Existing IV access. If IV access is not present, insert of IV cannula *(Refer to procedure - 6 of this Unit for insertion of IV cannula)*
- Prescribed medications, normal saline bottle or ampule, ampule of sterile water for injections
- Syringe of different sizes as needed, syringe pump and PMO line, needleless access device and IV fluid set
- IV tubing cap, as needed to maintain sterility of tubing
- Alcohol swabs, sterile gloves pack
- Fluid stand to hang the IV medication bag/bottle, if needed
- Treatment sheet, Medication card
- Waste disposal containers
- Documentation sheet of IV medications.

Assessment and Preparation

- Assess the child's weight, height, age, hydration status, vital signs and risk factors to consider when calculating medication dosage and fluid requirement. Assess child's previous experiences with receiving IV medications and history of drug allergy

- Assess existing vascular access for the patency and signs of complications with the IV line (redness, swelling, fluid leakage from IV site, signs of phlebitis or infiltration). If the IV line is not patent or signs of complications exist, then establish new vascular access before administering IV medications
- Assess the child and parent for level of understanding for the requirement for IV medications to be administered and ability to cope with the situation

- Self preparation should be done with hand hygiene and practice of aseptic technique
- Environment should be clean, calm, well lighted and well ventilated
- Articles preparation: Necessary supplies should be collected and arranged in medication room for preparation of IV medications. Prepared IV medication and medication card/treatment sheet only to be taken at child's bedside to administer medication. Aseptic technique and handling of sterile items should be done carefully to prevent contamination of IV medication and infections of vascular access/catheter
- Preparation of parent: Explain the procedure of IV medication, its purpose and possible complications. Encourage the parent to support the child to cope with the procedure
- Preparation of child: Explain the procedure of IV medication in age-appropriate simple language. Provide distraction and play materials to the child to reduce fear and anxiety. Make the child comfortable and answer to the questions, as appropriate.

Performing the Steps of Procedure with Rationale/Point of Emphasis

1. Verify the medication order with the medical record to detect possible transcription errors.
2. Perform hand hygiene to reduce transmission of microorganisms.
3. Assemble all necessary supplies in the medication room for time management and organized approach.
4. Obtain prescribed IV medications and read the label to verify with the order. Check the expiration date, if expired, do not administered. This helps to decrease the chance of medication error by ensuring "right drugs".
5. Bring the medication to room temperature before IV administration, if storage was in refrigerator. Cold medication increases discomfort during infusion.
6. Determine the best method of administration of IV medications for the particular child. It is determined by the volume to be infused, type of medications, required therapeutic effects, and amount of time for infusion, infusion site and size of the child. Whatever method is used, the medication must be completely infused within one hour, unless otherwise specified. It is required to maintain therapeutic drug levels with optimum rate of infusion of IV medications and to ensure that the medication does not degrade before administration.
7. Perform hand hygiene. Don gloves to maintain standard precautions to prepare IV medications and to prevent contamination.
8. Prepare the medication in the medication/procedure room, as sight of needle can increase fear and anxiety of the child.
9. Draw up correct amount of medication into the syringe to prevent dosing error.
10. Reconstitute the powder medication, as per unit policy or as indicated. Follow manufacturer's recommendations or reference manual for type and amount of fluid to dilute with. Some medications are diluted in specific solutions to avoid incompatibility or with specific fluid amounts to obtain the correct dose.
11. Use separate needle to draw medication up from the ampule or rubber-topped vial to prevent small particles of glass or other substances from entering the syringe.
12. Verify the medication again from treatment record. Take and carry the prepared syringe with IV medication in a sterile knife dish/kidney dish to the child

for administration along with medication card/record.

- Verify the child's identity by comparing name on medication record with child's identification band and any other patient identifier/parent to ensure right patient with proper identification of the child, thus to prevent medication error.

13. Explain to the child and family that you are going to administer the IV medication, as previously explained.
14. Verify the IV access is patent and without any complications (e.g., edema, swelling, redness, tenderness, discoloration), to ensure IV access is without infiltration.
15. *If the child has an intermittent lock* - (a) Cleanse the needleless injection cap with 70% alcohol swab and allow it to dry, thus to reduce transmission of organisms, (b) Insert the syringe with 1 mL normal saline using appropriate needleless system adapter, (c) Slowly infuse 1 mL normal saline to flush the tubing and verify IV patency, (d) Connect to initiate IV medication infusion.
16. *For medication administration through IV push* - (a) Cleanse the top of needleless injection cap with 70% alcohol swab (if not cleaned previously) and allow it to dry, (b) Insert the syringe with prepared prescribed medication, using appropriate needleless system adapter, if required, into the port closest to the IV insertion site. Using the port closest to the insertion site allows IV medication to be administered in proper time. Using a site high up on the IV tubing may result slow infusion that may take place more than one hour time, (c) Inject the IV medication slowly as IV push over the specified time. Injecting the IV medication slowly reduces pain and decreases adverse reactions.
17. *For IV medication administration through syringe pump* - (a) Obtain the prepared diluted, prescribed medication in the appropriate sized syringe in calculated amount. Children can develop fluid overload, if too much fluid is infused, (b) Prime the IV infusion tubing with the infusate, if needed, and attach infusion tubing to the syringe. This removes air from IV tubing and initiate the infusion of IV medication, (c) Attach the syringe to the IV-controlled infusion device to allow the small volumes to be infused over a specific period of time, (d) Cleanse the port closest to the IV infusion site with 70% alcohol swab and allow it to dry, (e) Connect IV medication tubing to IV line or at "Y" connector closest to IV site, (f) Set the IV controlled infusion device to infuse IV medication volume, rate of infusion and correct time, (g) Start infusion with specific flow rate (mL/hour) of IV medication. Rapid infusion of IV medication may cause adverse effects associated with high serum drug level.
18. *For IV medication administration through a small-volume container* - (a) Cleanse the volume container diaphragm/port used for medication insertion with 70% alcohol and allow drying, (b) Inject the prescribed medication into the bag/bottle using sterile syringe and needle or obtain premixed medication bag/bottle to ensure correct medication for infusion, (c) Connect IV administration tubing to small volume bag/bottle to initiate the medication infusion. Flush the IV line with the fluid/infusate, if not already primed, (d) Cleanse the port closest to the IV insertion site with 70% alcohol and allow drying, (e) Connect medication administration tubing to main IV line at "Y" connector closest to IV site. Infusing into port closest to child allows quicker infusion and prevents further dilution of the medication, (f) Set the infusion rate to infuse required medication volume and flush over the desired time (antibiotics are typically administered over 30–60 minutes), (g) Start infusion and check medication is infusing. To indicate medication is infusing, label the chamber with name of medication, dose, date, time, rate of flow, total amount to flow, and initials of medication administering personnel.

19. Observe the flow of IV medication and appropriate functions of the IV system. Rapid infusion of IV medication should be avoided to prevent adverse effects related to high serum drug levels.
20. Provide comfort to the child and praise for cooperation. Ask for presence of any discomfort, pain at infusion site and any other adverse reactions related to initiation of IV medication. Allow parent with the child to get cooperation during IV medications.
21. Dispose all wastes in appropriate containers. Perform hand hygiene to prevent infections.
22. Monitor the child's condition initially and then every 15 minutes during the infusion for presence of any adverse reactions, such as respiratory distress, changes in vital signs, hemodynamic instability and so on. Continuous monitoring provides early detection of adverse reactions. As IV medication enters into the vascular system rapidly, onset of anaphylaxis or toxic side effects may occur at any time.
23. Flush the medication from the IV tubing on completion of medication administration. Amount of flush solution is dependent on tubing volume. This facilitates infusion of all medication into the child, so none is left in tubing that could interact with other medications or solutions.
24. After completion of IV medication infusion and flush, disconnect infusion tubing and attach sterile tubing cap to the end of infusion tubing. This maintains sterility of the tubing until next infusion of medication. Tubing used for intermittent infusions should be replaced when the main line tubing is changed or whenever the integrity of either line is compromised.
25. Document the procedure of IV medication and related observational findings in the treatment sheet or child record.

Evaluation and Documentation

- Evaluate child's response to the procedure of IV medication, any infiltrations of fluid, any allergic reactions and presence or absence of any other side effects.
  - Evaluate the child for change in vital signs and in hemodynamic status or presence of any other abnormal signs related to the procedure of IV medication
  - Evaluate child's and family's understanding of IV medications and their ability to participate during the procedure of IV medication, if required
- Document the followings: the type of IV medication administered, dose and route, date and time of administration of IV medication, appearance of IV access site, dilution and flush fluid amount (these amounts must be included in calculation of child's 24 hours fluid intake), monitoring findings, presence or absence of side effects, child's response and tolerance of the procedure and information given to child and parents.

Communication and Teaching for Homecare

- Communicate with child and parents about child's health condition, precautions during IV medication, plan of further treatment for existing illness and for questions as asked
- Teach the parents about hygienic practices, health promotion activities and prevention of illness, diet and fluid intake, routine care of the child at hospital and home, continuation of treatment after discharge, potential complications, long-term drug effects, need for medical help and plan of follow-up schedule.

PROCEDURE–14: ADMINISTRATION OF NASAL MEDICATIONS TO CHILDREN

Clinical Guidelines

- Follow the Principles of Pharmacologic Management *(Refer Unit - 1 of this Manual for the Principles).*
- Follow at least "Ten Rights" for administration of medications to the children

- Nasal medications are required in case of upper respiratory tract infections, sinusitis, rhinitis, allergic rhinitis, nasal congestion, nasal surgery and nasal injury
- Commonly used nasal medications are nasal drops or spray as nasal decongestants, antihistaminic, antiallergic, steroids, and antibiotics
- Nasal medications must be water based and not oil based. This prevents possibility of aspiration pneumonia and facilitates absorption through nasal mucosa
- Follow the manufacturer guidelines for use and storage of nasal drop containers or nasal spray canisters. Do not share or use nasal drop containers or nasal spray canisters with other child to prevent cross contamination. The child should have personal supplies of nasal medications in hospital and at home
- Teach the parents about nasal medications and its precautions for continued care at home.

Equipment Required

- Hand hygiene supplies for hand wash and hand rub to prevent cross contaminations
- Nonsterile gloves as standard precautions of infections control
- Tissue paper or soft cloth or gauze pieces to remove nasal secretions, as needed
- Disposable suction device or mechanical suction devices with disposable suction catheter and other supplies to remove nasal secretions, whenever required
- Prescribed correct nasal medications (with dropper or sprayer, as prescribed)
- Waste disposal containers as per BMW rules.
- Documentation sheet for nasal medication and child's treatment sheet.

Assessment and Preparation

- Assess child's present health condition, previous experience with receiving nasal medications, history of any drug allergy and any other medication related information. Assess child's and parent's understanding of importance of administration of nasal medication and their ability to perform the procedure whenever needed
- Self preparation should be done with practice of standard precautions and hand hygiene
- Environment should be calm, clean, well lighted and well ventilated
- All necessary supplies should be arranged at child's bedside for easy accessibility
- Preparation of parents: Explain the procedure of nasal medications, its purpose and necessary precautions during administration. Allow parent participation to help the child to cope with the procedure of application of nasal drops or spray
- Preparation of child: Give age-appropriate simple explanation for nasal medication to the child. Provide comfort and reply to the area of concern, whenever needed.

Performing the Steps of Procedure with Rationale/Point of Emphasis

1. Verify the medication order with the medical record to detect possible transcription errors.
2. Check for drug allergy history of the child. If present, do not administer and notify the physician. Allergic reactions to any medication may be life threatening.
3. Perform hand hygiene to reduce transmission of microorganisms.
4. Wear gloves to prevent cross contamination and cross infections.
5. Assemble all necessary supplies near the child/treatment room for organized approach.
6. Obtain prescribed nasal medication and read the label to verify with the treatment order. Check the expiration date of nasal medication, if expired, do not administered. This helps to decrease the chance of medication error by ensuring "right drugs".
7. Identify the correct nostril (right, left, or both) in which medication to be administered.
8. Bring the nasal medication to room temperature before administration,

if it was stored in refrigerator. Do not administer cold nasal medication. Warm the solution by gently rotating the bottle of nasal medication in your hand before administration. Cold medication increases discomfort when medication is administered nasally.

9. Verify the nasal medication again from treatment record. Take the nasal medication tray with all supplies to the child for administration along with medication card/record.
10. Verify the child's identity by comparing name on medication record with child's identification band and any other patient identifier/parent to ensure right patient thus to prevent medication error.
11. Ask the child to blow his or her nose before administration of nasal medications. If the child is not old enough to cooperate, use suction device to clear nasal secretions. Clearing of nose allows proper absorption of nasal drops or spray.
12. ***Administer nasal drops with following steps (Fig. 3.6):***
    i. Place the child in supine position with the head tilted back or place a rolled towel or pillow under the child's neck and shoulder. An older child can extend the head over the side of the bed so that it is lower than the trunk. This allows the nasal medication drop to coat nasal mucosa
    ii. Instill the prescribed nasal drops into nostrils (both or right or left) with the tip of dropper toward the nasal passage. This helps to deposit the drug within the nose rather than in the throat and ensures administration of correct dose. Be careful not to touch the sides of the nostril to prevent contamination of dropper
    iii. Have the child to remain in that position for several minutes, if possible, to give time for absorption of nasal medication.

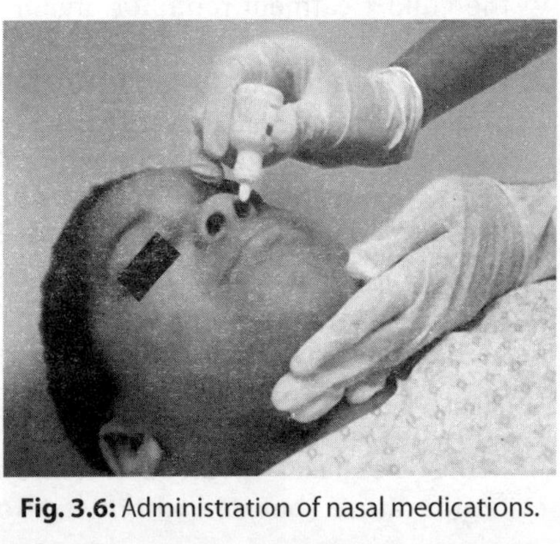

Fig. 3.6: Administration of nasal medications.

13. ***Administer nasal spray with following steps:***
    i. Place the child in semi-Fowler position with the head tilted slightly back. This allows the nasal spray to coat the nasal mucosa
    ii. Instill the nasal spray by holding one nostril closed while the medication is sprayed into the other nostril. Direct the spray to the side away from the nasal septum and toward the top of the nose on that side. This allows full administration of the spray into the nostril.
14. Have the child take a deep breath slowly through the nostril while the medication is being administered to facilitate absorption of medication.
15. Repeat the procedure for other nostril, if indicated. Repeat number of spray, as prescribed.
16. Remove gloves and perform hand hygiene to prevent cross infections.
17. Recap the nasal medication drop container or spray canister and arrange to preserve in safe storage area (as per manufacturer instructions).
18. Make the child comfortable and praise for cooperation. Clear all supplies from child's bedside. Allow the parent to remain with the child. This promotes positive nurse-patient relationship and decreases long-term negative effects of painful procedure.
19. Discard all waste. Take care of all reusable supplies for next use.
20. Document the procedure administration of nasal medications and related findings.

Evaluation and Documentation

- Evaluate the child's reactions after medication and presence of any potential side effects. Evaluate the child for change in vital signs and in hemodynamic status or for any other abnormal signs related to the procedure to identify the effects of nasal medication
  - Evaluate child's and family's understanding of nasal medication and their ability to perform the procedure at home, if required
- Document date and time, type and dose and route (one or both nares) of administration of nasal medication. Record presence or absence of adverse effects, response and tolerance of the procedure. Keep record of the teaching and demonstration given to parents.

Communication and Teaching for Homecare

- Communicate with child and parents about child's health condition, importance of nasal medications and further plan of treatment
- Teach the parents about preventive measures for upper respiratory infections, rhinitis, nasal injury, hygienic practices, routine care of the child at hospital and home and about plan of follow-up visits
  - Demonstrate and take return demonstration of technique of nasal medications with necessary precautions. Instruct about signs of adverse reactions, safe storage of nasal drops and spray and need for emergency medical help, whenever required.

PROCEDURE–15: ADMINISTRATION OF OTIC (EAR) MEDICATIONS

Clinical Guidelines

- Follow the Principles of Pharmacologic Management *(Refer Unit - 1 of this Manual for the Principles).*
- Follow at least "Ten Rights" for administration of medications to the children
- Otic medications are administered for the treatment of infections (external ear or middle ear) and allergic conditions of ear, otorrhea, wax, and mastoid and ear surgery. Common aural/otic medications are antibiotic ear drops, antifungal ear drops, corticosteroid drops and cerumenolytic ear drops
- Use any ear drops container within one month after opening or follow the instruction on the label. If any irritation persists after administration of ear drops, discontinue that otic medication and inform the prescriber for further decision.

Equipment Required

- Hand hygiene supplies for hand wash and hand rub to prevent cross infections
- Nonsterile gloves as standard precautions
- Otic medication with dropper, as prescribed, in a small tray
- Sterile cotton balls in a covered container
- Wipes or gauze pieces, if needed to clean any ear discharge
- Treatment sheet or medication card and child case sheet
- Waste disposal containers as per BMW rules
- Medication documentation/record sheet.

Assessment and Preparation

- Assess child's present health condition, previous experience with receiving aural/otic medications, history of any drug allergy and any other medication related information. Assess child's and parent's understanding of importance of otic medications and their ability to perform the procedure whenever needed, especially at home
- Self preparation should be done with practice of standard precautions and hand hygiene
- Environment should be clean, well lighted and well ventilated
- All necessary items should be arranged at child's bedside for time management
- Preparation of parents: Explain the procedure of otic medications, its purpose and

necessary precautions during administration of ear drops. Ask the parent to hold the young child to allow easy application of ear drops

- Preparation of child: Give age-appropriate simple explanation for medication in the ear of the child and related discomfort. Provide comfort and ask for cooperation. If feasible, allow play materials and answer to the questions, as needed, for effective coping.

Performing the Steps of Procedure with Rationale/Point of Emphasis

1. Verify the medication order with the medical record to detect possible transcription errors.
2. Perform hand hygiene and don gloves to reduce transmission of microorganisms.
3. Assemble all necessary supplies near the child/procedure room for organized approach.
4. Obtain prescribed medication and read the label to verify with the order. Check the expiration date of the medication, if expired, do not administered. This helps to decrease the chance of medication error by ensuring "right drugs".
5. Bring the otic medication to room temperature before administration, if it was kept in refrigerator. Do not administer cold otic medication. Warm the solution by gently rotating the bottle of otic medication in your hand before administration. Cold otic medication may cause discomfort and produce vomiting or vertigo in the child.
6. Verify the otic medication again from treatment record. Carry the otic medication in a small tray with all necessary supplies to the child for administration to the child along with medication card/record.
7. Verify the child's identity by comparing name on medication record with child's identification band and any other patient identifier or parent to ensure "right patient" thus to prevent medication error.
8. Place the child in supine position with his or her head turned to the affected side up, or as appropriate. The young child can also lie across parent's lap with affected side ear up. This allows entry of ear drops into the ear canal.
9. Distract the child with play materials and soothe the child to keep him or her quiet while the otic medication is instilling. This facilitate instillation of otic drops.
10. Pull the earlobe down and back, for children younger than 3 years of age for instillation of medication in the ear. For older children, pull the pinna of the ear up and back. This helps to straighten the ear canal and facilitates entry of ear drops into the ear canal.
11. Administer prescribed amount of ear drops into the ear canal, holding the dropper ½ inche above the ear canal. Be careful not to contaminate the dropper of otic drug. Avoid touching the nozzle tip to external ear. This prevents transmission of microorganisms onto the dropper from the child's ear.
12. Gently massage the tragus (area anterior to the ear canal), unless contraindicated due to pain. Massage of tragus facilitates entry of otic medication into the ear canal.
13. Have the child to remain in supine position with head turned for 2–3 minutes. This gives time for the medication to enter the ear canal.
14. Insert a small cotton ball, preferably sterile, into the entry to the ear canal. This prevents the medication from leaking out the external ear. Moistening the cotton ball with sterile water (can be warm with suitable temperature) or otic medication prevents the cotton ball from absorbing the medication in the ear canal.
15. Repeat the instillation of ear drops to other ear, if prescribed only.
16. Recap the otic medication drop container and preserve in safe storage area (as per manufacturer instructions).
17. Clear all supplies from child's bedside. Discard all waste as per BMW rules.
18. Remove gloves and perform hand hygiene to prevent nosocomial infections.
19. Make the child comfortable and praise for cooperation.

20. Allow the parent to remain with the child. This promotes positive nurse-patient relationship and decreases long-term negative effects of painful procedure,
21. Document the procedure administration of otic medications and related findings. Report about presence of any abnormal findings to appropriate authority.

Evaluation and Documentation

- Evaluate the child's response to the otic medication and presence of any discomfort. Observe the child after administration of ear drops for any potential side effects, such as dizziness or vertigo. Evaluate child's condition related ear problems about improvement or any other associated abnormalities
  - Evaluate child's and family's understanding of otic medications and their ability to perform the procedure of giving ear drops at home, if required
- Document date and time, type and dose and route (one or both ear) of administration of otic medication. Record presence or absence of adverse effects, response and tolerance of the procedure. Keep record of the teaching and demonstration given to parents for instillation of ear drops.

Communication and Teaching for Homecare

- Communicate with child and parents about child's health and ear condition, importance of otic medications and further plan of treatment. Determine whether the child and family have additional areas of concern to discuss
- Teach the parents about preventive measures for ear infections (such as swimming in dirty water, putting finger or stick in the ear), hygienic practices, routine care of the child at hospital and home, and about follow-up visits
- Demonstrate and take return demonstration of technique of administration of otic medications with necessary precautions. Instruct about signs of adverse reactions, safe storage of ear drops and need for emergency medical help, whenever required.

PROCEDURE–16: EAR IRRIGATION OF THE CHILDREN

Clinical Guidelines

- Ear irrigation is the cleansing of ear canal by flushing with sterile water or normal saline or other fluids. The cleansing solutions should be sterile. Irrigation should be given gently with minimum amount of pressure
- Ear irrigation in children is performed to remove material or foreign bodies that blocks the external ear canal or to clean drainage from the ear canal and to reduce local discomfort
- Cerumen or earwax is the most common cause of ear pain, dizziness, and hearing deficits in the children. Impacted cerumen may need treatment by ear irrigation with or without cerumenolytic pretreatment to soften the cerumen
- If a foreign object is visualized in the ear canal or suspected to be in the ear canal, the procedure of ear irrigation should not be attempted until the healthcare prescriber or physician has been consulted
- If the tympanic membrane is not intact, do not perform ear irrigation. This avoids transmission of fluid into the middle ear and prevents further complications.

Equipment Required

- Hand hygiene supplies for hand wash and hand rub to prevent cross infections
- A tray containing – Pediatric size Otoscope, nonsterile gloves, cotton-tipped applicators, cotton balls, gauze pieces, washcloth, sterile normal saline in covered container, mild antiseptic irrigating solution (as indicated), bulb syringe or irrigating tip, towel, sterile blunt ear curette size 00 or cerumen spoon in a sterile covered container, if needed
- Waterproof pad or sheet to protect the child's bed or procedure table
- Sheet or blanket for wrapping or restraining the child

- Torch or focus light source for good visualization
- Emesis basin/kidney dish and waste disposal containers
- Documentation sheet for ear irrigation and child's treatment sheet.

Assessment and Preparation

- Assess the child's present ear pathology, definite indication of ear irrigation, vital signs, history of previous experience of any ear interventions and any other abnormalities.
  Assess the child and parent for their understanding level and anxiety for presence of ear problem of the child for planning to provide necessary support
- Self preparation should be with practice of standard precautions of infection control and hand hygiene
- Environment should be clean, calm, well lighted and well ventilated. Usually ear irrigation is performed in procedure room. It can be also done on child's bed. Privacy should be maintained with use of screen around the child's bed, thus to avoid fear and anxiety of other child. Parent will be allowed at bedside to help the child to cope with the procedure of ear irrigation
- Articles preparation should be done following standard guidelines. All supplies should be collected and arranged conveniently for organized approach at procedure room or at child's bedside
- Preparation of parents: Explain the procedure of ear irrigation, its purpose and possible side effects. Encourage the parents to stay with the child during the procedure to reduce fear and anxiety of their child
- Preparation of child: Explain the procedure of ear irrigation, its need and possible discomfort during the procedure in age-appropriate simple language. Make the child comfortable during positioning. Ask for cooperation to reduce risk of trauma.

Performing the Steps of Procedure with Rationale/Point of Emphasis

1. Perform hand hygiene and gather necessary supplies in procedure room for time management and organized approach to the procedure
2. Prepare irrigating solution at tepid temperature. Solution should be at body temperature because variations in other temperature stimulate the inner ear and can cause dizziness and nausea
3. Raise the child's bed to working height to prevent back strain for the nurse or position the child on a procedure table with the head of the bed elevated at 45-degree. The child may also sit in a chair or on parent's lap for the procedure of ear irrigation
4. Have the child sit up or lie with head tilted toward the side of affected ear. Sitting up allows easier access to the child's ear and prevent dripping down the side of the face, neck and back
5. Place a waterproof sheet/pad under the child's head to prevent the bed becoming wet. Have another towel available to dry the child's face, neck and back, as needed
6. Have an assistant to immobilize the head and extremities of the child, as required. The highly mobile or combative child may need to be further immobilized during the procedure to ensure safety. Use of sheet or blanket to apply mummy restraints to the younger child can help in immobilization. But precautions should be taken for use of restraint for the child to prevent any injury
7. Perform hand hygiene and don gloves for prevention of cross infections
8. Assess child's ear canal and pinna for redness, lesions and drainage by visual inspection and ask for pain
9. Use an otoscope to assess the inner canal and integrity of the tympanic membrane. This step may need to be done by the physician or healthcare prescriber, as per unit or institutional policy
   Large accumulations of cerumen may not allow visualization of the tympanic

membrane. If the tympanic membrane is red and bulging and no light reflex is exhibited, that indicates presence of otitis media

10. Clean the outer ear, if necessary, using cotton swabs or a warm wet washcloth. This prevents the spread of debris from outer ear to ear canal
11. Place emesis basin/kidney dish below the child's ear to receive the irrigating solution
12. Fill the bulb syringe/irrigating tip with prescribed solution. Filling the syringe with irrigating fluid decreases the amount of air forced into the ear canal and provides a steady irrigating system. Expel the air from the syringe so that bubbles will not forced into the ear as it produces loud sound and cause great discomfort
13. Pull the ear auricle down and back in the child 3 years of age or younger. Pull the ear auricle up and back in children over the age of 3 years. Keep the tragus forward in both groups. This allows for maximum straightening of the ear canal and also provides good view of the eardrum
14. Place tip of bulb syringe/irrigating tip about one (1) cm above the opening of ear canal and gently squeeze the syringe toward the roof of the ear. Do not "flood" the ear canal with fluid. Do not occlude the ear canal with the irrigating nozzle
    i. Allow the solution to flow out unimpeded. Continue slow stream of fluid until the ear canal is cleansed or all prescribed solution has been used
    ii. It is important to be gentle with the use of syringe in the ear because the epithelium lining the bony portion of ear canal is very thin and sensitive. Directing the solution toward the roof prevents injury to the tympanic membrane. Obstructing the outflow of fluid may cause the pressure to rise in ear canal and on eardrum, thus causing ear pain
    iii. During the irrigation process, if the child begins to scream and complains of pain in the ear or bloody discharge is noted, then stop the irrigation immediately and notify the problems to physician or healthcare prescriber
15. If a curette is needed to remove the cerumen, use a blunt ear curette, size 00, or wire curette (called as cerumen spoon). With an otoscope, visualize the ear canal and advance the curette beyond the point of the cerumen accumulation, resting medial to the occlusion. Pull the cerumen out of the ear canal carefully
    i. As per institutional policy, use of the ear curette may need to be completed by a healthcare prescriber or physician or ENT specialist.
    ii. Precautions must be taken to prevent trauma to the eardrum and ear canal during use of curette in children. The child's head must be immobilized to avoid nicking or irritating the tympanic membrane and ear canal, as trauma risk is high in children.
16. On completion of irrigation, dry the child's outer ear and insert cotton ball loosely into ear canal opening. Instruct the child to lie on the affected side or ask the parent to place the child on affected side for a few minutes to continue the draining of fluid. A cotton ball absorbs fluid from the ear canal and gravity allows the remaining solution in the ear canal to escape out from the ear
17. Repeat the procedure on other ear, if prescribed and needed. Do not automatically irrigate both ears, if not indicated. Only affected ear should be treated and irrigated
18. Clear away all equipment and supplies. Clean up the area after ear irrigation
19. Make the child comfortable and praise for cooperation. Ask for feeling any problems
20. Return the child to his or her bed, if procedure was done in treatment room. Adjust the child's bed to lowest position to promote child's comfort and safety.
21. Clean and dry the bulb syringe. Allow it to air dry. Take care of all other reusable items

22. Dispose single use items and all waste in appropriate containers as standard precautions
23. Remove gloves. Perform hand hygiene to reduce transmission of microorganisms
24. Document the procedure of ear irrigation and related findings.

Evaluation and Documentation

- Evaluate the child's health status, condition of the affected ear and reassess the ear using otoscope to determine whether amount of cerumen has diminished
- Document the date and time of ear irrigation, type of solution used for ear irrigation, color and amount of discharge during irrigation, size of the cerumen and other observational findings before and after the procedure of ear irrigation. Note and report child's tolerance to the procedure and current level of comfort.

Communication and Teaching for Homecare

- Communicate with child and parents about condition of the ear before and after the ear irrigation. Discuss about future plan of management and precautions to be followed to prevent ear problems. Additional areas of concern to be discussed
- Teach the parents and child about prevention of incidence of foreign body in the ear and upper respiratory infections, hygienic practices, routine care at hospital and home, continuation of medication at home, technique of instillation of ear drops, signs of ear problems, need for contact with medical professionals and plan of follow-up visits.

PROCEDURE–17: ADMINISTRATION OF RECTAL MEDICATIONS TO CHILDREN

Clinical Guidelines

- Rectal route of administration of medication is not the preferred route for the children because of potential emotional trauma to the child and unpredictable absorption of drugs from the colon. Absorption of medication given in rectal route can be affected by the presence of stool in the colon and rectum. If infant's or child's rectum is full of stool, then do not administer rectal medication and notify the healthcare prescriber
- The rectal route may be the best choice for a child who cannot tolerate oral medication and in whom parenteral route is not available
- Administration of rectal medications are contraindicated in children who are thrombocytopenic or immunosuppressed, because the risk of bleeding and infections is more in those children
- Rectal suppositories are the most frequent form of rectal medication, although occasionally other medications may be administered in an enema form
- Follow the Principles of Pharmacologic Management *(Refer Unit – 1 of this Manual for the Principles)*.
- Follow at least "Ten Rights" for administration of medications to the children.

Equipment Required

- Hand hygiene supplies for hand washing and antiseptic hand rub for prevention of cross contaminations
- Nonsterile gloves as standard precautions of infection control measures
- Prescribed rectal medication or rectal suppository
- Rectal catheter (age-appropriate) and syringe to administered liquid medication
- Water soluble lubricant, if needed for easy introduction of rectal catheter
- Waste disposal container as per BMW rules
- Medication documentation sheet and child's treatment sheet.

Assessment and Preparation

- Assess child's present health condition, previous experience with receiving rectal medications, history of any drug allergy and any other medication related information

- Assess child's and parent's understanding of importance of rectal medications and their ability to perform the procedure whenever needed, especially at home
- Self-preparation should be done with hand washing and practice of standard precautions
- Environment should be clean, well lighted and well ventilated
- All necessary supplies should be arranged at child's bedside for organized approach
- Preparation of parents: Explain the procedure of rectal medications to the child, its purpose and necessary precautions during administration of rectal medication. Ask the parent to hold and support the young child to allow easy administration of rectal medication and to get cooperation from the child
- Preparation of child: Give age-appropriate simple explanation for rectal medication the child and its related discomfort. Provide comfort to the child; ask for cooperation, if feasible. Allow therapeutic play materials, if child's condition permits. Reply to the area of concern, as needed, for effective coping.

Performing the Steps of Procedure with Rationale/Point of Emphasis

1. Verify the medication order with the medical record to detect possible transcription errors
2. Check for drug allergy history with the prescribed medication to prevent drug reactions
3. Perform hand hygiene to reduce transmission of microorganisms
4. Assemble all necessary supplies near the child or in procedure room for organized approach and time management
5. Obtain prescribed medication and read the label to verify with the treatment order. Check the expiration date of the rectal medicine. If expired, then do not administer that drug. This helps to decrease the chance of medication error by ensuring "right drugs"
6. Check the form of medication to ensure that it is appropriate for the rectal administration of the child, as prescribed
7. Bring the medication to room temperature before administration to prevent discomfort, if storage was in refrigerator
8. Verify the rectal medication again from treatment record. Take the rectal medication tray with all supplies to the child for administration along with medication card/record
9. Verify the child's identity by comparing name on medication record with child's identification band and any other patient identifier/parent to ensure right patient thus to prevent medication error
10. Wear gloves to protect the administrator's hand from contamination with fecal material, thus reducing transmission of microorganisms
11. Prepare the rectal medication or suppository for administration.
    - Avoid cutting suppository, if possible. If it requires cutting the suppository to obtain prescribed dose, then it must be cut lengthwise. Cutting suppository lengthwise helps absorption at the required time
    - Liquid rectal medication can be administered using small rectal catheter (age-appropriate size) and appropriate size syringe depending upon the amount of medication to be administered
12. Place the child in left lateral position with the right leg flexed or in knee-chest position. These positions exposes the anus and helps to relax the external anal sphincter for easy insertion of rectal suppository or rectal catheter for introduction of medication
13. Remove the suppository packaging and lubricate the suppository with water soluble lubricating jelly. This reduces friction with rectal mucosal surfaces
14. Gently insert the apex (pointed end) of the rectal suppository beyond the internal anal sphincter, placing the medication

against the rectal wall. In an infant or toddler, suppository can be inserted with the help of little finger, if required. Index finger can be used for older children, whenever needed. Suppository must be placed beyond the internal sphincter to prevent expulsion of it.

i. Liquid rectal medication can be administer using small rectal catheter and disposable single use syringe (with measured amount of prescribed medication) in same technique mentioned above for rectal suppository

15. Instruct the child to pant like a puppy slowly. This provides distraction and relaxes the anal sphincter. Distraction helps to administer medication easily and avoid expulsion of it
16. Hold the child's buttock's until the child relaxes or loses the urge to push out. This prevents expulsion of rectal medication. If the child has a stool within 30 minutes, examine the stool for the presence of the suppository
17. Remove gloves and dispose in appropriate container. Discard waste as per BMW rules
18. Make the child comfortable. Praise for cooperation. Allow parent to support the child
19. Perform hand hygiene. Document the procedure of rectal medication and related findings.

Evaluation and Documentation

- Evaluate the child's response to the administration of rectal medication and discomfort. Observe the child after administration of rectal suppository or rectal medication for any potential side effects
  - Evaluate child's health condition and presence of any other abnormalities
  - Evaluate child's and family's understanding for administering rectal medications and their ability to perform the procedure of application of rectal suppository at home, if required and indicated
- Document date and time, type and dose of administration of rectal medication or rectal suppository. Record presence or absence of adverse effects, discomfort, response and tolerance of the procedure. Note the passage of stool and expulsion of suppository, if it happened. Keep record of the teaching and demonstration given to parents for application of rectal suppository.

Communication and Teaching for Homecare

- Communicate with child and parents about child's health condition, importance of rectal medications and further plan of treatment. Determine whether the child and family have additional areas of concern to discuss
- Teach the parents about hygienic practices, routine care of the child at hospital and home, continuation of medication, as needed, at home and about follow-up visits
  - Demonstrate and take return demonstration of technique of application of rectal suppository with necessary precautions. Instruct about signs of adverse reactions, and need for emergency medical help, whenever required.

PROCEDURE–18: ENEMAS TO THE CHILDREN

Clinical Guidelines

- Enema is the introduction of solution into the rectum and colon to stimulate bowel activity. It helps in emptying the lower intestine and to relieve from distention and flatus
- Enemas are commonly administered as (i) therapeutic enema (e.g., retention enema with prescribed medication), or (ii) diagnostic enema (e.g., barium enema with use of barium sulfate solution as a contrast agent to facilitate X-ray and fluoroscopic examination of the colon), or as (iii) cleansing enema (with liquid soap solution)

- Enema is administered for the purpose of instillation or slowly pouring of liquid into the large bowel to soften feces, assist peristalsis and evacuate rectum and colon. It is given for preparation of surgical interventions and for diagnostic procedure
- The type and amount of enema solution to be instilled varies with the age and size of the child and with the reason for the enema
- *Types of enema:* It can be administered as—(a) Cleansing enema: Remove feces from the colon, (b) Hypotonic or isotonic enema: Large-volume cleansing enema, (c) Hypertonic enema: Small-volume cleansing enema, (d) Oil retention enema: Lubricates the stool and intestinal mucosa, making defecation easier, (e) Carminative enema: Helps to expel flatus from the rectum and relieve distention secondary to flatus, (f) Medicated enema: Used to administer medication rectally, (g) Anthelmintic enema: Used to remove or to destroy intestinal parasites, (h) Nutritive enema: Replenishes fluids and nutrition rectally, and (i) Return-flow enema: Allows small amount of solution to be administered and then allowed to return to the container. This process is repeated for several times to stimulate the peristalsis and to help in expelling flatus
- Recommended *amount of solution for administration of enemas*: (a) *For saline enema or plain water enema:* (i) in 2–6 years age group - 6 oz or 180 mL, (ii) in 6–12 years age group - 12 oz or 360 mL, and (iii) for more than 12 years of age - 16 oz or 480 mL, and (b) *For mineral oil enema* - (i) in 2–6 years age group - 2 oz or 60 mL, (ii) in more than 6 years of age - 4.5 oz or 135 mL
- Recommended *lengths of advancement of rectal tube/catheter for enemas* are as follows - for (a) Infant - 1 inch/2.5 cm, (b) Small child - 2 inches/5 cm, (c) Large child - 3 inches/7.5 cm, (d) Adolescent - 4 inches/10 cm
- Administration of enema is contra-indicated for children with recent colon or rectal surgery, in acute abdominal conditions and/or bleeding disorders or low platelet count
- Enema is very private and scary experience for the children. Psychosocial concerns and child's developmental level should be taken into consideration in regards to explanations of the procedure of enema, parental presence and privacy.

Equipment Required

- Hand hygiene supplies for hand wash and hand rub to prevent cross infections
- Enema solution, as prescribed or manu-facturer's prepackaged enema solution
- Enema bag/can/container with tubing, clamp, connector, and rectal catheter
- Nonsterile gloves, water-soluble lubricant, gauze pieces, and swab sticks
- Waterproof protective sheet, towels, toilet papers, cotton balls/tow, bowl of water
- Irrigating stand, lotion thermometer (if available), screen/curtains
- Bedpan, waste disposal containers
- Documentation sheet for enema and child's treatment sheet.

Assessment and Preparation

- Assess the child's health history, present health conditions and physical findings to determine the reason and underlying factors for administering enema (e.g., constipation, preparation for surgery or diagnostic procedure). Assess psychological concerns and level of understanding of child and family in relation to administration of enema
- Sel-preparation should be done with practice of standard precautions of infection control
- Environment should clean, calm, well lighted and well ventilated. Enema can be given at child's bed with privacy and necessary precautions. It can also be administered in the procedure room as convenient
- Articles preparation should be done depending upon the requirements and child's developmental age. Necessary

supplies should be arranged at child's bed or in procedure room, as per feasibility for organized approach

- Preparation of parents: Explain the procedure, its importance, effects and necessary assistance from parents. Take help of the parents during use of toilet or bedpan, if needed
- Preparation of child: Explain the procedure, purpose and expected results of enema in age-appropriate simple language. Ensure the child's privacy. Ask for cooperation. Encourage the child to drink one or two glasses of water before the procedure of enema

Performing the Steps of Procedure with Rationale/Point of Emphasis

1. Perform hand hygiene to reduce transmission of microorganisms.
2. Arrange the necessary supplies in procedure room or at child's bed for organized approach and time management.
3. Review the type of enema and amount of enema solution prescribed by the physician with its indications.
4. Prepare the enema solution. Select appropriate amount, as prescribed and warm the solution to temperature of 100°F or 37.8°C. Too much fluid can cause cramping and retention of fluids, leading to systemic absorption. Too little solution will reduce the success of administering enema to the child.
5. For prepackaged enema solutions – open the package. Follow the manufacturer instructions for warming the fluid and remove the cap on the enema tip.
6. For self-prepared solutions: (a) Close the clamps on the enema container tubing, (b) Fill the can with the warmed prescribed enema solution, (c) Prime the tubing by opening the clamp and allowing the solution to free-flow through the entire length of tubing. Priming the tubing evacuates air from the tubing. If air enters into the intestinal tract, it may produce abdominal cramping, (d) Close the clamp after all air has been removed from the tubing to prevent spilling.
7. Provide privacy to the child. Close the curtains around the child's bed and drape towels over the child, exposing only the anal area. Privacy can improve the child's comfort level.
8. Don gloves as standard precautions to prevent potential cross contamination.
9. Place the child's bed in high flat position and place the child in one of the following positions that is most comfortable for his or her – (a) On the left side in the lateral recumbent position with knees drawn up to the chest, (b) On the back of the child with the legs together lifted to expose the anal orifice (best position for infants), (c) Left Sim's position, with the right thigh flexed about 45-degree to the body axis and positioned at the edge of the bed, (d) Knee-chest position with the child balancing on knees and forearms, resting the head on a pillow so that the buttocks are angled upward off the bed. Knee-chest position helps to distribute the solution throughout the lower intestinal tract **(Figs. 3.7A to D)**
10. Place waterproof protective sheet/pad under the child's buttocks to protect the bed.
11. Lubricate the rectal tube/catheter or enema tip up to the length to be introduced in rectum.
12. Insert the rectal tube or catheter or enema tip as follows: (i) Separate the child's buttocks, (ii) Gently touch the anus, observing for anal contraction followed by relaxation. Relaxation of the anus will ease the insertion of the enema tube or catheter or enema tip, (iii) Insert the enema tube or catheter or enema tip of prepackaged container with the tip pointing in the direction of the child's umbilicus to the appropriate length for advancement and hold in place. Inserting the tip toward the umbilicus decreases the chance of the tube scraping the rectal wall.
13. Never force the catheter into the anal canal. If a well lubricated catheter does not advance easily, then remove the tube and stop the enema. Forcing the tube may injure the intestinal mucosa wall.

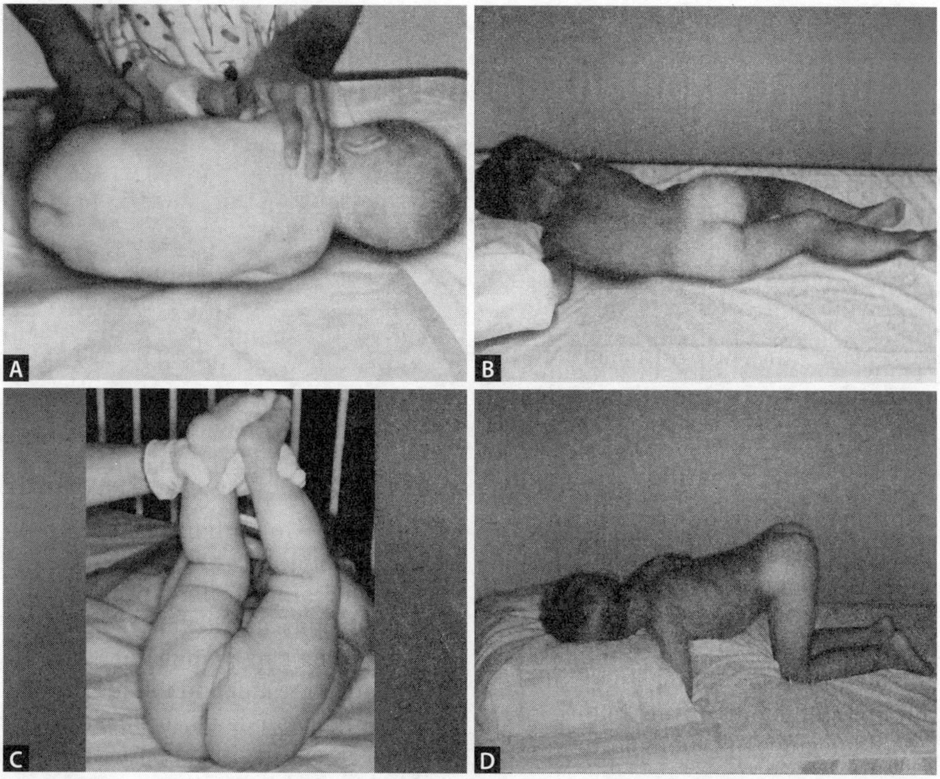

Figs. 3.7A to D: A. Left lateral position for giving enema. B. Position for administering enema in infant. C. Sim's position for administering enema. D. Knee - Chest position for administering enema.

14. Elevate the enema solution container about 10 cm/4 inches above the anus. Unclamp the tubing and administered the fluid as tolerated by the child. The height of the container determines the amount of pressure of the solution. Too much pressure may cause discomfort or premature expulsion of the solution.
15. Squeeze and roll the prepackaged enema container or bag toward the child's rectum until all the solution is administered. Rolling the container or bag assists in dispensing the solution into the intestines.
16. Practice the following techniques to reduce cramping during enema administration: (a) Encourage the child to relax, breathe deeply and let his or her breath out rapidly through the mouth. This promotes relaxation, distraction and comfort. (b) For moderate cramping, pinch off the enema tube or catheter to interrupt the flow of solution temporarily. This permits to equalize the pressure, thereby minimizing the cramping. (c) For severe cramping, lower the enema bag or container below the level of the bed. Flatus pockets are often broken in this manner.
17. Administer the full amount of enema solution, if no such problem occurs. Do not end the enema until at least three-fourths of the solution is given (unless any serious problems occurred) to fulfill the purpose of enema and to ensure that the complete large bowel has been filled with the enema solution.
18. If resistance is met while inserting the enema tube, then permit a small amount of solution to enter, after that withdraw the tube slightly and then continue to reinsert the tube. Resistance may be due to intestinal spasms or failure of the internal sphincter to open. The small amount of solution may help to reduce the spasms and relax the sphincter. Ask the child to

take deep breaths because this may also help to relax the anal sphincter.

19. If the child cannot retain the enema solution for an adequate amount of time, then modify the amount and length of administration of enema. The child may need to be placed on a bedpan in supine position while receiving the enema. Elevate the head of child's bed 30-degree to provide more comfort to the child.
20. On completion of administering enema, remove the rectal tube or container tip by pressing the buttocks together and quickly withdrawing the tube. The urge to defecate is diminished with this approach.
21. Instruct the child to retain the solution as long as possible. Holding the buttocks of the infant or small child together, by the parent or nurse will assist to retain the solution. The evacuation reflex is stimulated by fluid retention.
22. Assist the child onto the bedpan or to the toilet. An upright sitting position facilitates in elimination of the solution and subsequent defecation.
23. Assist the child for cleaning or washing using wet cotton balls to maintain perianal hygiene, as necessary. Washing the child's buttocks decreases skin irritation and prevents the spread of microorganisms. Teach the child to cleanse the perianal area always from front to back to prevent contamination of the urinary meatus.
24. Make the child comfortable. Praise for co-operation during the procedure of enema.
25. Dispose the used supplies and waste in appropriate containers as standard precautions.
26. Remove gloves and perform hand hygiene to reduce contaminations and cross infections.
27. Document the procedure of enema and findings related to the procedure.

Evaluation and Documentation

- Evaluate the child for general health status and determine the presence of any complications of enema such as abdominal cramp, excessive irritation of colonic mucosa, electrolyte abnormalities, arrhythmias due to vasovagal stimulation and water intoxication
  Evaluate child's psychological concerns and provide age appropriate emotional support. Allow parents with the child to cope with the situation. Evaluate parent's understanding
- Document the followings: Date and time of enema given, types of enema, amount of fluid administered, amount of output after enema, child's response to enema, complaints of unusual pain, symptoms of shock and any other abnormal reactions.

Communication and Teaching for Homecare

- Communicate with the child, especially with the older child and parents about child's general health condition, effects of enema, presence of any problems and plan of continuation of treatment
- Teach the parents, if possible to child also, about hygienic practices, dietary habit, and amount of water intake and use of laxatives, if required. Discuss about continuation of treatment at home, need for emergency medical help and plan of follow-up schedule.

PROCEDURE–19: INSERTION AND REMOVAL OF INDWELLING URINARY CATHETER IN CHILDREN

Clinical Guidelines

- Indwelling urinary catheter facilitates continuous bladder drainage that remains in situ for longer period of time until the child is able to void voluntarily without any problems
- Patients with chronic difficulty in spontaneous urination, sometimes are given indwelling urinary catheter; as an alternative, they may be instructed in the technique of clean, intermittent self-catheterization to empty the urinary bladder
- Older children can do intermittent self-catheterization or parents can do for their children with appropriate teaching, demonstration and return demonstration.

For most patients/children, this technique requires to be done for 4–5 times daily

- Indications of indwelling urinary catheter in children are mainly considered as urinary obstructions, urinary retention, urinary surgical interventions, neurogenic bladder incontinence of urine in unconscious patients or spinal cord injury or quadriplegic or paraplegic child
- Selection of urinary catheter is based on the child's age and gender, construction material of the catheter and the internal and external diameter of the catheter. Recommended urinary catheter size for children are: (a) up to 2 years of age – 6 F, (b) 2–5 years of age 6–8 F, (c) 5–10 years of age 8–10 F, and (d) 10–16 years of age 10 – 12 F
- When self-retaining balloon catheters are used, they should be made of silicon or coated with Teflon to reduce irritation and inflammation of urethral mucosa
- Use of water-soluble lubricant, 2% lidocaine gel is effective in reducing discomfort associated with insertion of urinary catheter. Lidocaine gel takes at least 8 minutes for the anesthetic effect to be completed. Use of lubricant must be considered based on child's age, level of anxiety and urgency of the procedure. The use of lidocaine lubricant may be more appropriate with older adolescents. In younger child it may increase the length of the procedure and therefore increase the child's anxiety.
  Total amount of lidocaine gel required in infant is – $\frac{1}{2}$ to $1\frac{1}{2}$ mL, in toddler it is – $1\frac{1}{2}$ to $2\frac{1}{2}$ mL, in school-aged – $2\frac{1}{2}$ to 5 mL and in adolescent it is 3–5 mL
- Sterile technique must be followed strictly during insertion of urinary catheter to prevent catheter related urinary tract infections, which is one of the most common HCAIs. Presence of another nurse may be necessary to assist during urinary catheterization to maintain asepsis and sterile technique throughout the procedure
- Carefully performed intermittent catheterization is less likely to cause urinary tract infections than the chronic indwelling urinary catheterization.

Equipment Required

For Insertion of Indwelling Urinary Catheter

- Hand hygiene supplies for hand wash and hand rub to prevent cross infections
- Prepackaged sterile urinary indwelling catheter insertion kit or obtain following sterile items in a covered sterile tray: (i) gloves, (ii) povidone-iodine swabs, (iii) water soluble lubricant, (iv) towels and drapes, (v) syringe filled with 3–5 mL of sterile water, (vi) gravity drainage and urine collection bag, and (vii) age-appropriate urinary catheter
- Transfer forceps or lifter in a sterile container to use for handling sterile items
- Nonsterile gloves, gown in a container and protective eyewear
- Applicator with 2% lidocaine water soluble lubricant, if prescribed
- Wash basin, soap and lukewarm water, washcloths and towels, if needed
- Sheet to drape the older child, may not be necessary for infant and small child
- Waterproof pad or mackintosh and towel to protect the child's bed
- Flashlight or examination light, if needed
- Adhesive tape to fix the urinary catheter
- Waste disposal containers and one small paper-lined waste receptacle/kidney dish
- Documentation sheet for catheterization and child's case sheet.

For Removal of Indwelling Urinary Catheter

- Hand hygiene supplies for hand wash and hand rub to prevent cross infections
- Nonsterile gloves, gown in a container and protective eyewear
- Sheet to drape the older child, may not be necessary for infant and small child
- Waterproof pad or mackintosh and towel to protect the child's bed
- Syringe to deflate the balloon of the indwelling catheter
- Wash basin, soap and lukewarm water, washcloths and towels, if needed

- Waste disposal containers and one small paper-lined waste receptacle/kidney dish
- Documentation sheet for removal of urinary catheter and child's case sheet.

Assessment and Preparation

- Assess the child for indications of indwelling urinary catheterization, presence of distended urinary bladder, inability to void, burning on urination, feeling of fullness and signs and symptoms of other urinary problems. Assess child's vital signs and general health condition. Assess cognitive level, readiness and ability to process information, level of understanding and anxiety of the family and the child, as appropriate
- Self-preparation should be done with meticulous hand hygiene and practice of sterile technique during catheterization. Assistance of another nurse may be necessary to maintain sterility of the supplies and to support the child during the procedure
- Environment should be clean, calm, well lighted and free of overcrowding. This procedure can be performed on the child's bed or in the procedure room. Privacy must be maintained especially for older children
- Articles preparation should be done for maintenance of strict aseptic technique. All supplies must be sterile for insertion of urinary catheter
- Preparation of parents: Explain the purpose of indwelling urinary catheterization, precautions and risks of placing an indwelling catheter. Assure the parents that the catheterization will not harm the child or damage the urethra or hymen, if all precautions and care are provided in due time. Provide the opportunity to ask questions
- Preparation of child: Explain the procedure of indwelling urinary catheterization in age-appropriate and simple language. Make the child clean and comfortable. Ensure privacy of older child. Provide the opportunity to ask questions and alleviate fears in older child. Reassure the older child that the catheter is flexible and will produce a feeling of pressure and a desire to urinate. Support the young child with participation of the parent and following gentle approach during the procedure.

Performing the Steps of Procedure with Rationale/Point of Emphasis

Insertion of an Indwelling Urinary Catheter

1. Perform hand hygiene to reduce transmission of microorganisms.
2. Gather all necessary supplies near the child to promote efficient time management and to provide an organized approach to the procedure of urinary catheterization.
3. Ensure selection of appropriate size catheter for the child. Small catheter sizes promote comfort. Use of shorter-length urinary catheter based on gender and age of the child can reduce incidence of knotting. For toddlers and younger females, insert the catheter two inches in the urethra. For male toddlers, insert 3–4 inches into the urethra.
4. Have extra catheter readily available during the procedure of urinary catheterization. If the catheter becomes contaminated or inadvertently placed in the vagina of female child or turns out to be incorrect size, then an extra catheter will be immediately needed to maintain sterility in catheterization and to complete the procedure in a timely manner.
5. Maintain privacy of the child during catheterization. Draw the curtains around the child's bed or close the door of the child's room.
6. Raise the child's bed to a comfortable height or stand on a step stool at the crib side. This reduces your back strain during performance of the procedure.
7. Perform hand hygiene. Don nonsterile gloves and protective apparel, as standard precautions to reduce transmission of microorganisms and cross infections.
8. Place a waterproof pad or mackintosh and towel under the child's/infant's buttocks

while positioning the child/infant. This prevents the bed linen being soiled.

9. Place the female infant/child in supine position with the heels of the feet together and the knees tilted outward (in frog-like position). Use rolled blanket, pillow or towels to support legs in this position. This position facilitates visualization of inner labia
   i. Place the male infant/child in supine position with legs together. Used rolled towels under the knees. Raise the penis and scrotal sac to rest on top of the thighs. This position facilitates visualization of the urethral opening. Bending the knees slightly may be more comfortable position for the child
   ii. Remind the older child to keep his or her buttocks on the bed or procedure table and to keep the perineal muscles relaxed. The child may need to be reminded this for several times during the procedure.
10. Place a drape over the child. In females, place the drape in a diamond configuration with one corner at the child's sternum, one corner over each knee and one corner over the perineum. In males, cover the child's chest and lower extremities with sheets, leaving only the genital area exposed. This allows exposure of the child's perineum while covering the rest of the body and maintaining child's privacy.
11. Clean the child's genital area with soap and lukewarm water. Rinse thoroughly and dry the area. This helps to remove secretions, dirt and feces.
12. Remove gloves and perform hand hygiene to prevent cross infections.
13. Don sterile gloves to maintain sterile technique during insertion of urinary catheter.
14. Take help from the assistant to maintain sterile technique.
15. Establish a sterile working area, using a sterile towel spreading open. It helps to establish a space/sterile field to gather sterile equipment and proceed with catheterization without contamination.
16. Using sterile technique, open the sterile catheter, sterile povidone-iodine swabs, sterile lubricant, sterile applicator, sterile prefilled syringe with sterile water, and place them on sterile working field
   i. Open the sterile gravity drainage and urine collection bag and keep it on a convenient place/container. This facilitates easy access to the equipment. If lidocaine gel is to be used, assemble lidocaine applicator according to the manufacturer's instructions and follow the procedure of use of lidocaine lubricant gel.
17. Aseptically place a sterile towel between the female child's legs under the perineum area or on the thigh of a male child. This provides extension of sterile working area.
18. Attach the prefilled syringe of water to the secondary lumen balloon port of the urinary catheter and inflate the balloon with the sterile water and then deflate the balloon, retaining the sterile water in the syringe only. Ensure that the balloon of the retention catheter is working and does not have a leak.
19. For insertion of catheter in female child, expose the urethral opening of the female child using the thumb and middle finger of your nondominant sterile hand to spread open the child's labia, while laying your nondominant arm across the midsection of the lower abdomen. This allows exposure and visualization of urethral opening. A flashlight or examination light may be helpful in locating the urethral opening
   i. For a male child, use your nondominant hand to position the child's penis perpendicular to child's body, while laying your nondominant arm across the midsection of the lower abdomen. In an uncircumcised male child, withdraw the foreskin just for enough to visualize the urethral opening. Do not pull back behind the glans penis. Withdrawing the foreskin further will be painful to the child and could cause tears that could lead to potential sites of infections.

20. Cleanse the area around the urethral opening using the sterile povidone-iodine swabs with the dominant sterile hand. Discard the used swabs in a nearby waste receptacle/paper lined kidney dish
    i. In females, using a separate povidone-iodine swab for each stroke, cleanse both right and left side of the inner labia with one downward stroke. Then clean midline, from the clitoris down to the rectum with one stroke
    ii. In males, cleanse the penis in an outgoing circular motion, from the urethral opening to the base of the penis, using a new povidone-iodine swab each time
    iii. This prevents contamination of the catheter by microorganisms present on the skin, thus prevents introduction of microorganisms into the patient's urethra and urinary bladder.
21. Lubricate the tip of the sterile catheter, using your sterile dominant hand, with water-soluble lubricant that has been squirted on the sterile field. Take help of the assistant to maintain asepsis. The catheter should be lubricated about 2 inches for a female child and about 6 inches for a male child. Lubrication decreases the friction between the catheter and the urinary tract during insertion of the catheter.
22. Lift the lubricated tip of the catheter with your dominant sterile hand and gently insert it into the child's urethral opening.
23. Collect sterile urine specimen at this time for laboratory examination, whenever indicated.
24. Do not touch the child's perineal skin or hair, during advancement of the catheter into the urethra. Skin or hair usually contaminates the urinary catheter.
25. In males, insert the lubricated catheter tip into the urethra without allowing the intraurethral lubricant (if lidocaine gel was used) to exit the urethral meatus. Because gentle pressure may cause an erection of penis in an adolescent male. If the adolescent has an erection of penis, stop the procedure until there is a non-erectile state and then continue with the procedure. Hold the penis firmly but not tightly. If held tightly, pressure will collapse the urethra and will prevent advancement of the catheter.
26. Ask the child to take a deep breath while inserting the catheter. Deep breath helps to relax the urinary tract.
27. Insert the catheter until urine begins to flow. If an obstruction is encountered, do not force the catheter. If the catheter is inadvertently placed in the vagina in females, leave it in place. Take the second catheter and insert it in the urethra. After second catheter is placed in the urethra, remove the first catheter from vagina. In males, if the prepuce is retractable, put it back in the natural position after inserting the catheter. This avoids possible painful swelling of the glans penis (paraphimosis)
    i. A "Rule of Thumb for Catheter length" in males is twice the length of the penis plus 4 cm. Insertion of the catheter too far into the bladder can cause irritation to the bladder wall and/or knotting of the catheter. Forcing the catheter can cause trauma, bleeding and possible scar formation, which can lead to strictures and obstruction of the urethra
    ii. If lidocaine gel is used it will increase the volume of intraurethral lubricant. Therefore urine return may not be as rapid as when minimal amounts of water-soluble lubricants are used for insertion of catheter
    iii. When the catheter reaches proximal urethra in males and mid-urethra in females, the child may vigorously contract the pelvic muscles, that temporarily stopping insertion of the catheter. Hold the catheter in place with steady gentle pressure. Assist the child to press the hips against the bed or procedure table and to relax the pelvic muscles, before gently advancing the catheter into the urinary bladder. If still unable to advance the catheter, discontinue the procedure and notify the healthcare prescriber.

28. After urinary flow is established, insert the catheter approximately 1–2 cm further and inflate the secondary lumen balloon port of the catheter with sterile water to the specified amount and disconnect the syringe. Use only the specified amount of sterile water to prevent over-inflation of balloon which can cause balloon rupture. Balloon prevents the catheter from slipping out and accidental dislodgement
    i. If the child complains of pain or burning sensation, it indicates that urinary catheter may not be fully seated in the urinary bladder. Then deflate the balloon, advance the catheter further and re-inflate the balloon.
29. Gently tug or pull back slightly on the catheter. It ensures that the catheter is securely seated in the urinary bladder and not floating.
30. Tightly connect the sterile gravity drainage and urine collection bag to the urinary catheter. Tape the connections and ensure that urine continues to flow out the tubing. It provides a closed-system collection of urine output.
31. Attach the urine collection bag to the frame of the child's bed or crib, below the level of urinary bladder, ensuring there are no kinks or obstructions in the tubing. Positioning the urine collection bag below the level of the bladder prevents reflux of urine through the tubing and back into the urinary bladder.
32. Cleanse the child's perineal area. Cleansing promotes the child's comfort and sense of well being, while removing the povidone-iodine solution from the area.
33. Ensure that foreskin of the uncircumcised male child is in its normal position. Failure to return the foreskin can lead to swelling of the penis and impairment of circulation.
34. Tape the catheter tubing to the thigh of the older child on the intact skin. For small male infants and neonates not using a balloon catheter, tape the catheter to the lower abdomen or upper perineum, allowing the penis to point upward toward the umbilicus. For small female infants or neonates not using balloon catheter, tape the catheter at its closest point outside on the left or right labia or thigh
    i. Taping prevents any tension from being placed on the catheter from inside the urinary bladder and avoids dislodgement from accidental pulling or tugging. Movements of the catheter in and out can lead to contamination from microorganisms.
35. Place the child in comfortable position on his or her bed. Praise the older child for cooperation. Ask the child for any discomfort in lower abdomen.
36. Observe for the flow and amount of urine output to the urine bag. Check the urine bag secure in place.
37. Set the child's bed to the lowest position or as age-appropriate, and secure the side rails to prevent accidental falls and injury.
38. Dispose all used supplies and waste in appropriate containers as BMW guidelines.
39. Remove gloves and perform hand hygiene to reduce transmission of microorganisms.
40. Document the procedure of indwelling urinary catheterization and related findings.

Removal of an Indwelling Urinary Catheter

1. Collaborate with the child, family and healthcare prescriber regarding time of removal of urinary catheter. Ensure child and family is prepared for the procedure.
2. Perform hand hygiene and collect all necessary supplies for removal of urinary catheter.
3. Provide privacy to the child during the procedure. Draw the curtains around the child's bed or close the door of child's room.
4. Adjust the child's bed in working height or stand on a step stool at crib side to reduce the strain placed on your back.
5. Perform hand hygiene. Don gloves, gown and protective eyewear as standard precautions.
6. Place a waterproof pad under the child's buttocks while positioning the child to prevent the bed linens from being soiled.

7. Place the child in supine position, legs spread apart, with access to the urinary catheter. This facilitates visualization of inner labia in females and the urethral opening. Boys should be placed in supine position with their legs straight for easy access.
8. Place a drape over the child to maintain privacy. Allow exposure to the child's perineum while covering the rest of the child's body.
9. Gently remove the tape holding urinary catheter in place, for easy removal of catheter.
10. Attach a syringe to the secondary lumen balloon port of the urinary catheter and deflate the balloon of its entire contents of sterile water. This allows atraumatic removal of the self-retaining catheter.
11. Gently remove the urinary catheter by withdrawing slowly and evenly. If resistance is felt, do not pull harder. Stop the catheter removal procedure and notify the healthcare prescriber. Any resistance to removal may suggest kinking, knotting, failure of balloon deflation or stone formation. Forceful pulling leads to irritation and trauma to the urethra.
12. Wash the child's genital area with lukewarm water and soap to remove secretions and leaked urine. Rinse and dry the area to reduce growth of microorganisms.
13. Remove the waterproof under-pad and cover the child as appropriate, to maintain privacy and sense of well being.
14. Make the child comfortable and ask for any discomfort or problems.
15. Adjust the child's bed in lowest position to prevent falls.
16. Dispose the used supplies and waste in appropriate containers as standard precautions.
17. Note the final amount of urine collected in the bag.
18. Remove gloves and perform hand hygiene to reduce transmission of microorganisms.
19. Monitor child's first void after removal of indwelling urinary catheter. Note the amount, color and presence of any sediment of the urine when the child does void. Decrease urinary bladder function may occur after the catheter is removed. Encourage the child to drink plenty of fluids. Assess the child for presence of dysuria, enuresis and hematuria for two days. A warm sitz bath may help to comfort the children who have voiding difficulties. Urinary tract infections can develop as a result of catheterization.
20. Document the procedure of removal of indwelling catheter and related findings.

Evaluation and Documentation

- Evaluate the amount, color, clarity, odor of urine and presence of any sediment. Evaluate the child for signs and symptoms of urinary tract infection including fever, tachycardia, nausea, vomiting, flank pain, foul-smelling urine, redness or irritation of urethral opening, urethral discharge, perineal discharge, cloudy or sedimented urine or urine discoloration. Evaluate child's general health status and level of anxiety
- Document the following: (a) date and time of urinary catheterization or removal of catheter, (b) amount, color, clarity, odor of urine and presence of any sediment, (c) size of the catheter, (d) amount of sterile water in balloon, (e) child's response, (f) presence of signs and symptoms of urinary tract infections, and (g) any other abnormal findings.

Communication and Teaching for Homecare

- Communicate with child and parents about the effectiveness of catheterization, presence of any complications and future plan of management
- Teach the parents and the child, as appropriate, about hygienic care, general cleanliness, perineal hygiene, routine care/self care by the child, frequent water intake (if not contraindicated), measurement of urine output, presence of blood in urine, features of urinary tract infections and any other abnormalities,

need for medical assistance and plan of follow-up schedule for continuation of further treatment.

PROCEDURE–20: CARE OF INDWELLING URINARY CATHETER OF CHILDREN

Clinical Guidelines

- Placement of indwelling urinary catheter or retention catheter is performed for many reasons. This is including but not limited to—(a) insertion before, for and after surgical interventions; (b) assisting the sick child in urinary elimination of those who are unable to void spontaneously; (c) maintaining an empty urinary bladder; (d) instilling medications in urinary bladder; (e) splinting the urethra; (f) preciously measuring urine output; (g) obtaining urine for analysis over an extended period; and (h) urinary incontinence
- Performance of hygienic care at least twice a day for children with an indwelling urinary catheter is important to prevent infections
- Privacy must be ensured for the child during care of urinary catheter
- Institutional policy is followed to determine how long the urinary catheter may remain in place without being changed or to be removed, when indicated
- Children with indwelling urinary catheter are observed for signs and symptoms of urinary tract infections as long as the catheter is in place and for several days after it is removed.

Equipment Required

- Hand hygiene supplies for hand wash and hand rub to decrease HCAIs
- Gloves to protect nurse's hand being contaminated
- Syringe, to check and inflate the balloon of the catheter, if needed
- Basin with soap and warm water, washcloths and towels
- Waterproof sheet or pad to protect the child's bed
- Sheet to drape the child, especially the older child
- Examination light or flush light, Curtains for privacy, if required
- Waste disposal containers as per BMW rules
- Documentation sheet for care of indwelling urinary catheter and child's case sheet.

Assessment and Preparation

- Assess the child for signs and symptoms of urinary tract infections or bladder infections including fever, burning sensation, and feeling of fullness, bladder spasms, foul-smelling urine, redness or irritation of urethral opening, urethral discharge, discomfort, pain and crying without consolation. Assess for distended bladder, lower abdominal distention and residual urine, if any, and for child's general health status
  - Assess the cognitive level, readiness and ability to understand the information by the child and family. The readiness to learn and process information may be impaired as a result of age, stress or anxiety
- Self-preparation should be done with practice of standard precautions of infection control
- Environment should be clean, calm, well lighted and free of overcrowding
- All necessary supplies should be collected and arranged at child's bed side
- Preparation of parents: Explain the procedure of catheter care, its importance and precautions. Provide opportunity to ask questions to reduce anxiety
- Preparation of child: Explain the procedure, as appropriate, for care of indwelling urinary catheter. Ensure privacy and comfort. Ask for cooperation and related questions.

Performing the Steps of Procedure with Rationale/Point of Emphasis

1. Perform hand hygiene to reduce the transmission of microorganisms.
2. Collect and assemble all necessary supplies near the child for efficient time management.

3. Draw the curtains around the child's bed or close the door of the child's room to maintain privacy of the child during care of urinary catheter.
4. Ensure that the child's bed is in comfortable height to reduce your back strain.
5. Don gloves as standard precautions to prevent cross contaminations and infections.
6. Place waterproof sheet or pad under the child's buttocks, while positioning for catheter care, to protect child's bed to become wet.
7. Place the girl child in supine position with their legs spread apart to facilitate visualization of inner labia and urethral opening. Boys should be placed in supine position with their legs straight for easy access.
8. Place a drape over the child to maintain privacy, with exposure of the child's perineum only. For girls, place the drape in a diamond shape with one corner at the child's sternum, one corner over each knee and one corner over the child's perineum. For boys, cover the child's chest and lower extremities with sheets, leaving only the genital area exposed.
9. Use a flash light or examination light to locate the urethral opening.
10. Ensure patency of the balloon of indwelling catheter. Sterile water within the balloon may leach out, causing the balloon to deflate and the urinary catheter may slip out of the bladder. Re-inflate the balloon with the manufacturer specified amount of sterile water to ensure patency, whenever required.
11. Wash the child's genital area with lukewarm water and soap. Cleanse around the urinary meatus and around the catheter itself. Cleansing helps to remove secretions, smegma and fecal matter. Be careful not to manipulate the catheter back and forth, as movement of the catheter can introduce microorganisms and lead to urinary tract infections
    - For boys, gently retract the foreskin of the uncircumcised child and cleanse the area. Then return the foreskin to its normal position. Failure to return the foreskin can lead to swelling of the penis and impair circulation.
12. Observe for any signs of irritation, trauma, secretions or incrustations on the urinary catheter. Assess for any foul smells emanating from the urethra. These signs indicate presence of urinary tract infections.
13. Rinse the perineum of the child with plain water and allow drying. This prevent growth of microorganisms in the perineal region.
14. Assess the drainage tubing for urine flow. Observe that there are no kinks or obstructions in the tubing. Make sure that all connections are tightly secured. This provides a closed system collection of urine output with free flow of urine and prevents entry of organisms into the urinary catheter.
15. Ensure the urine collection bag or drainage bag is attached to the frame of the bed or crib below the level of the urinary bladder. It prevents reflux of urine through the tubing and back into the urinary bladder.
16. Ensure that the catheter is taped to the thigh of the child. Taping is done to prevent any tension from being placed on the catheter from inside the bladder and to avoid dislodgement from accidental pulling or tugging. Movement of the catheter in and out can lead to contamination from microorganisms. Ensure there are no pressure points or areas of skin break-down before taping or re-taping to the thigh or leg of the child.
17. Remove the waterproof under-pad or sheet and re-cover the child to promote sense of well-being. Make the child dry and comfortable.
18. Return the child's bed to the lowest position to prevent potential injury from falls.
19. Dispose all used supplies and waste in appropriate containers for standard precautions.
20. Remove gloves. Perform hand hygiene to reduce transmission of microorganisms.

21. Document the procedure of care of indwelling urinary catheter and related findings.

Evaluation and Documentation

- Evaluate the child's general health condition and signs and symptoms of urinary tract infections including fever, tachycardia, pain, foul-smelling urine or perineum, perineal discharge, cloudy or sedimented urine or urine discoloration and amount of urine. Evaluate child's response and reactions to the procedure of urinary catheter care
- Document the following: Time of completion of hygienic catheter care, catheter size in place, color, odor and clarity of urine, condition of child's skin in and around genital area, intactness of balloon, presence of signs and symptoms of urinary tract infections and child's response to the catheter care.

Communication and Teaching for Homecare

- Communicate with the child and parents about child's current health status and condition related to indwelling urinary catheter. Discuss about further plan of treatment and about the questions asked by the parents and the child
- Teach the parents and child (age appropriate) about hygienic practices, water intake, diet, routine care of the child at hospital and home, continuation of treatment, precautions to prevent catheter related urinary infections, possible complications in future, need for medical assistance and plan of follow-up visits.

PROCEDURE–21: URINE SPECIMEN COLLECTIONS FROM CHILDREN

Clinical Guidelines

- Urine sample collection for examination can be done as clean-catch (midstream) specimen, or routine voided specimen, or 24-hour period specimen, or indwelling catheter specimen, or straight catheter specimen (one-time catheter) or suprapubic aspiration specimen
- A clean-catch (midstream) urine specimen is collected when a urinary tract infection is suspected and uncontaminated urine is needed for urine culture and sensitivity or for routine examination. Confirmation of diagnosis of urinary tract infection is completed using transurethral bladder catheterization or suprapubic aspiration. This method is usually followed for older children
- Routine voided urine specimens are usually collected for routine urinalysis and can be used to examine the urine for color, specific gravity, pH, protein, glucose, acetone, bilirubin or the presence of blood or pus cells. It can also be used to check for presence of bacteria in the urine; however, it is not used to make a final determination of presence of the bacteria in urine
  - Routine urine sample collection for examination is done on child's admission to the hospital, before surgery or during routine check up for well-child visit
  - Methods of collection of routine voided urine specimen can be done using a clean bedpan or urinal or toilet specimen container for the toilet-trained child. For the child who is not toilet-trained, collect urine sample using an adhesive urine collection bag, or urine collection pad or cotton balls or foil bowl
- Urine is collected over a 24-hour period to examine and determine the excretion rate of certain hormones, proteins and electrolytes.
- Urine specimen from indwelling catheter is collected when a urinary tract infection is suspected and a sterile specimen is needed for urine culture and sensitivity test
- To confirm the diagnosis of urinary tract infection, suprapubic aspiration or transurethral bladder catheterization urine sample may be obtained, if a child with unexplained fever is assessed as being

sufficiently ill and warrant immediate antimicrobial therapy

- Whenever possible, collect the child's first voiding in the morning, because bacterial counts are the highest in this voiding. Such a specimen is more likely to reveal abnormalities than a later voiding
- The diagnosis of urinary tract infection cannot be established by culture of urine collected in a urinary bag.

Equipment Required

- Hand hygiene supplies for hand wash and hand rub to prevent cross contaminations
- Nonsterile gloves as protective barrier
- Basin with soap and warm water, wash-cloth and towel
- Sterile urine specimen container, adhesive urine collection bag, cotton balls
- Antimicrobial perineal wipes, swabs or sponges
- Waterproof sheet of pad, diaper and diaper changing requirements, if needed
- Adhesive specimen label or marker, appropriate laboratory requisition form
- Biohazard bag for transporting the urine specimen to the laboratory
- Waste disposal containers as per BMW guidelines
- Documentation sheet for urine specimen collection and child's case sheet.

Assessment and Preparation

- Assess child's health condition, presence of urinary problems or infections, indications for urine specimen collection, method to be followed for urine specimen collection, self-care ability of the child, readiness to follow instructions for urine collection, and present history for age-appropriate toilet training. Assess understanding level of both the child and parents to perform the urine specimen collection by themselves
- Self-preparation should be done with hand hygiene and standard precautions
- Environment should be clean, well lighted, and free of overcrowding
- All necessary supplies should be arranged at child's bedside for easy availability. Older child can do urine specimen collection at toilet or bathroom/washroom
- Preparation of parents: Explain the method and purpose of urine specimen collection. Allow the parent to help young toilet-trained child to collect the urine sample. Explain about hygienic measures and hand washing to follow during the urine sampling
- Preparation of child: Explain the child about method of urine specimen collection in age-appropriate simple language. Instruct the older child about the technique of midstream urine sampling and hygienic measures. Reply to the questions and area of concerns. Maintain privacy, whenever required for older children. Provide opportunity to ask questions for clarifications about the procedure. Offer the child to drink water or any other liquid before the procedure to encourage voiding.

Performing the Steps of Procedure with Rationale/Point of Emphasis

Clean-Catch (Midstream) Urine Specimen Collection

1. Perform hand hygiene to reduce the transmission of microorganisms.
2. Collect and assemble all necessary supplies for organized approach to the procedure.
3. Draw curtains around the child's bed or close the door of child's room to provide privacy, as appropriate. Use urinal for urination at bedside or assist to child to the use toilet/bathroom.
4. Don gloves to prevent transmission of microorganisms.
5. Remove the lid of the sterile specimen container and place it with the inside of the lid facing up, on clean surface within easy reach. Touching the inside of the lid causes contamination.
6. If parent is assisting or older child is performing self-care, he or she should

perform hand hygiene and don gloves (optional). This helps to prevent contamination of specimen.

7. Clean around the child's urethral opening with antimicrobial wipes, swabs or sponges and discard them in a nearby open waste receptacle. Allow the area to dry. This prevents specimen contamination by microorganisms on the skin
Instruct the parent or child how the clean the urethral opening area and assist, as needed.
8. Instruct the child to void a small amount of urine into the toilet or in urinal. This helps to cleanse the meatus of any remaining bacteria. Run water in the sink to trigger voiding.
9. Have the child urinate 10–20 mL directly into the sterile specimen container during midstream of urine. The child can then finish urinating in the toilet or urinal. Urinating directly into the specimen container decreases the possibility of specimen contamination.
10. Place the lid back on the specimen container. Avoid touching the inside of the lid or of the container. Wipe off the outside of the container.
11. Assist the child with wiping or cleansing the perineal area after voiding is complete, as needed to promote cleanliness.
12. Assist the child to return to bed after disposing of gloves and performing hand hygiene.
13. Label the specimen and place it in biohazard bag to send to the laboratory for examination with filled up laboratory requisition form.
14. Send the specimen to the laboratory immediately. Urine analysis results may alter, if the specimen is more than 1 hour old. If the specimen is not fresh, bacteria may enter into the urine and other components can break up and disintegrate.
15. Dispose the used supplies and waste in appropriate containers as standard precautions.
16. Remove gloves and perform hand hygiene.
17. Document the procedure of midstream urine specimen collection and related findings.

Routine Voided Urine Specimen Collection using Urine Collection Bag

1. Perform hand hygiene and don gloves. Ensure all supplies are within reach.
2. Position the child on back with legs in a frog-like position. This position exposes the genitalia to facilitate cleansing of the area and proper placement of urine collection bag.
3. Remove the diaper and clean the perineum or prepuce of the infant to prevent contamination of urine specimen.
4. Apply chemical adhesive (e.g., tincture benzoin or as prescribed) to maintain seal between the urine collection bag and child's skin. Do not use chemical adhesive on preterm infants or neonates to prevent skin irritation and transdermal tearing.
5. Attach the urine collection bag to the infant by removing the protective backing from the adhesive. Make sure that the bag does not cover anus. Proper placement of the bag avoids having to repeat the procedure
   - For boys, insert the penis and scrotum into the bag opening. Adhesive should adhere to perineum and symphysis. For girls, position lower half of adhesive on bag on perineum first and then press on adhesive up toward symphysis.
6. Cut a hole in the diaper, pulling the urine bag through the opening. When the child voids, it is easily visible and the urine bag can be removed immediately.
7. Replace the diaper and wait for the child to void. Child may not void immediately.
8. Remove gloves and perform hand hygiene to prevent cross contaminations.
9. After the child has voided, don gloves and remove the urine bag from the infant. Transfer urine to specimen container by holding the urine bag over open specimen container (without lid) cautiously.
10. Make the child clean and comfortable. Answer to the questions as asked.

11. Label the urine specimen and send the laboratory immediately for examination with filled up laboratory requisition form.
12. Dispose all waste in appropriate containers. Take care of reusable items.
13. Remove gloves. Perform hand hygiene.
14. Document urine collection procedure and about urine sample send for examination.

Refer: For Sterile Urine Specimen Collection during insertion of Plain or Indwelling Urinary Catheter, Procedure-19.

Evaluation and Documentation

- Evaluate child's health condition and reactions for the procedure of urine specimen collection. Evaluate the child's or parent's ability and how they have done the procedure of urine specimen collection and any problems occur in between
- Document the amount, color, odor of urine, presence of signs and symptoms of urinary infections or any other abnormalities. Document about the type of urine specimen send for laboratory examination and type for examination asked for. Document child's response about the procedure.

Communication and Teaching for Homecare

- Communicate with child and parents about child's urinary problems and purpose of urine specimen collection. Discuss about further plan of management and about areas of concern
- Teach the parents about hand washing, hygienic practices, water intake, routine care at hospital and home, continuation of treatment, as required, emergency health problems, need for medical help, and plan of follow-up visits.

PROCEDURE–22: BLOOD SAMPLING BY VENIPUNCTURE FROM PERIPHERAL SITES OF CHILDREN

Clinical Guidelines

- Blood specimens are collected for various laboratory examinations to detect underlying pathophysiology of disease conditions and considered as most common diagnostic approach. Usually venous and capillary blood sampling are done for the children, but arterial blood sampling also may required as diagnostic procedures
- Blood sampling should always be done using aseptic technique and standard precautions. Appropriate skin preparation with antiseptic agents before venipuncture must be followed as it is very significant to prevent entry of microorganisms directly into the blood stream. Hand washing and use of sterile gloves should be practiced to reduce cross contamination
- Precautions must be followed to prevent contamination of blood specimen containers
- Blood specimens should be sent to the specific laboratory immediately to prevent alteration of examination findings due to delay. Filled up requisition form with required investigations should be clearly mentioned
- Most commonly used venipuncture sites are veins in the upper extremities such as cephalic vein, dorsal arch, fifth interdigital vein, median antebrachial vein, basilic vein, median basilic vein
- Avoid veins above where an IV line is in place or any scars or lesions are present. IV fluids alter the test results findings. Scars make the entry into the vein more difficult. Lesions are avoided to prevent the transfer of microorganisms.

Equipment Required

- Hand hygiene supplies for hand wash and hand rub to prevent cross contaminations
- Sterile gloves, dry sterile gauze pads, cotton swabs/wipes in a sterile container
- Alcohol 70% or alcohol wipes or chlorhexidine for skin preparation at venipuncture site
- Venous access device: Vacuum container needle and vacuum holder with needle protection system (for blood sampling)

or appropriate size syringe and needle, if vacuum container is not available
- Appropriate blood specimen tubes for blood tests, as prescribed
- Tourniquet, if needed and topical anesthetic, if prescribed
- Small adhesive tape or bandage
- Label for blood specimen tubes or marker
- Appropriate laboratory requisition form
- Biohazard bag for transporting the specimen to the laboratory
- Waste disposal containers as per BMW rules
- Procedure Documentation sheet for blood specimen collection and child's case sheet.

Assessment and Preparation

- Assess severity of child's illness and previous venipuncture experiences. Assess child's total blood volume and associated pathology (e.g., anemia, blood loss, shock) to determine necessity of limiting the amount of blood to be taken. Check with the laboratory to determine the minimum amount of blood needed for tests
  - Determine whether there is time for use of topical pain relief and amount of time that can be devoted to explain of procedure. Determine whether fasting or after food or timing of medication administration need to be consider for the test being performed
- Self preparation should be with hand hygiene and practice of aseptic technique
- Environment should be clean, calm, well lighted and free of overcrowding
- Articles preparation should be done following aseptic process for venipuncture
- Preparation of parents: Explain the procedure, its purpose and necessary precautions for the procedure, Encourage parents to remain with the child during the venipuncture to practice distraction techniques and to help the child to cope with the pain of venipuncture
- Preparation of child: Explain the child as appropriatc for developmental age. Ask for cooperation. Instruct the child to stay still but he or she can cry if desired so. Do not give false information regarding pain. Distract the child with play materials. Make the child clean and comfortable.

Performing the Steps of Procedure with Rationale/Point of Emphasis

1. Verify the child's investigation instructions for blood sampling and laboratory requisitions to avoid unneeded venipuncture and to collect required supplies for the procedure.
2. Identify the child using two patient identifiers to ensure correct patient for blood specimen collection for required laboratory tests.
3. Perform hand hygiene to reduce transmission of microorganisms.
4. Gather necessary supplies based on size of the child, method of collection and required blood tests to be done. This promotes efficient time management and provides organized approach. Too large needle may damage valves in the vein
   - Use of the syringe and straight needle to draw blood is not suitable and not recommended, because the amount of pressure exerted to draw blood sample cannot be controlled. The vein may collapse and damage may occur. It is better to use vacuum container needle and vacuum holder with needle protection system for blood sampling.
5. Select puncture site, using the distal veins first. Veins most commonly used are the antecubital fossa veins. The median antecubital vein may not always be visible, but it is usually large and palpable. It is well supported by subcutaneous tissue and least likely to roll. Other veins also can be used especially as per child's choice **(Fig. 3.8)**.
6. Place the venipuncture site in dependent position to facilitate blood flow to that area.
7. Position the child comfortably. Young child can lie down and a second person or parent can assist to stabilize the venipuncture site. Older child may cooperate better with detailed explanations. He or she can sit up with the arm well supported on a pillow.

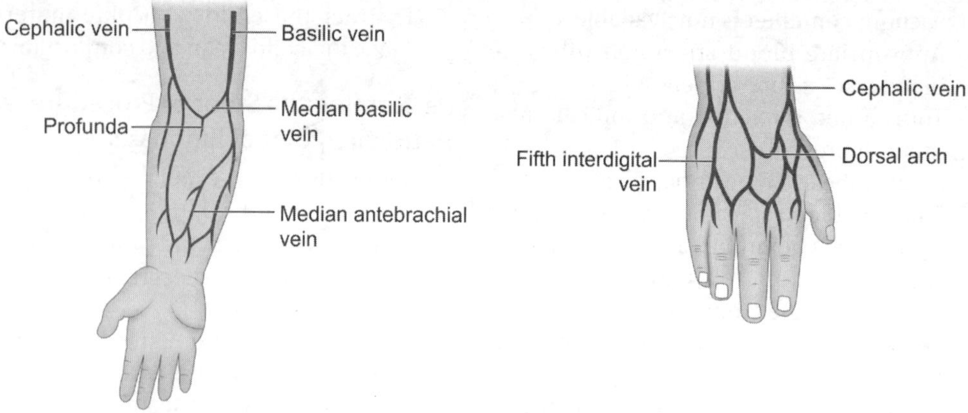

Fig. 3.8: Venipuncture sites of upper extremities for blood sampling.

8. Don gloves as per standard precautions to reduce transmission of microorganisms.
9. If the child is able to follow the instructions, ask the child to make a fist. This helps in vein distention for older child.
10. Apply tourniquet around child's extremity above the venipuncture site. This obstructs venous blood flow and causes vein distention so that the vein is easier to see and palpate.
11. Cleanse the venipuncture site with alcohol or chlorhexidine using circular motion from puncture site outward. When using alcohol, scrub the site for 20 seconds and allow drying. If using chlorhexidine, allow to dry for at least 30 seconds. Always use chlorhexidine when obtaining blood culture sample
    - Cleansing with antiseptic agents removes microorganisms from the selected venipuncture site, thus decreasing the transfer of microorganisms into the bloodstream. Alcohol is less effective than chlorhexidine in decreasing bacterial colonization and can cause tissue damage.
12. Do not touch the cleansed area again with your fingers or any other unsterile object after cleansing with antiseptic agent.
13. Remove the needle shield. Anchor the child's selected vein with thumb of your nondominant hand. This helps to prevent rolling of the vein.
14. Hold the needle bevel up, positioned at a 45-degree angle over the vein. This allows placement of the needle parallel to the vein.
15. Puncture the vein at selected site. If unsuccessful after two attempts, ask another practitioner or care provider to perform the procedure of venipuncture.
16. Obtain required amount of blood using a vacuum container. If the needle is in the vein, the tube will begin to fill with blood. Stabilize the vacuum holder and push in on the specimen tube to puncture the stopper. When first specimen tube is full, remove it from the vacuum holder while stabilizing the holder, insert succeeding tubes in holder, making sure that the stoppers are punctured on each tube to initiate blood flow. Gently invert tubes containing additives for 8–10 times.
17. If no blood flows into the specimen tube or ceases to flow before an adequate blood sample is collected, the following steps to be done: (a) Confirm correct needle position, change the angle of needle insertion by a few degrees, (b) Remove specimen tube and replace with a new specimen tube, (c) If the new tube does not fill with blood, remove the needle, (d) Evaluate the need for repeat venipuncture.
18. Release the tourniquet to prevent blood entering surrounding tissue.

19. Note the total amount of blood withdrawn to keep record of how much blood has been taken for laboratory tests.
20. Remove the tourniquet to allow venous blood flow to resume.
21. Apply dry sterile gauze pad and withdraw the needle. Apply pressure to venipuncture site until bleeding stops. Keep the child's arm straight and elevate the extremity above the level of the heart. This helps to stop bleeding. Elevation of extremity promotes negative pressure in vein and facilitates clotting.
    Do not bend the child's arm after drawing blood because it promotes hematoma formation. Children with cardiac disease should not raise their extremities, because this action creates negative pressure in veins and can lead to complications.
22. Place blood specimen in appropriate tube to ensure adequate preparation and stabilization of specimen for accurate analysis.
23. Invert all tubes containing additives for 8–10 times, before specimen collection in next tube, to ensure mixture of additives. Do not shake tubes. Rough handling of tubes such as forceful injection or shaking may damage erythrocytes and alter laboratory results.
24. Dispose the sharps immediately to prevent accidental needlestick injuries with contaminated sharps.
25. Apply small adhesive bandage, as appropriate to prevent further bleeding. This reassures the children as feel that all their blood will not leak out.
26. Make the child comfortable and praise for cooperation, as appropriate.
27. Label the blood specimen tubes or containers with child's name, medical record number, date and time of collection of blood sample, test to be done, unit/ward and initials of person collecting. This ensures correct specimens are tested for correct child.
28. Place the blood specimen in biohazard bag to prevent contamination and transport to the laboratory along with filled up laboratory requisition form.
29. Dispose all waste in appropriate container to prevent cross infections.
30. Remove gloves and perform hand hygiene to reduce transmission of microorganisms.
31. Recheck the venipuncture site for any bleeding or hematoma.
32. Document the procedure of blood sampling, plan of laboratory tests for the child and presence of any problems during the procedure.

Evaluation and Documentation

- Evaluate child's health status and reactions after venipuncture for blood sampling. Evaluate child and family understanding of venipuncture and coping during the procedure
- Document date, time and site of venipuncture, specimen obtained for laboratory tests, amount of blood loss and child's response to pain during procedure.

Communication and Teaching for Homecare

- Communicate with the child and parents about child's health condition, expected date and time of receiving laboratory results and plan of continuation of treatment
- Teach the parents about the care of venipuncture site, routine care of the child at hospital and home including hygienic practices, dietary intake, activity limitations, signs of complications (e.g., bleeding, infections), need for medical help, transport, referral facility available and follow-up schedule for long-term management.

PROCEDURE–23: CAPILLARY BLOOD GLUCOSE MONITORING OF CHILDREN BY GLUCOMETER

Clinical Guidelines

- Blood glucose monitoring helps to detect hypoglycemia and hyperglycemia in various childhood health problems. This helps the child with diabetes to reach

a desired level of glycemic control and management of the disease condition
- For the child with diabetes, it is important to perform the blood glucose monitoring at the prescribed time for the assessment of insulin requirements and treatment of hypoglycemia. Strict glycemic control is important to prevent diabetes-related complications. For other health problems in which hypoglycemia or hyperglycemia is concern, blood glucose monitoring is performed based on clinical signs and symptoms
- Capillary whole blood glucose level is measured with Glucometer and reagent strips to do rapid assessment of child's metabolic state at bedside, at triage or at home. Venous blood can also be used for blood glucose estimation by the laboratory test
- Test result from glucometer is not as accurate as laboratory results and does not distinguish between true hypoglycemia and low-normal reading. The diagnosis of diabetes or verification of hypoglycemia must be made using laboratory blood glucose results, not glucometer results. Venous and capillary blood glucose concentration may differ, depending on how long after a meal the blood sample is collected. Plasma and serum reading may be 10% higher than whole blood
- Puncture site of capillary blood glucose (CBG) monitoring usually vary with the age of the child, for example heel stick is common for neonates and finger stick is common for older children
- Follow strict aseptic technique and standard precautions for the needle stick procedure
- CBG estimation must be taught to the older children with diabetes and to their parents, so that they can perform the procedure at home or whenever necessary with necessary precautions.

Equipment Required

- Hand hygiene supplies for hand wash and hand rub
- Glucometer and test strips
- Lancets, lancet device or 25 or 26 gauze needle
- Sterile cotton swabs, sterile gauze pieces in a sterile covered container
- Sterile gloves to prevent transmission of organisms
- A bottle of 70% alcohol for skin preparation
- Waste disposal containers as per BMW guidelines
- Procedure Record sheet for CBG estimation and child treatment sheet.

Assessment and Preparation

- Assess the child's health status and comfort level. Assess child and parents for level of understanding of the procedure and its significance and readiness to learn the monitoring of blood glucose using Glucometer, if needed to be performed at home
- Self-preparation should be done by hand hygiene and practice of standard precautions
- Environment should be clean, stress free and well lighted
- All necessary articles should be assembled near the child's bed
- Preparation of parents: Explain the procedure and its purpose. Involve them during the use of glucometer. Parent can hold the child securely during puncturing the site to collect blood sample
- Preparation of child: Explain the procedure in age-appropriate simple words. Older child can assist and learn the procedure. Make the young child clean and comfortable. Allow toys or dolls to the child as diversional measures to get cooperation during the procedure. Ask for cooperation to prevent pain and discomfort.

Performing the Steps of Procedure with Rationale/Point of Emphasis

1. Review the child's treatment sheet or prescription to determine the rational and timing for blood glucose estimation using glucometer.

2. Perform hand hygiene and assemble all necessary items near the child for organized approach and efficient time management.
3. Ensure glucometer is functioning correctly and verify that quality control of the glucometer has been done.
4. Check the expiry date and any discoloration of the reagent strips. Make sure that the cap is always kept on to cover the reagent strips container, as strips are sensitive to light and humidity and may become inactivated.
5. Check the matching of code on the glucometer to the code on the test strip container to ensure accurate reading.
6. Load the lancet in lancet device according to manufacturer's instructions. Lancet device is more comfortable for the child because it may not penetrate the skin as deeply as using the lancet alone. Lancet sizes vary for use with neonates, children and adults. Use a new lancet for each procedure. Needle can be used if lancets are not available.
7. Perform hand hygiene and don gloves. Follow standard precautions to protect against exposure to blood or body fluids.
8. Select a puncture site for CBG estimation:
   i. In neonates, infants and children who are not walking, heel stick is commonly used
   ii. In infants and toddlers with diabetes, the toe pads can be used
   iii. In older children and adolescents, the end or lateral aspect of the fingertips (middle-fingers or ring-fingers) is the most common site. Do not use the very center of the finger pad, because it is very sensitive to pain. Use a site just lateral to the center that can help to reduce the child's discomfort (Refer **Figs. 3.9A and B**).
   iv. Alternate sites can be used for testing such as finger pads, heel of hand on thumb side or finger side, forearms, upper arms, thighs, or abdomen. Alternate site testing is not as accurate as testing fingertips, heels and toes.
9. Warm the puncture site, if needed. Use warm water or warm cloth. This promotes vasodilation, which helps to obtain an adequate-sized blood sample.

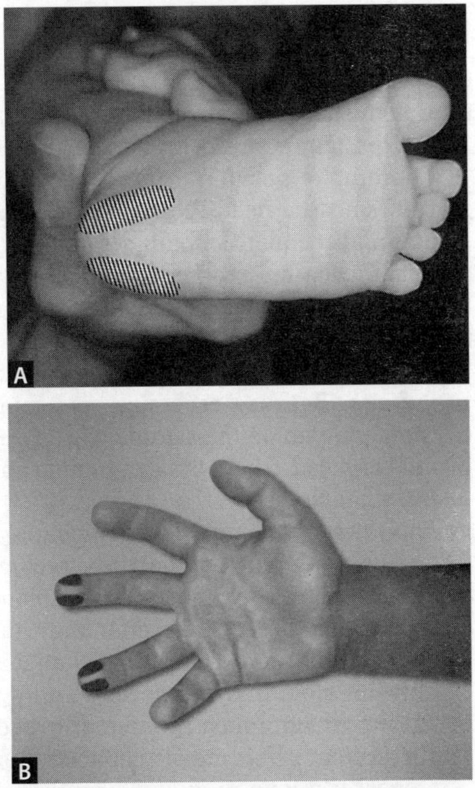

Figs. 3.9A and B: Sites for heel stick and fingertip for capillary blood sampling. A. Posterolateral aspect of heel for children younger than 18 months. B. Sides of third or fourth finger near the tip for children older than 18 months of age.

10. Turn on the glucometer. Place test strip into the glucometer. Follow manufacturer instructions to use glucometer.
11. Hold the child securely and place the puncture site in the appropriate position. For example, place extremity in dependent position to facilitate blood flow to the area. Infants can be swaddled during the procedure, leaving the chosen extremity uncovered for access. Older child can be supported by nondominant hand while performing the procedure to prevent pulling away of limbs.
12. Use diversional and recreational measures to reduce pain perception.
13. Wipe the puncture site with 70% alcohol swab and allow the site to dry or remove

the alcohol using sterile gauze piece. Presence of alcohol can influence the accuracy of result.

14. Hold the lancet perpendicular to the skin and puncture site using lancet device. Continue to position the site below the child's heart level to allow increase blood flow and adequate amount of sample.
15. Ensure that an adequate-sized drop of blood is obtained before applying it to the test strip and glucometer. Too little blood may give false low reading. Do not squeeze the site. Because excessive squeezing can contaminate the sample with tissue fluid and cause hemolysis of sample and trauma to the site.
16. Apply first or second drop of blood to the test strip, as per manufacturer recommendations. Usually second drop of blood is taken into the test strip after removing out the first drop of blood. A "hanging drop" of blood may be needed and the finger may not touch the test strip/pad. The accuracy of results is dependent on proper technique.
17. Apply sterile cotton ball or gauze to the puncture site and apply pressure to stop bleeding.
18. Wait for developing time of test results and note the reading on the glucometer.
19. Compare the test and pad color scale on the bottle label from which the test strip is taken, if color chart is available.
20. Turn off the glucometer. Ensure test strip container is capped tightly.
21. Dispose all wastes in appropriate container as per standard precautions.
22. Remove gloves and perform hand hygiene.
23. Document the CBG estimation and its findings. Inform the procedure and test results to healthcare prescriber to take decision about further treatment.

Evaluation and Documentation

- Evaluate child's response to the procedure and compare test results with the previous findings. Immediate treatment must be initiated, if the child is having hypoglycemia or hyperglycemia. Evaluate older child's or parents ability to perform blood glucose monitoring using glucometer
- Document the test result finding of capillary blood glucose with date and time of the procedure. Any problems found during the procedure should also be noted and informed.

Communication and Teaching for Homecare

- Communicate with the child and parents about the CBG estimation results and plan of management. Answer to their concern in simple language
- Teach the parents and the child (as feasible) about the followings:
  - Discuss importance of blood glucose monitoring especially for diabetic child
  - Describe the signs and symptoms of hypoglycemia and hyperglycemia in children
  - Demonstrate the correct technique for use of glucometer and storage of strips
  - Inform about the place (shop, market) of availability of glucometer and reagent strips
  - Instruct for immediate management at home, if the child demonstrates signs of hypoglycemia or hyperglycemia and to contact healthcare providers or community health workers (ASHA, ANM, CHO), as feasible
  - Discuss about hand hygiene, other hygienic care, recommended diet, water intake, rest and activity, continued medications at home, disposal of sharps, need for emergency medical help and plan of follow-up care.

Refer: Blood Glucose Monitoring in Neonates as Procedure – 15, in the Unit – 2 of this Manual.

PROCEDURE–24: INCENTIVE SPIROMETRY IN THE CHILDREN

Clinical Guidelines

- Spirometry is the most common type of pulmonary function or breathing test. This test measures how much air one

individual can breathe in and breathe out of the lungs. It also measure how quickly and easily one can blow the air out of the lungs. It measures the air flow and lung volumes using an apparatus known as spirometer
- Incentive spirometry is a procedure in which visual and vocal stimuli are given to the patient to produce maximum effort during deep breathing. It may be incorporated in addition to deep breathing, coughing, turning, positioning, early mobilization, and ambulation. It helps the patients to improve their lung function by their own efforts.
- There is no evidence that the use of incentive spirometry is associated with any harmful side effects. Incentive spirometer is a handhold device that helps the lungs to recover after a surgery or pulmonary illness. This device assists to expand the lungs by helping to breathe more deeply and fully
- The objectives of this procedure are to increase transpulmonary pressure and inspiratory volumes, improve inspiratory muscle performance and reestablish or stimulate the normal pattern of pulmonary hyperinflation and promote expectoration of secretions
- Common indications of spirometry include severe pneumonia, chest injury, and post-cardiothoracic surgery. It is used most often in postoperative patients to prevent fluid accumulation in lungs, hypostatic pneumonia and atelectasis
- Children may perform this procedure while supervised by a trained staff member or adequately trained family member. Once the child has demonstrated mastery of the technique of incentive spirometry, then direct supervision may not be necessary
- The child should use the spirometer 5–10 breaths per session at a minimum of every hour while awake or as prescribed.

Equipment Required

- Hand hygiene supplies for hand wash and hand rub
- Incentive spirometer with mouthpiece
- Tissue paper or gauze pieces and a container for sputum
- Extra pillow or folded bath blanket
- Waste disposal containers as per BMW guidelines
- Documentation sheet for incentive spirometry and child's treatment sheet.

Assessment and Preparation

- Assessment: Obtain baseline respiratory assessment, indications of spirometry, present respiratory problems, including previous incentive spirometry measurements and arterial blood gas results, if available. Assess child's ability to perform the procedure independently. Determine both child and family members readiness to learn and presence of any barriers for learning
- Self-preparation should be done by practicing standard precautions of infection control
- Environment should be clean, calm, well lighted and well ventilated
- Required articles should be assembled near the child. Clean the spirometer as per manufacturer's instructions to prevent contaminations and further infections
- Preparation of parents: Explain the purpose and technique of use of spirometer in simple language. Involve the parent during the procedure of spirometry. Answer to questions as asked by the parents and other family members
- Preparation of child: Explain the procedure and importance of incentive spirometry in age appropriate language. Preoperative teaching, demonstration and instruction to use the spirometer to the older child and family members should be done to facilitate use of the incentive spirometer postoperatively in case of surgery.

Performing the Steps of Procedure with Rationale/Point of Emphasis

1. Perform hand hygiene. Collect and assemble all items near the child.

2. Ensure that the spirometer is used only by one child. Label it with child's name to prevent nosocomial transmission of respiratory infections.
3. Place the child in semi-Fowler's or high-Fowler's position. Raise the bed to a comfortable level and lower side rails. Provide comfort, as appropriate for the child.
4. If the child has an abdominal incision, instruct the child to splint the abdomen with pillow or bath blanket. It will provide support and comfort of incision area while simultaneously allowing for maximum expansion of chest and lungs.
5. Demonstrate the breathing techniques to the child. It will prepare the child for active participation to perform the spirometry. Ask to follow "step 6" and "step 7" as stated below of this procedure.
6. Instruct the child to exhale "until there is no more air to come out". Exhaling purges air of the lungs before sustaining maximum inhalation
   - Then direct the child to place the mouthpiece of the spirometer in his or her mouth and sealing the lips around the mouthpiece. Effectiveness of the incentive spirometry is enhanced when adequate seal is made around the mouthpiece, thus preventing leakage of exhaled air.
7. While ensuring that the child maintains the seal around the mouthpiece, then direct the child to inhale slowly and deeply through the mouthpiece of the spirometer. Instruct not to inhale through nose. Watch the indicator of the spirometer
   - During inhalation, the child's goal should be to keep the ball or indicator in the optimal region on the spirometer or to move the ball or indicator to its highest level
   - Inhaling through the nose or through mouth and nose diminishes the child's ability to move the ball or indicator to the highest level.
8. Instruct the child to hold his or her breath for 3–5 seconds and to remove the mouthpiece and then to exhale normally in slow and even fashion. Holding the breath ensures optimum lung expansion by allowing the alveoli to re-expand. Normal slow exhaling prevent collapse of the alveoli.
9. Note the highest level the volume indicator reaches. Mark this on the device. Volume on incentive spirometry should increase with practice as the child reaches maximum lung capacity. Marking the baseline helps the child, as he or she seeks improvement during future attempts.
10. Direct the child to take two to four normal breaths and then repeat the process 5–10 times per session, at a minimum, every hour while awake. If appropriate, encourage the child to perform the procedure independently, with new and increasing volumes established each day. When the procedure is repeated on a regular basis, airway patency is maintained and lung atelectasis can be prevented or reversed
    - Have tissue paper available near the child and encourage to cough, as needed, to facilitate expectoration of secretions.
11. Monitor the child for any untoward effects such as dizziness, hyperventilation or shortness of breath. If such symptoms occur, stop the procedure and notify the physician.
12. When the session is complete, place the child to a comfortable position and return the bed to its lowest position. Assess child's safety and raise side rails, if appropriate.
13. Remove the mouthpiece from the spirometer and rinse with soap and water to cleanse it from sputum. It helps to reduce transmission of microorganisms during future use. Reattach the mouthpiece after drying and store the spirometer at child's bedside within easy reach for easy access.
14. Discard all waste in appropriate containers. Perform hand hygiene.
15. Document the procedure of incentive spirometry and related findings in child's record.

Evaluation and Documentation

- Evaluate the child's respiratory status, sputum production, other health problems and level of comfort after the incentive spirometry. Evaluate the ability to perform the procedure and need for support to both child and family members
- Document date, time, number and frequency of repetitions of spirometry, child's respiratory status, and volume level achieved during inhalations, sputum productions, if any, and presence of any untoward effects.
  - Keep record of teaching and demonstration given along with understanding level, anxiety and ability to perform incentive spirometry by the child and assistance provided by the family members.

Communication and Teaching for Homecare

- Communicate with child and parents about child's health and respiratory conditions and plan of future management. Answer to questions as asked by the child and parents
- Teach the parents about hand hygiene, respiratory hygiene, diet and fluid intake, comfort and routine care at hospital and at home. Demonstrate about the use, cleaning and storage of spirometer with mouthpiece and take return demonstrations. Instruct the family members about home care after discharge from hospital and to contact healthcare providers, if the child experiences shortness of breath, dizziness, extreme exacerbation of coughing or extreme fatigue associated with use of incentive spirometer. Explain the plan of follow-up visits to healthcare institutions.

PROCEDURE–25: CHEST PHYSIOTHERAPY OF THE CHILDREN

Clinical Guidelines

- Physiotherapy is a treatment method that focuses on the science of movement and helps the individual to restore, maintain and maximize physical strength, function, motion and overall well-being by addressing the underlying physical issues
- Physiotherapy is a form of physical therapy for therapeutic interventions of diseases and disorders by using physical and mechanical means such as therapeutic exercise, movements, massage, hydrotherapy, use of thermal modalities and electricity, performed by trained the physiotherapist. This also includes conducting examination, alleviating impairments and functional limitations along with preventing injury and disability
- Chest physiotherapy facilitates the removal of excess secretions from the peripheral parts of the lungs. It is indicated in case of bronchiectasis, neuromuscular diseases, atelectasis from mucus plugs, cystic fibrosis and hypersecretory states. The method and position of chest physiotherapy should be selected considering that which will fit best for the child's needs. This procedure can be performed by well-trained nursing professionals
- Chest physiotherapy should not be performed for at least one hour after feeding or meals to prevent vomiting and aspiration
- Chest physiotherapy is withheld when the child has episodes of hemoptysis, pulmonary hemorrhage, or in case of fracture ribs, vertebral compression fractures or increased intracranial pressure
- Mechanical percussor or cupped-hand technique is used for chest physiotherapy. When mechanical percussor are used, then vibration is not necessary because mechanical percussor are more effective for loosening secretions than the hand technique
- Generally, bronchodilators and mucolytic medications are administered before chest physiotherapy procedures to assist with airway clearance, whereas inhaled corticosteroids and antibiotics are administered after airway clearance procedures to allow for maximal penetration of the medications into the lungs.

Equipment Required

- Hand hygiene supplies for hand washing and antiseptic hand rubbing
- Stethoscope, mechanical percussor, if indicated
- Extra pillows, blanket and sheet
- Container for sputum and tissue paper or gauze pieces
- Suction apparatus to remove excessive secretions
- Oxygen delivery setup and resuscitation articles
- Diversional activities such as music therapy, videos, if needed
- Chest X-ray report, if already done
- Waste disposal containers as per BMW guidelines
- Documentation sheet for chest physiotherapy and child's case sheet.

Assessment and Preparation

- Assess child's general health status and vital signs. Perform respiratory assessment using visual inspection of respiratory status and by auscultation of breath sounds with stethoscope. Determine when the therapy was given last and child's response
- Self-preparation should be done with hand hygiene and practice of standard precautions
- Environment should be clean, calm, well lighted and well ventilated
- Articles preparation: All necessary items should be collected and arranged near the child
- Preparation of parents: Explain the importance of the chest physiotherapy and its technique to the parents. Allow them to participate during the procedure to reduce stress and anxiety of the child
- Preparation of child: Explain the procedure in age-appropriate simple language. Determine when the child had last oral intake. Administer pain medication before the procedure, if needed. Initiate diversional activities before the procedure. Ask for cooperation and to follow the instructions during chest physiotherapy.

Performing the Steps of Procedure with Rationale/Point of Emphasis

1. Review physician's direction to determine the lung fields where chest physiotherapy should be administer. Review the latest chest X-ray report.
2. Check for medications or any other therapy, that to be administered in conjunction with chest physiotherapy.
3. Perform hand hygiene to prevent cross infections. Gather all necessary supplies near the child to perform chest physiotherapy efficiently and without interruptions.
4. Place the child in upright sitting position with his or her back toward the performer of chest physiotherapy. Placing the child's body in this position allows gravity to assist drainage of mucus from the lung periphery to the segmental bronchus and upper airway.
5. Percuss over the lung field in a successive rhythmic motion over each lung segment, using a mechanical percussor or with a cupped hand. Each position should be percussed for at least 3–10 minutes, based on child's tolerance and underlying disease process. Percussion dislodges secretions from the bronchial wall. In conjunction with positioning, the secretions drain into the larger airways and are expectorated or swallowed, depending on the child's age. Percussion over bony prominences is not effective in vibrating the chest wall to loosen secretions. *(Refer **Fig. 3.10**: Positions of chest physiotherapy)*
   i. When a mechanical percussor is not available or preferred, then use of cupped hand creates an air cushion, which in turns vibrates through the chest wall
   ii. Postural drainage in head-down position is contraindicated for infants because it increases gastro-esophageal reflux.
6. Perform percussion procedure with vibration over each lobar area using hand technique. Use an open flat hand

to provide a shaking motion on the chest wall, synchronized with exhalation to loosen the secretions. This technique provides additional vibrations to help in mobilization of secretions.

7. After percussion and vibration, allow the child to sit up, take a deep breath and cough up and spit out the mucous into a sputum container or tissue paper. Sitting up allows for maximal diaphragmatic excursion for expelling mucous and clearing the airway.
8. Perform suctioning, as indicated and if the child is intubated or unable to generate an effective cough. Mechanical removal of secretions is necessary, when required.
9. Reposition the child in alternate positions (Refer **Fig. 3.10**) and repeat percussion/

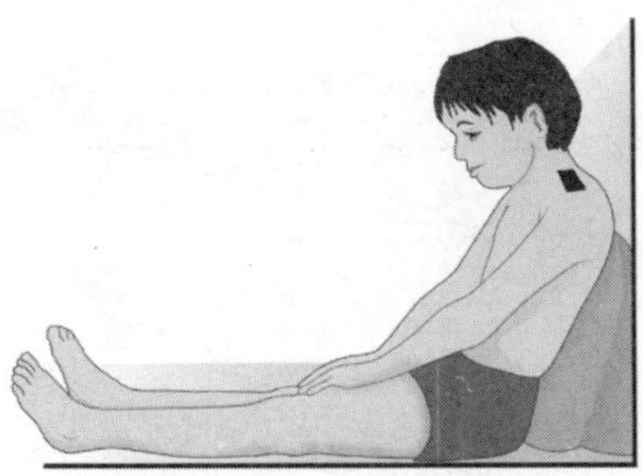

Position #1
Upper lobes, apical segments

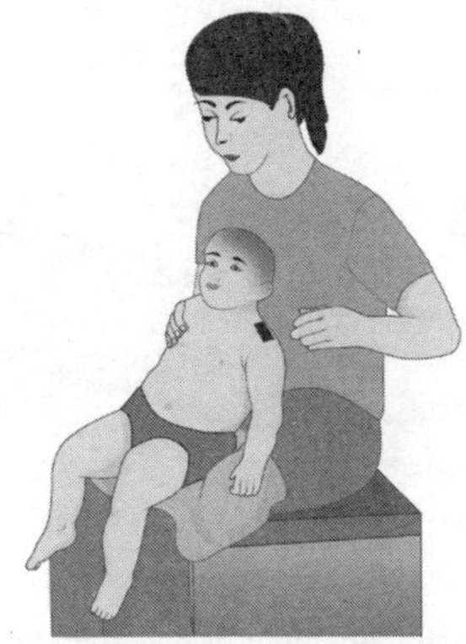

Position #1, for infant
Upper lobes, apical segments

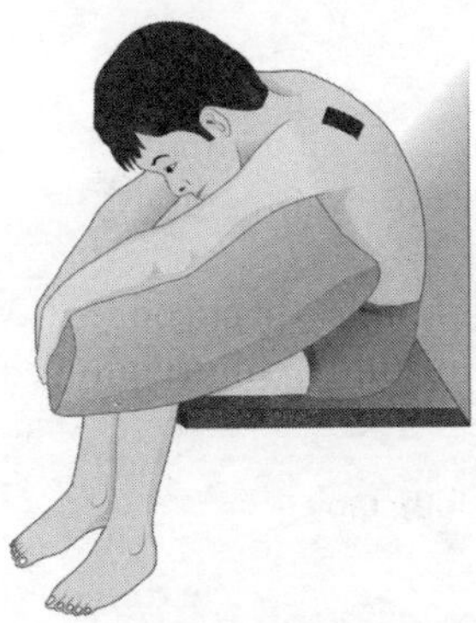

Position #2
Upper lobes, posterior segments

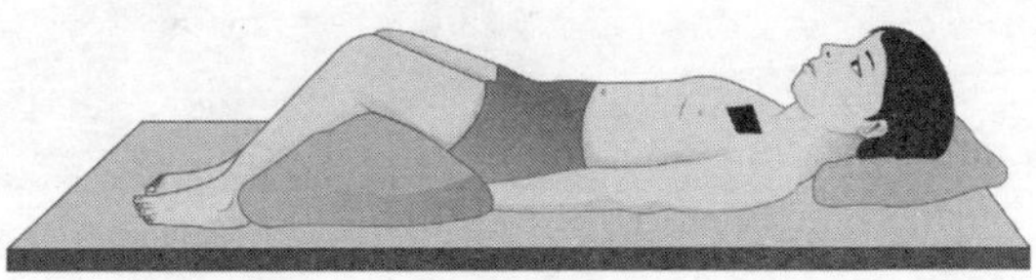

Position #3
Upper lobes, anterior segments

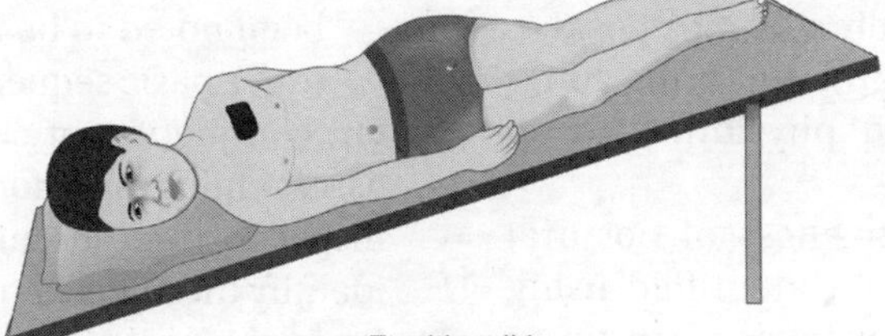

Position #4
Lingula

Fig. 3.10 *(Contd...)*

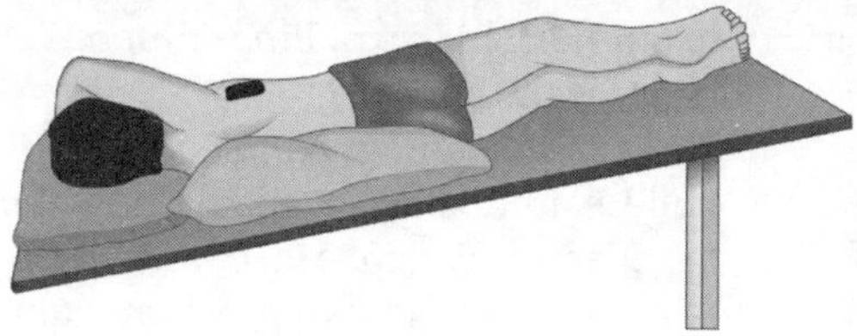

Position #5
Middle lobe

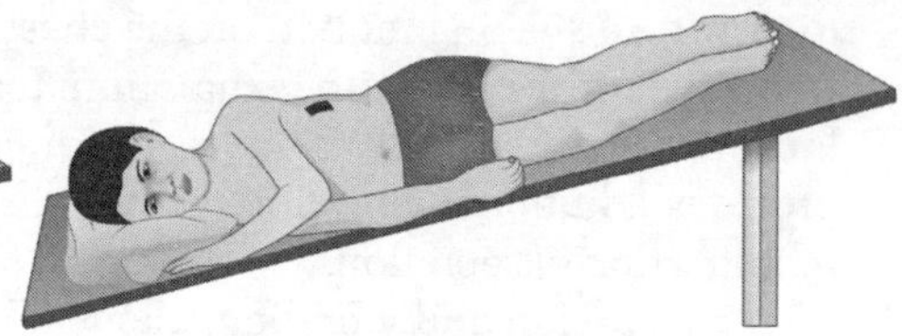

Position #6
Lower lobes, anterior basal segments

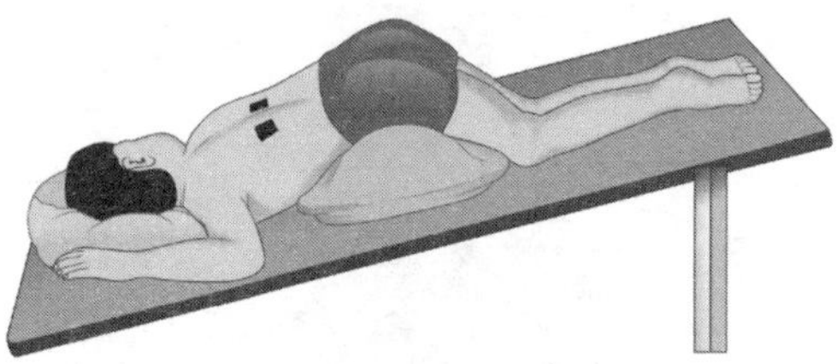

Position #7
Lower lobes, posterior basal segments

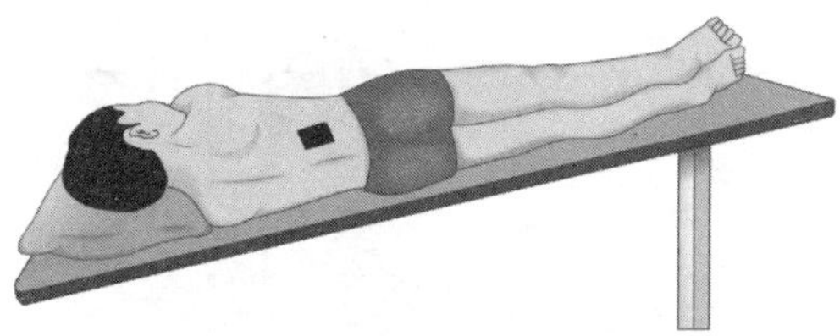

Position #8 and 9
Lower lobes, lateral basal segments
(For both left and right lungs)

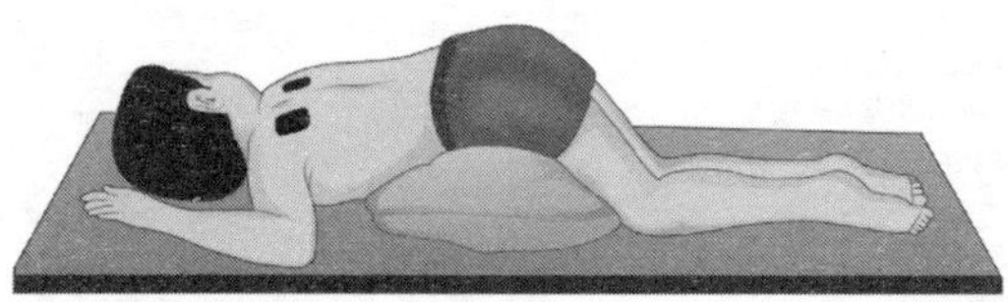

Position #10
Lower lobes, superior segments

Fig. 3.10: Ten recommended positions for chest physiotherapy.

vibration/cough therapy. Modifications may be necessary based on child's tolerance and health condition. Allow rest to the child in between two positions, if needed. Systematically changing position ensures that all segments of the lungs receive the needed physiotherapy to loosen secretions

- Increased effectiveness of postural drainage has been identified using the following sequences of postures: supine, 45-degree rotative prone with left side up, 45-degree rotative prone with right side up, and return to supine. The positions of 10-degree right side up supine and 45-degree rotative prone with head raised 45-degree have been noted to be helpful when added to the basic sequence.

10. On completion of chest physiotherapy, assess child respiratory status using visual inspection and auscultation techniques to identify the effectiveness of therapy.
11. Place the child in comfortable position with side rails up to provide rest after the therapy.

12. Provide oral care and assist the child to rinse out his or her mouth. It is required to clean the mouth and to increase child's comfort, when the child expectorated a lot of mucus.
13. Praise the child for cooperation during the procedure and inform about the time of next session of chest physiotherapy.
14. Dispose waste. Take care of reusable items. Perform hand hygiene.
15. Document the procedure of chest physiotherapy and medications administered along with related findings.

Evaluation and Documentation

- Evaluate the child's respiratory status, noting respiratory rate, breathing patterns, symmetric chest expansion, breath sounds and skin color. Evaluate improvement of child's health status, therapeutic effects and response to chest physiotherapy
- Document date, time and duration of chest physiotherapy, findings of respiratory assessment of the child before and after the procedure, child's response on completion of chest physiotherapy and adjunctive treatments given concurrently (e.g., nebulization or inhaled medications) with child's response to these treatments.

Communication and Teaching for Homecare

- Communicate with child and parents about child's health condition, need for chest physiotherapy and plan of further treatment
- Teach the parents about routine care of the child at hospital and at home after discharge. Demonstrate deep breathing exercise and positions of chest physiotherapy to family members according to their ability and understanding level, if the chest physiotherapy to be continued at home. Instruct about signs of worsening of child's respiratory condition, need for emergency medical help and plan of follow-up visits.

PROCEDURE–26: PEDIATRIC BASIC LIFE SUPPORT MEASURES

Clinical Guidelines

- Basic life support (BLS) is the life-saving method used when there is limited access to advanced interventions such as medications and monitoring devices. In general, BLS is performed until the Emergency Medical Services (EMS) arrives or available to provide a higher level of care. In every healthcare setting, availability of high quality cardiopulmonary resuscitation (CPR) is the foundation of both BLS and pediatric advanced life support (PALS) interventions. High quality CPR gives the child or the infant the greatest chance of survival by providing circulation to the heart, brain and other organs until return of spontaneous circulation
- CPR or BLS is indicated in any situation in which breathing, heartbeat or both are absent
- CPR must be initiated in all children who do not have "Do Not Resuscitate" (DNR) order
- Age-appropriate resuscitation equipment should remain easily accessible in all areas of the healthcare facility where pediatric patients may be seen or treated
- For children and infants, ***if two rescuers are available to do CPR, the chest compression to breathe ratio is 15: 2. If only one rescuer is available, the chest compression to breath ratio is 30: 2 for all age groups. But in neonates it is 3:1 with two rescuers.***
- Neonatal Resuscitation Program (NRP) has different recommended algorithm to follow
- Infant CPR guidelines are appropriate for victims younger than approximately one year of age. Child CPR guidelines are appropriate for victims from about one year of age to the onset of adolescence or puberty (about 12–14 years of age). However the size of the child should be taken into consideration to decide the techniques

- Check the child's pulse using the carotid artery on the side of the neck or femoral artery on the inner thigh in the crease between the leg and groin. For checking infant's pulse use brachial artery on the inside of the upper arm between the infant's elbow and shoulder. Femoral artery pulsation can also be checked for infants
- Perform chest compressions using one or two handed chest compressions technique depending on the size of the child. Perform chest compressions on the infant using two thumbs with hands encircling the infant's chest (with two rescuers) or using two fingers (if you are only one rescuer)
- Chest compression depth should be one third of the chest depth. For most children more than one year of age, this is about two inches and for the infants this is about 1.5 inches
- If you are only one person at the scene and find an unresponsive child or infant, perform CPR for 2 minutes before you call for EMS or go for an Automated External Defibrillator (AED). Use AED after 5 cycles of CPR. AED is usually not recommended for infants (< 1 year of age)
- If you witness a cardiac arrest in a child or infant, call for EMS and get an AED before starting CPR
- High quality CPR for BLS should have: (a) Rate at least 100 chest compressions per minute, (b) Chest compression depth one-third diameter of chest, (c) Allow chest recoil between compressions, (d) Minimize chest compression interruptions, (e) Do not over-ventilate, (f) If there is definite pulse, administer one breath every three seconds. Add compressions, if pulse remains less than 60 breaths per minute with poor perfusion despite oxygenation and ventilation. Assess pulse every 2 minutes. (g) If no pulse, **one rescuer**: Begin cycles of 30 compressions and two breaths. **Two rescuers**: Begin cycles of 15 compressions and two breaths
- AED/Defibrillator arrives, assess for shockable rhythm. Shockable, then administer one shock and resume CPR immediately for 2 minutes. Nonshockable, then resume CPR immediately for 2 minutes. Assess rhythm every 2 minutes. Continue until more advanced help arrives or until the individual child shows signs of return of circulation.

Equipment Required

- Hand sanitizers for hand hygiene
- Protective apparels such as gloves
- Hard flat surface, such as cardiac board or the headboard
- Suction equipment and suction catheters
- Barrier or Bag-valve mask device
- Oxygen source, and oxygen delivery system
- Automated external defibrillator (AED)
- Emergency drugs and medications administration tray
- Cardiac monitor, pulse oximeter
- IV fluids, IV access, IV administration supplies
- Nasogastric tube to deflate stomach during prolong breathing support
- Endotracheal intubation equipment and supplies
- Mouth wipes, gauze pieces, cotton rolls, as required
- Waste disposal containers as per BMW rules
- Documentation sheet for CPR and for cardiac/respiratory arrest.

Assessment and Preparation

- Assess the child's life threatening condition promptly to initiate the CPR without delay. Assess the family's emotional needs and anxiety to provide necessary support, as needed
- Self-preparation should be done with prompt response to perform life support measures following necessary precautions
- Environment should be calm, well ventilated, well lighted and free from overcrowding
- Preparation for required equipment and supplies should always be done before hand, as it is an emergency procedure.

Anticipation should be made for the need of CPR in emergency situations in the children at-risk of cardiac or respiratory arrest

- Identified children at-risk for cardiac or respiratory arrest should be placed on a unit where access to resuscitation equipment and trained resuscitation personnel is immediately available
- Preparation of parents: Maintain frequent communication with the family during this stressful time and allow the family members to be with the child, regardless of the outcome of the resuscitation efforts. Anticipatory guidance can be provided to the family depending upon the child's emergency conditions. If family members choose not to be present, then ongoing updates of the child's health condition can be provided by the support staff, if available and feasible
- Preparation of child: Prompt assessment of child's airway, breathing and circulation must be done to perform effective resuscitative life saving measures.

Performing the Steps of Procedure with Rationale/Point of Emphasis

Assessing and Managing Airway during Cardiopulmonary Resuscitation (CPR) in Children

1. Use hand sanitizer or hand rub before touching the child, if feasible.
2. Assess child's ability to respond. Gently tap on the shoulder to arouse the child and loudly call for help. This helps to determine whether the child is sleeping or unconscious and need of assistance. These actions may startle a conscious child.
3. If the child is unresponsive and you are alone, follow "***Phone fast***": start CPR immediately, continue for 1 minute and then call for help. If the child (8 years of age or older) is unresponsive and you are alone, follow "***Phone first***": call immediately for help and then start begin CPR
   - The "***Phone first***" and "***Phone fast***" sequences are applicable only when one rescuer is present. If two rescuers are present, one rescuer always stays with victim and initiates CPR while other calls for help
   - Most children have arrest because of respiratory difficulties. Initiating CPR and opening the airway may be all that is necessary to revive those children. Older children may have a cardiac origin of arrest and ensuring the quickest arrival of a defibrillator improves chance of survival.
4. Place the child on a firm, flat surface, in a horizontal supine position, turning the body as a whole unit. The child must be on his or her back for the rescuer to perform CPR. It is important to prevent movement of the head and neck when positioning the infant/child to prevent possible neck injuries. A firm, flat surface is optimal for facilitating proper compression of the chest. Supine position facilitates blood flow to the brain.
5. Decide whether to open the airway with head-tilt/chin-lift or the jaw-thrust method. If neck or cervical spine injury is suspected, then use the jaw-thrust method
   - In an unconscious child, the tongue relaxes and falls against the back of the throat, blocking air entry to the lungs. Sometimes, just opening the airway is enough to get the infant or child breathing again.
6. To perform ***the head-tilt/chin-lift method***, tilt the head back by gently pressing the forehead into a neutral position with the palm of one hand that is closest to the child's head (i.e., to make sniffing position). Infants have small flexible airways and hyperextending the head may occlude the airway (Refer **Fig. 3.11**)
   - Place fingertips of your other hand on the bony part of the child's jaw near the chin and lift upward and outward. This prevents fingers from pressing on the soft tissue under the chin and occluding the airway.
7. Remove the foreign body or vomitus, if it is visible in the mouth. Use suction if

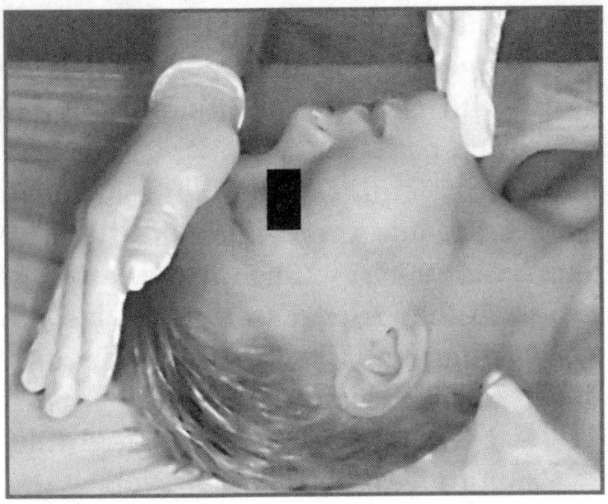

Fig. 3.11: Head tilt-chin lift method.

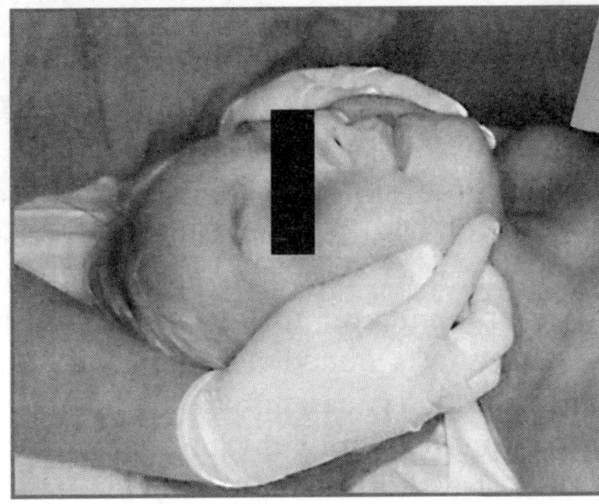

Fig. 3.12: Jaw-thrust method.

available. Do not perform blind sweep of the mouth. This technique may push the foreign body further into the back of throat.

8. To perform ***the jaw-thrust method*** on infants and children (> 1 year of age) who may have a neck or cervical injury, rest your elbows above the child head on the hard surface and place two or three fingers under each side of the lower jaw at an angle and lift the jaw upward and outward. If a second rescuer is available, that rescuer should immobilize the spine (Refer **Fig. 3.12**)
   - This opens the airway by moving the tongue and epiglottis away from the back of the throat. Do not close the mouth completely or press on the soft area under the chin. This may further occlude the airway
   - If the jaw-thrust maneuver alone does not open the airway, a slight head-tilt maneuver may be added in patients with no evidence of cervical spine injury. This minimizes the child's neck movements.
9. To determine whether the child is breathing, place your ear near the child's mouth, face and chest. This enables you to feel presence of any air movement
   - Look to see whether the chest and abdomen are moving. Listen and feel for air movement from the mouth and nose. Chest may be moving up and down, but there may not be any air movement into the lungs because of obstruction.
10. If the child is breathing, maintain the open airway and continue to monitor. Giving breaths to a breathing child is unnecessary and could damage the child's respiratory tract.
11. Check for breathing for 5–10 seconds. This minimizes the time for the child without oxygen.
12. Call for help for breathing support to the child.

Implementing Rescue Breathing during Cardiopulmonary Resuscitation (CPR) in Children

1. Use hand sanitizer or hand rub before touching the child, if feasible.
2. Use bag-mask and oxygen, as available, for a breathless child, and deliver two slow breaths (1–1.5 seconds' duration of inspiration). Delivering breaths provides oxygen to the child. Use bag-mask as barrier device to avoid contact with body secretions.
3. Adjust volume of breath to the size of the child. Watch for normal chest rise with each breath and allow the chest to fall as the infant/child exhales between breaths
   - Gastric distension may occur if the breaths delivered too fast and the volume of air is too large for the size of the child. The chest wall will rise if the breath was adequate enough

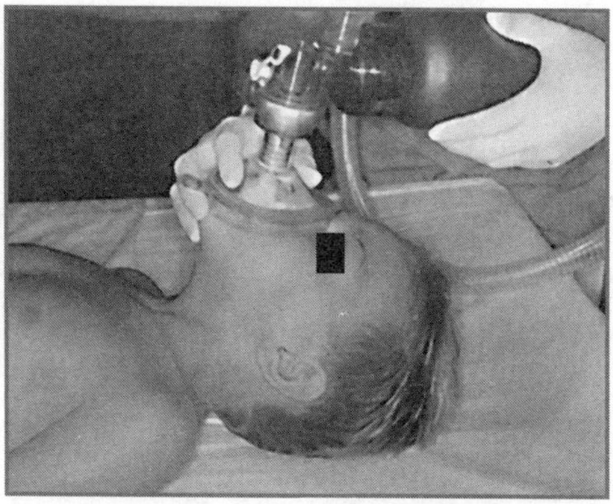

Fig. 3.13: Use of bag mask ventilation.

to ventilate the child. Pause between breaths help to increase oxygen concentration and to decrease carbon dioxide retention.

4. Make complete seal by covering the nose and mouth with the mask. Complete seal must be maintained to ventilate the infant/child. Properly performed bag-mask ventilation is safe and effective way to provide breathing (Refer **Fig. 3.13**).

Note: There is risk of contact with body secretions and transmission of microorganisms, when the rescuer is performing "Mouth-to-Mouth or Mouth-to-Nose Rescue Breathing". A barrier device must be used during rescue breathing.

Managing Circulation during Cardiopulmonary Resuscitation (CPR) in Children

1. Use hand sanitizer or hand rub before touching the child, if feasible.
2. Check the pulse for 10 seconds
   - Use the carotid artery (located on the side of the neck between the trachea and the sternocleidomastoid muscle) to check pulse in children > 1 year old. It is most accessible pulse to find. Palpate femoral pulse as an alternative
   - In infants, use brachial artery (located on the inside of the upper arm between the elbow and shoulder) or femoral artery to check pulse. Infants are having short neck, making it difficult to palpate the carotid artery.
3. If pulse is present and respiration are absent, give breaths at the rate approximately 20 breaths/minute for the infant and child >1 year of age as long as necessary. This breathing rate is adequate for short-term oxygenation. Without breathing, the child will not be oxygenated and his or her heart will soon stop
   - It is very important to maintain oxygenation to prevent cardiac arrest and to promote oxygen perfusion to the brain and other vital organs.
4. If there is no pulse, or pulse is less than 60 beats/minute and signs of poor perfusion present, then begin chest compression. If you are uncertain that pulse is present and the child is not breathing, then it is better to start chest compressions. Chest compressions provide more blood supply to the vital organs including lungs and brain.
5. Ensure that the child is on firm flat surface to facilitate effectiveness of chest compressions.
6. Place the child (> 1 year old) on AED or cardiac monitor/defibrillator, if available. Children > 1 year old, are at greater risk of cardiac arrhythmia as the primary cause of cardiopulmonary arrest.
7. Perform chest compressions and ventilation cycle for the child > 1 year old, in 30:2 by single rescuer or 15:2 by two rescuer.
8. To provide chest compressions to the child (>1 year old), place the heel of your one hand over the lower half of the sternum between breast nipples. Avoid compressing the xiphoid process. This facilitates adequate cardiac output and minimizes chances for injuries to the sternum and ribs
   - To perform chest compression to the infant, use two-thumb technique. Place both thumbs side by side on the lower third of sternum and encircle the chest with your hand. Take precaution to prevent injury of ribs.
9. Press straight down during chest compressions to a depth of one third to one half of the depth of the chest. Chest of

the children is smaller and more flexible than that of an adult and does not require much pressure to compress.

10. Release the pressure in between compressions and allow the chest to expand fully. This allows time to the heart to refill. Keep fingers in contact with the chest to maintain proper positioning and to minimize injury.
11. Provide chest compression at the rate 100 per minute approximately. This provides perfusion to vital organs.
12. Give two rescue breaths. Each breath should take one second for inspiration. Watch for normal chest rise while delivering breaths. This provide oxygen to the child.
13. After 1 minute of CPR, stop 5 seconds to recheck pulse. This helps to determine whether there is pulse or whether you need to continue CPR.
14. Call for help if you are alone. Once calling for help has been initiated and there is still "No pulse" present, resume 30:2 for single rescuer or 15:2 for two rescuer cycle of chest compressions and ventilations. This allows for oxygenation and ventilation at proper ratios to maintain optimal recovery.
15. Repeat pulse check every few minutes and then continue CPR as indicated. Determine resumption of spontaneous breathing and circulation and whether you need to continue CPR or not.
16. During the chest compressions - ventilations cycle, if unable to ventilate the infant or the child, then reposition the infant's head and try to ventilate again. If still unable to ventilate, the airway may be obstructed with a foreign body.
    - In infant, repositioning of the head may be all that is necessary to open the airway. To remove foreign body in infant, use combination of "five back slaps and five chest thrusts" to dislodge the foreign body. Chest thrusts are similar to chest compressions. Chest thrusts produce an "artificial cough" to dislodge the foreign body
    - In a child (> 1 year old), make sure that the child is positioned on his or her back on a firm flat surface. Look for foreign body in the mouth and back of the throat. If an object is visible, remove it. Do not do a blind finger sweep. Then open airway with head-tilt/chin-lift and attempt to give rescue breaths. If unable, then reposition and reattempt ventilation. Foreign-body checks should be performed before delivering another breath
    - If the child is unconscious, clearing obstructed airway should be done by placing the child on the ground. Then kneel down and straddle the child's legs. Place one hand directly over the other and place the heel of your hand in the middle of the abdomen a little above the navel. Press quickly inward and upward into the abdomen toward the head for five times in rapid succession
    - Use the Heimlich maneuver to clear obstructed airway for the conscious child (> 1 year old). The Heimlich maneuver for children is the same as for adults except less force is used for the thrusts.

Care to the Children in Post-CPR Phase

1. Use hand sanitizer or hand rub before touching the child or wash hand, if feasible.
2. Perform frequent assessment and reassessment of cardiac and respiratory function to monitor for systemic chest expansion, equal breath sounds, oxygenation, heart rate, respiration rate, body temperature, skin color, tissue perfusion and BP to detect deterioration or improvement of child's health condition promptly.
3. Perform ongoing resuscitation efforts and stabilization of the child, as indicated.
4. Continue to maintain normal ventilation without hyperventilation using bag-mask ventilation and compressions at the appropriate ratios. This provides oxygenation for the vital organs. Bag-mask ventilation has been shown to be highly

safe and effective. Hyperventilation is not recommended to be used routinely, as it reduces cerebral blood flow and may create cerebral ischemia.

5. Administer emergency medications and IV fluids, as indicated to provide circulatory support. Establish IV access promptly, as needed. Use precalculated medication dosage, amount of fluid volume replacement, and endotracheal tube sizes to prevent errors and malpractice in therapeutic interventions. Infants and children in cardiac or respiratory arrest are often hypovolemic, and require rapid fluid boluses to manage that condition.
6. Use AED in the treatment of cardiac arrest in children > 1 year old, as indicated. Pediatric ventricular fibrillation (VF) may be more common than previously suspected. Early defibrillation of VF and pulseless ventricular tachycardia (VT) are important and highly successful treatment. Ideally, the rescuer should use a pediatric dose-attenuating system.
7. Transfer the child to an area, as soon as possible, where trained and skilled personnel are available to perform PALS techniques, whenever indicated. Management of pediatric emergencies with continued evaluation, stabilization and treatment may be required as life-saving measures for some children.
8. Place the child on cardiac or apnea monitor and on pulse oximeter. Pulse oximeter is a non-invasive technique used to measure arterial saturation and heart rate. The oxygen saturation reading may not be reliable if the heart rate does not correlate with the cardiac monitor or if the infant's/child's tissue perfusion is poor.
9. Arrange for endotracheal intubation and mechanical ventilation, as indicated, for stabilization of the child's condition. Tracheal intubation must be performed only by the trained healthcare professional, who has frequently practiced this skill.
10. Administer medications (such as epinephrine, atropine, etc.) in endotracheal route, if IV access is difficult to establish or if it is not functioning properly.
11. Ensure peripheral IV line is functioning appropriately. An intraosseous (IO) line may be inserted, if required. An IO line is also a reliable route to infuse fluids, drugs and blood products. There is no upper age limit to use an IO route for fluids and medications.
12. Maintain neutral thermal state of the infant/child. Both hypothermia and hyperthermia can complicate the health status of the infant/child.
13. Assess blood glucose level to ensure that normal level is maintained. Hyperglycemia and hypoglycemia can have detrimental effects to the infant and child. Alterations of blood glucose level must be detected for prompt initiation of therapeutic management.
14. Perform brief neurological examination of the child including level of consciousness and pupillary response. This helps to obtain baseline information after cardiac arrest and to detect the extent of brain injury, which may occur due to insufficient cardiac output to provide oxygen to the brain.
15. Perform continue ongoing assessments and necessary interventions to ensure optimal health outcomes for the child who requires CPR.
16. Follow the universal precautions for prevention of infections during the procedure.
17. Dispose all waste and take care of reusable supplies and equipment, as per standard guidelines and institutional policy.
18. Document the procedure of CPR performed for the infant/child including findings of assessments and other interventions required, both in child's record and hospital record.

Evaluation and Documentation

- Evaluate the infant's/child's response to resuscitation efforts. Evaluate family's anxiety and understanding related to the situation, the need for resuscitation measures and outcomes after resuscitation efforts

- Document the date and time of the event, findings of vital signs and other assessments, medications and fluids administered, required specific interventions, healthcare personnel involved or present during CPR and child's responses to resuscitation efforts. Keep record of parental presence during the performance of CPR and their response to resuscitation efforts.

Communication and Teaching for Homecare

- Communicate with child and parents: Debriefing of the resuscitative efforts should be done to the family members after completion of the procedure, whether it is successful or not. Explain about child's present health condition and further plan of management
- Teach the parents about signs of life-threatening emergency conditions and routine care of the child at hospital and at home. Instruct about community help and transport facility, as available, for immediate transfer to healthcare facility. Discuss about continuation of treatment after discharge from hospital and plan of follow-up visits.

PROCEDURE–27: CARE OF CHEST TUBE AND CHEST DRAINAGE IN CHILDREN

Clinical Guidelines

- Chest tube placement in children is performed for the purposes of: (a) removal of air or fluid (blood, pus, or serous fluid) from the pleural cavity or mediastinum, (b) re-expansion of lungs, (c) restoration of negative pressure to the pleural space, (d) relief of respiratory distress associated with collapsed lung and (e) improvement of ventilation and perfusion of the lungs
- Common indications of chest tube insertion and drainage include pneumothorax, hemothorax, pleural effusion and empyema. Other indications include malignant effusions, chylothorax, and thoracic surgery
- Placement of chest tube is a surgical procedure performed by a surgeon, intensivist or emergency medicine specialist in strict aseptic/sterile technique. It should be done in operating room (OR), but in emergency it can be done in the pediatric unit with all special precautions for prevention of infections
- Generally, chest tube is placed in the midaxillary to anterior axillary line. In case of pneumothorax, the chest tube is inserted through the second intercostal space at the midclavicular line. For removal of fluid, the chest tube is inserted through the fifth to seventh intercostal space at the midaxillary line
- Before chest tube insertion, preparation of child must include the following: (a) obtain baseline data, i.e., vital signs, respiratory rate, respiratory efforts and patterns, skin color, tissue perfusion, level of consciousness, oxygen requirements, and hemodynamic stability of the child, (b) administer sedation or pain medication as prescribed by physician/healthcare prescriber, (c) position the child as appropriate, exposing the selected site for chest tube insertion, (d) restrain child's limbs to ensure sterility of the procedure, and (e) assist the physician/healthcare prescriber during preparation of sterile working field and administration of local anesthetic agent
- During insertion of chest tube, assist the physician/healthcare prescriber as required and monitor the child's vital signs continuously to detect any acute changes promptly
- On completion of chest tube insertion, assist to secure the chest tube with suture material and to attach the disposable sterile chest drainage unit to the chest tube. Allow the large effusions to drain slowly to prevent post-thoracentesis pulmonary edema. Assist to apply gauze pressure dressing over chest tube insertion site. Ensure that the drainage tubing has

a straight flow to chest tube drainage collection device and has no dependent loops or kinks which may obstruct the flow of drainage

- Nurses are responsible to prepare the child for chest tube insertion and to assist the physician/surgeon during the insertion procedure. Nursing responsibilities include providing care during chest tube therapy, evaluating respiratory and thoracic functions and assessing vital signs that reflect effectiveness of chest-tube placement. Nurses are also responsible to identify complications related to chest tube, perform appropriate interventions, make clinical decisions regarding changes in the child's chest tube therapy and inform immediately to the appropriate authority.

Equipment Required

- Hand hygiene supplies for hand wash and antiseptic hand rub
- For chest tube drainage system collection device: (a) single-use, disposable, sterile chest drainage collection unit (water-suction system or dry suction system), (b) sterile water, (c) suction source and wall regulator suction device, (d) suction connection tubing, and (e) chest tube clamp
- For chest tube insertion –
  - A clean tray containing - local anesthetic agent lidocaine (0.5% or 1%), disposable single use mask, cap, protective eye gear, disposable sterile syringes packs (1 mL, 3 mL, 5 mL), disposable single-use sterile 22–24 gauge needle packs, adhesive tape, and antiseptic agents (chlorhexidine, alcohol 70%)
  - A sterile chest tube insertion tray containing (a) sterile gown, gloves, (b) sterile drapes, and sterile swabs for skin preparation, (c) hemostats, scalpel, trocar, Kelly clamps, scissors, suture materials, sterile connectors, (d) sterile gauze dressing. swabs and sponges, (e) appropriate size sterile chest tube catheter, (f) chest tube clamps, (g) transparent dressing, and (h) sterile water in sterile small bowl/container
- For chest tube removal – nonsterile gloves, sterile gloves, sterile gauze dressing, chest tube clamp, adhesive tape, topical analgesic cream
- Transfer forceps or lifter to handle sterile items by the assistant
- Cardiac monitor, pulse oximeter, according to the child's condition
- IV access of the child for medications and fluid therapy, as required
- Emergency medications, syringes, needles for emergency management
- Waste disposal containers as per BMW rules
- Documentation sheet for chest tube care and child's case sheet.

Assessment and Preparation

- Assess child's vital signs, clinical features of respiratory distress including tachypnea, decreased or absent breath sounds, dyspnea, cough, cyanosis, asymmetric chest expansion, shortness of breath, restlessness, tachycardia, anxiety, hypotension, dysrhythmia, sudden sharp chest pain, oxygen saturation, and abnormal chest X-ray or blood gas findings
  - Assess child's history of previous lung disease, spontaneous pneumothorax, pulmonary diseases or procedures requiring and indicating chest tube placement
  - Assess the child and family for cognitive level, stress and anxiety, readiness and ability to process information regarding chest tube
- Self-preparation should be with hand hygiene and use of PPE, as needed
- Environment should be made clean, calm and well lighted and well ventilated
- All necessary equipment and supplies should be arranged near the child. Strict sterile technique must be followed
- Preparation of parents: Explain the purpose of chest tube insertion and chest tube drainage for the child. Encourage to ask questions and answer accordingly. Allow one parent with the child as per facility rules to help the child to cope with

the conditions. Written informed consent with signature must be taken from the parent or legal guardian

- Preparation of child: Explain the procedure in age appropriate simple language. Administer pain management medication, as prescribed and position the child comfortably during chest tube insertion, removal and ongoing care. Encourage to express feeling and ask for cooperation to the older child.

Performing the Steps of Procedure with Rationale/Point of Emphasis

Chest Tube Drainage System Collection Device Setup

1. Perform hand hygiene to prevent transmission of microorganisms.
2. Collect and assemble all necessary equipment and supplies near the child for effective time management and organized approach to the procedure.
3. Open single-use sterile chest drainage unit. Fill the water-seal chamber to the specified level according to the manufacturer's instructions, using sterile water.
   - The water-seal chamber acts as a one-way valve to allow air to pass out of the lung, down through a narrow channel and bubble out through the bottom of the water-seal. Because air must not return to the child, a water-seal is considered one of the safest means for protecting the child.
4. Maintain sterile patient connection tube with the cap in place and set aside. This allows for later connection of chest tube catheter to chest tube drainage system collection device.
5. Fill the suction-control chamber with sterile water to 20 cm of water or as ordered by the healthcare prescriber/pediatrician. The addition of suction (10–20 cm of water) increases the negative intrapleural pressure and helps to overcome air leakage by improving the rate of airflow out of the child as well as improving fluid removal.
6. If dry-suction chest drainage system is used, this step will not require. The dry-suction systems use a bellows device and suction wheel to adjust amount of suction. It does not require the addition of water to a suction control chamber.
7. Connect the chest drain to the child first, before initiating suction.
8. After chest tube drainage system has been connected to child's chest tube, then connect the short end of the drainage collection system to the suction source and apply wall regulator chamber suction-to-suction outlet until gentle bubbling appears in the suction control chamber. This connects the suction source to the water-seal and activates suction.
9. Place the chest tube drainage collection device at the child's bedside, at least 30 cm below the child's chest in the upright position. Placement of the device below the chest allows for gravity, in addition to negative pressure, to drain the tube for optimum results. Avoid accidental knock-over of the device by hanging the system on the crib or bed-frame with the hangers provided.
10. Take care of all used items. Discard all waste. Perform hand hygiene.
11. Document about the chest tube drainage system collection device setup for the child.

Chest Tube Maintenance and Troubleshooting

1. Perform hand hygiene to prevent transmission of microorganisms.
2. Maintain sterility of the equipment and insertion site to prevent infections.
3. Check water-seal for bubbling and fluctuation every 4 hours or more often as required. Bubbling indicates air leaving the system and is normal for the child with pneumothorax, but it could indicate an air leak in a child without pneumothorax. Fluctuation of water in the water-seal chamber is normal reflection of pressure changes in the pleural cavity during respirations.
4. Observe the integrity of the drainage tubing and chest tube at least once every shift. This ensures that the system is intact,

with no air leaks and helps to prevent formation of kinks or clots.

5. Check water-seal and suction level every shift. This ensures that system is being used properly and maintains child safety while the equipment is in use.
6. Keep the chest tube clamps readily available at bedside. Clamps are used to replace the drainage system or to locate the source of an air leak if bubbling occurs in the water-seal bottle while the system is on suction.
7. Never clamp the chest tube to get the child out of bed or during transportation of the child. Whenever the chest tube is clamped, air or fluid cannot escape from the pleural space. This puts the child at risk for a tension pneumothorax.
8. Troubleshoot the system as needed when problems arise (**Table 3.1**). Early and prompt attention to the difficulties will minimize the child's complications.
9. Take care of used items. Dispose all waste. Perform hand hygiene.

TABLE 3.1: Troubleshooting problems with chest tubes on children.

Problem	*Possible causes*	*Interventions*
Water level in water-seal chamber does not rise and fall with breathing	Clot in chest tubing or patient's chest	Gently pinch the tubing around the clot and do milking carefully to move it into collection chamber
Do	Dependent loop or kink in patient tube with fluid occlusion	Straighten the catheter and tubing along its length to its connection with the collection device
Do	Dislodgement of catheter from patient/ child	If chest tube pulls out accidentally, the insertion site should be immediately sealed with sterile gauze dressing to prevent air entry in pleural cavity. Notify the responsible physician immediately
Do	Disconnection of patient's tube from chest tube connector	Quickly clamp the chest tube to prevent sucking air injury and notify physician immediately. Always keep a chest tube clamp for each tube at bedside
Do	Chest drain is not positioned sufficiently below patient's chest	Lower the chest tube to allow for gravity drainage
Do	Patient tube clamp may be closed	Clamp only when indicated, otherwise leave the chest tube open
Do	In-line connectors not properly secured, allowing for an air leak	Ensure that in-line connectors are properly secured and sealed at all times. Check for any loose connections periodically
There is constant bubbling in the water-seal chamber	This confirms an air leak is present	To determine source of air leak (patient or catheter connection), momentarily clamp the chest tube close to the chest drain and observe the water-seal. If the bubbling stops, the air leak may be from catheter connections or patient's chest. Check catheter connections and patient dressings for a partially withdrawn catheter. If catheter is dislodged, follow procedure as above. If bubbling continues after temporary clamping the patient's tube, this indicates a system leak, which require system replacement

Contd...

Contd...

Problem	*Possible causes*	*Interventions*
Overfilled water-seal level(water above 2 cm limit line) or over-filled suction control chamber	Too much water was added to the chamber	Press and hold the negative-pressure relief valve at the top of the chest drainage system to vent excess negative pressure in the water-seal chamber. Release the valve when the level of water returns to the 2 cm mark. To remove water from the suction control chamber, insert syringe and withdraw excess water
Not enough water in the water-seal or suction control chamber	Evaporation versus under-fill or spillage of water	Add additional water to the suction control chamber by temporarily turning off the suction source, removing the rubber stopper and adding water to the desired level. Additional water may be added to water-seal chamber with a syringe by quickly and temporarily clamping the patient's tube and injecting water to the desired level
Suction control chamber is not bubbling or bubbling too vigorously	Disconnection or too much suction source pressure in the system	Check and ensure that the suction tubing is connected and the suction source is turned on. A constant, gentle bubbling is the norm. Vigorous bubbling causes quicker evaporation. Adjust the suction control source for gentle bubbling
Chest drainage system has accidentally been knocked over	Human error	Set the system upright and check the fluid levels in the water-seal and suction control chambers for proper volumes. Adjust accordingly. Arrange a baffle system, if feasible, that prevents fluid from mixing between chambers, allowing for proper function after setting upright again
Specimen collection required of chest drainage fluid	Laboratory analysis of chest drainage fluid is indicated	Remove fluid with needle and syringe from the self-sealing portion of the drainage tubing after following the guideline for cleaning the tubing at fluid collection site
Patient needs transport or leaves the unit	As situation indicates, e.g., surgery, CT scan	Do not clamp the catheter tubing. Disconnect the suction tubing from the suction source. The system continues to collect fluid (by gravity) or air (by water-seal)

10. Document the observational findings related to chest drainage in child's record.

Chest Tube Removal

1. Perform hand hygiene to prevent cross infections.
2. Gather all necessary supplies for efficient time management and organized approach.
3. Apply topical anesthetic cream to the chest tube wound site, as prescribed. Administer sedation and analgesics, if prescribed. This reduces child's pain during the procedure of chest tube removal.
4. Position the child comfortably and for easy access of the chest tube for swift removal.
5. Maintain strict sterile technique during the procedure of removal of chest tube.
6. Wear nonsterile gloves and remove old dressing from chest tube insertion site. This allows access to the chest tube catheter for removal by healthcare prescriber.
7. Clamp the chest tube catheter (if not already done) about 1 to 2 inches from the insertion site. This minimizes dead space and stops air from entering and exiting catheter.
8. Instruct the child to exhale and hold his or her breath, as appropriate. This allows maximum positive pressure in pleural space.
9. Remove nonsterile gloves. Perform hand hygiene. Don sterile gloves.

10. Prepare sterile dressing to be placed over the chest tube site after removal. This prevents wound contamination. Sterile petrolatum gauze can be placed immediately over the chest tube insertion site followed by sterile gauze (4 × 4), because this seals the insertion site from any untoward air entry.
11. Assist the physician/healthcare prescriber to pull out the chest tube quickly and smoothly.
12. Instruct the child to breath normally. This allows removal of air and fluid.
13. Closely monitor the child's vital signs, respiratory rate, pattern and effort, skin color, perfusion, level of consciousness, oxygen requirements, hemodynamic stability and chest X-ray findings. This helps to identify the response to chest tube removal.
14. Dispose all waste in appropriate containers as standard precautions.
15. Remove gloves. Perform hand hygiene as standard precautions.
16. Document the procedure of chest tube removal in child's case sheet.

Evaluation and Documentation

- Evaluate child's vital signs and note changes in respiratory rate, effort or pattern and presence of any abnormal features at least every 2 hours on the special chest tube care chart as per institutional guidelines.
  - Evaluate the chest tube drainage system for water-seal bubbling or fluctuation every 4 hours or more frequently as symptoms warrant. Notify the physician/healthcare prescriber immediately for any unusual findings. Mark the drainage level on the disposable chest drainage collection device every 2–4 hours or as needed
  - Evaluate the child's and parent's level of understanding and anxiety related to the chest tube insertion and drainage
- Document the following at the time insertion – date and time of chest tube insertion, assessment findings, name of the person who inserted the chest tube, insertion site position and placement, chest tube size inserted, medications administered during chest tube insertion, amount of water-seal suction, prescribed water level for suction or suction level on dial of dry suction and child's response to the procedure
  - Document findings of vital signs and respiratory assessment, amount of drainage, its color and consistency, presence of any complications, troubleshooting problems related to chest tube and interventions required
  - Document chest tube removal with date, time, and amount of drainage, skin condition at insertion site and child's condition at the time of chest tube removal.

Communication and Teaching for Homecare

- Communicate with child and parents in simple local language about benefits and possible complications related to chest tube drainage and about further plan of management of child's health problems. Discuss about the areas of concern of the child and family members
- Teach the parents about precautions to be followed during handling of the child with chest tube, general routine care of the child, hand hygiene and other hygienic practices, signs and symptoms of infections at the wound site, breathing difficulties and any other complications. Explain about continued care at home after discharge from the hospitals, continuation of medications, emergency medical assistance and about follow-up care.

PROCEDURE–28: BLOOD AND BLOOD PRODUCT TRANSFUSION TO THE CHILDREN

Clinical Guidelines

- Blood or blood product transfusion is the replacement of whole blood or one of its components, having definite indications related to medical conditions (such as thalassemia, leukemia, hemophilia, thrombocytopenia, severe anemia, Rh or ABO isoimmunization, etc.) and surgical problems (such as cardiac or other major surgical interventions, accidental injury with massive blood loss, burns, etc.)

- Effective and safe transfusion therapy requires a thorough understanding of the clinical conditions being treated. Most patients require blood components rather than whole blood
- Transfusions are given using whole blood or blood products such as packed red blood cells (PRBC), saline washed RBCs, frozen deglycerolized RBCs, fresh frozen plasma (FFP), albumin (a plasma protein available in 5% or 25% solutions), platelets, cryoprecipitate, granulocytes, factor VIII concentrate, and factor IX complex
- The following measures should be followed during transfusion therapy:
  - Always donor's blood must be screened for transmissible diseases (HIV, HBV, HCV, Malaria) and for pathogens (such as syphilis or other sexually transmitted diseases)
  - Ensure that cross-matched blood products are given to correctly identified patient/child. The child must be identified from both hospital identification and blood bank records or with identity bands. Two healthcare professionals verify child's ABO and Rh blood type, its compatibility, expiry date, type of blood product, and amount and rate of transfusion
  - Avoid unnecessary transfusion, volume overload during transfusion therapy, hypothermia, electrolyte and clotting disorders
  - For young infants below three months of age, the blood to be transfused should be cross matched with mother's blood/maternal serum
  - Intervene promptly to transfusion reactions to the child and inform to all authority
  - Keep detailed record for transfusion therapy with all related findings
- Signs and symptoms of transfusion reaction include fever, chills, restlessness, headache, chest pain, abdominal or lower back pain, diaphoresis, rash, hives, urticaria, swelling, tachycardia, hypotension, respiratory distress, oliguria, shock, anaphylaxis
- Obtain informed written consent for blood product administration from the parents or legal guardian, unless in an emergency situation.

Equipment Required

- Hand hygiene supplies, and protective gear (mask, eye shield, gown, sterile gloves)
- Blood transfusion set, and IV fluid stand
- Syringe infusion pump, (if needed) and sterile 50 mL syringe
- Blood or blood componented for transfusion, as prescribed
- IV access with needle 22 G or more for older children and in neonates 24 G
- Blood-warming coil and blood warmer, as indicated and if available
- Sterile container/tray with sterile gloves, sterile cotton swab, gauze pieces and small bowl
- Emergency medication tray with drugs, normal saline, syringes and three-way cannula
- Stethoscope, BP monitor, Thermometer
- Bottle of 70% alcohol, adhesive tape, scissors, as required
- Waste disposal containers as per BMW guidelines
- Blood transfusion documentation sheet and child's case sheet.

Assessment and Preparation

- Assess child's vital signs for baseline information before starting blood or blood product transfusion. Assess child's transfusion history and presence of transfusion reactions. Assess ability to process information, anxiety and understanding level of both child and parents to provide necessary support to them

- Self-preparation should be done with hand hygiene and wearing of protective devices
- Environment should be clean, calm, well lighted and well ventilated
- All required articles and supplies should be arranged at child's bedside
- Preparation of parents: Explain the importance and procedure of blood product transfusion. Obtain written consent signed. Encourage participation of parents or any other family members during the transfusion therapy. Inform about potential features of transfusion reactions and precautions to be followed during transfusion
- Preparation of child: Explain the purpose and procedure of blood product transfusion, time requirement and possible transfusion reactions in simple age-appropriate approach. Allow the child to empty the bladder before transfusion. Follow the physician's direction for transfusion regarding medications to be administered and diet or food intake.

Performing the Steps of Procedure with Rationale/Point of Emphasis

1. Verify healthcare prescriber's/physician's direction for transfusion to ensure the correct blood product and correct amount for transfusion therapy.
2. Ensure blood specimens were sent to blood bank for typing and cross matching .
3. Perform hand hygiene and assemble all necessary items near the child's bed.
4. Make the child comfortable and allow the parents with the child.
5. Verify patency of IV infusion site or establish new IV access.
6. Ensure blood product is received from blood bank. Do not store it in the unit or ward where storage conditions may not be adequate to maintain integrity of the blood product.
7. Inspect the blood product visually for discoloration, separation of products and signs of contamination. If any inconsistencies found, notify and return the blood product to the blood bank immediately. This is important to prevent lethal transfusion reactions.
8. Check the blood product label against original order, transfusion record and child's identification with another qualified health personnel to prevent risk for incorrect administration. Verify the following information: Child's name and medical record/hospital registration number, type of blood component, child's ABO group and Rh factor, blood product unit number, expiration date of blood product, and special test report of diseases/pathogens.
9. Do signature on transfusion record after verification. Both the personnel must signed.
10. Ensure everything is ready to initiate blood product transfusion.
11. Administered prescribed medications. Antihistamine may be given to reduce allergic reactions to blood product. Furosemide may be needed for the child with cardiac diseases or in some other disease conditions.
12. Perform hand hygiene. Don appropriate protective apparel; mask, eye shield, gown, and sterile gloves, as standard precautions to reduce transmission of microorganisms.
13. Open the tubing of transfusion set with blood filter or use appropriate blood product filter and take precautions to prevent contamination during handling the tubing.
14. Ensure blood or blood product is in normal temperature before starting transfusion. Use blood-warming coil and blood warmer, if available and as indicated.
15. Attach transfusion set tubing with blood product bag carefully keeping all roller clamps close before fixing the tubing with IV access.
16. Open the roller clamp between blood product and drip chamber and fill drip chamber, covering blood filter. This allows for filtering of blood product. Then open roller clamp on tubing on infusion set

and prime the tubing. This prevents air embolus.

17. Close roller clamp when tubing is primed and place the tubing into IV-controlled infusion device. This prevents blood spillage and makes ready for administration.
18. Use syringe pump for small amount transfusion of blood product. Aspirate the required amount of blood into sterile 50 mL syringe, then connect to tubing with PMO line and put the syringe into syringe pump, then fix with IV access.
19. Avoid blood spillage during filling the syringe and priming the tubing and PMO line with blood product.
20. Cleanse the infusion port of child's venous access catheter and insert primed blood tubing. Follow institutional policy for cleaning of infusion port. Usually 70% alcohol swab is used to cleanse the port to reduce transmission of infectious agents.
21. Set the rate of transfusion, as directed by the physician/healthcare prescriber, open roller clamp of controlled infusion device/ set or set on the syringe pump (mL/hour). Start transfusion slowly and proceed.
22. Stay with the child and monitor continuously for signs of transfusion reaction for first 15 minutes. Explain signs and symptoms of transfusion reactions to the child and parent. Instruct them to notify immediately, if these occurs. Usually transfusion reactions occur within first 15 minutes of starting of transfusion, but it may occur at any time.
23 Stop the transfusion immediately if reaction occurs to minimize the amount of blood infused and potentially reduce the severity of the reactions. Notify the event to physician and blood bank and return the unused portion blood product to the blood bank, as per hospital policy.
24 Intervene promptly to manage transfusion reactions and maintain venous access catheter with normal saline infusion or as directed by the physician.
25. Monitor vital signs (temperature, respiratory rate, heart rate, BP) every 15 minutes for 1 hour and every 30 minutes thereafter and compare with baseline. These enable the early detection of complications related to blood product transfusion
    Monitor for signs of fluid overload. During transfusion, if the child develops tachycardia, labored breathing, dry cough and rales at lung bases that indicate signs of fluid overload. Then slow the transfusion rate of blood product and notify the physician immediately.
26. Complete total prescribed amount of transfusion within 4 hours of initiation of transfusion or faster if directed. Blood begins to clot after 4 hours and the likelihood of bacterial contamination markedly increases after 4 hours.
27. On completion of blood product administration, clamp the tube of transfusion set and venous access catheter, then disconnect the tubing carefully. This helps to prevent spills.
28 Change the tubing after completion of each blood product transfusion procedure. When administering two or more blood products, change the tubing between the products. When administering two units of PRBCs, the same tubing can be used for transfusing two units.
29. Flush the venous access catheter with normal saline to prevent clotting and to maintain patency for later use. Start maintenance fluid therapy, if prescribed.
30. Make the child comfortable. Praise for cooperation. Ask for presence of any problem.
31. Dispose all waste in appropriate BMW containers. Take care of reusable items.
32. Perform hand hygiene. Document the procedure of blood product transfusion details.

Evaluation and Documentation

- Evaluate child's vital signs, intake and output, patency of venous access, signs and symptoms of blood or blood product transfusion related reactions
    - Evaluate the child's response to the treatment with blood product. Assess

for post-transfusion hemoglobin and hematocrit levels, increased BP, decreased heart rate, increased urine output, improved oxygenation and respiratory status
- Evaluate the child for hyperkalemia because stored blood develops a high potassium level due to red blood cells lysis and for hypocalcemia because citrate ions in stored blood bind with calcium and are excreted by the body fluids
- Evaluate child's and family's understanding of the treatment with blood product administration and determine whether they have any area of concern to discuss.

- Document the followings in child's case sheet and hospital record:
  - Pre-transfusion and post-transfusion vital signs assessment findings (for baseline and serial recording)
  - Blood group, Rh type and blood product unit number that was transfused. Preserve the blood bank document of the transfused blood product in the child case sheet as legal record and for further reference
  - Name of the two personnel verifying the blood product and child's identity
  - Date and time of initiation and discontinuation of blood product therapy
  - Amount of blood product transfused hourly and total time required for transfusion
  - Any transfusion reactions occur and any interruption during therapy
  - Medications administered before, during and after the transfusion
  - Overall response of the child and family members/parents.

Communication and Teaching for Homecare

- Communicate with child and parents about indications and purposes of blood product transfusion, child's health status and plan of further management
- Teach the parents about precautions to be followed during blood product transfusion, routine care of the child with hygienic practices, recommended diet and fluid intake, continued care at home after discharge from hospital, medications, need for emergency medical help and follow-up visits
  - Instruct the family to contact healthcare provider if signs of delayed transfusion reactions occur (such as fever, jaundice, infection, or anemia)
  - Instruct the parents to preserve the record of child's blood group, Rh-type and date of blood product transfusion along with other medical records.

PROCEDURE–29: BONE MARROW ASPIRATION IN CHILDREN

Clinical Guidelines

- Bone marrow aspiration is a special invasive procedure performed to obtain specimens of bone marrow using a special aspirating needle for the purpose of examination. The material is usually obtained from the upper portion of the sternum or the iliac crest. Examination of the stained bone marrow is helpful in diagnosing a great number of blood disorders, infections and malignant diseases
- The iliac crest is the most common site of bone marrow aspiration. The sternum is not preferred in children because of associated pain and risk of injury of underlying vital structures. Bone marrow aspiration can be done from the proximal tibia, medial to the tibial tuberosity, in infants less than one year old. This site is preferred for bone marrow biopsy in infants as iliac crest is small and there is risk of pelvic visceral injury
- Bone marrow is the soft tissue in the marrow cavities of long bones (i.e., yellow marrow) and in the spaces between trabeculae of spongy bone in the sternum and other flat or irregular bones (i.e., red marrow). Yellow

marrow is mostly fat and stored energy. Red marrow produces all types of blood cells
- Bone marrow aspiration is performed by healthcare prescriber/physician with specific indications in strict aseptic technique. Nursing personnel are responsible for preparation of procedure, medications, monitoring of child's health status and assisting the physician during the procedure of bone marrow aspiration and collection of specimens
- Informed written consent form must be signed by the parents before the procedure.

Equipment Required

- Hand hygiene supplies and PPE to reduce transmission of microorganisms
- A sterile covered bone marrow aspiration tray or drum containing all sterile items such as gloves and gowns for physician and assistant, cotton balls or gauze pieces, gauze pads of various sizes, dressing forceps, small bowls, draping sheets/ cut sheet, two 5 mL or 10 mL syringe for marrow aspiration,, bone marrow aspiration needle (sized appropriate for the child), syringe and needle for giving local anesthesia, pressure dressing, bandage, specimen containers and slides (10–12)
- A clean tray or trolley containing bottles of antiseptic solutions for skin preparation (alcohol, povidone-iodine), adhesive tape, scissors, stethoscope
- Lifting or transfer forceps for handling sterile items by the assistant during procedure
- Pulse oximeter, BP monitor and age-appropriate resuscitation equipment
- Medication administration tray for local anesthesia (lidocaine 1% injection and cream) and emergency medicine tray (syringe, needle, IV cannula, IV fluid, emergency drugs, etc.) for emergency conditions
- Oxygen delivery supplies and supplies for vital signs assessment
- Small towel roll or pillow for positioning the child, if needed
- Specimen form and labeling items for the specimens
- Waste disposal containers as per BMW rules
- Consent form, child case sheet and documentation sheet for bone marrow aspiration.

Assessment and Preparation

- Assess child's vital signs, health status, platelet count and coagulation status to anticipate bleeding complications and presence of any other abnormalities. Assess anxiety, and level of understanding of child and parents
- Self-preparation should be done with hand hygiene and use of PPE
- Environment should be clean, calm, well lighted and well ventilated. Bone marrow aspiration should be done at procedure/ treatment room or in OR
- Articles preparation: All necessary equipment and supplies should be arranged for easy access near the procedure table at treatment/procedure room or in OR
- Preparation of parents: Explain the purpose and procedure of bone marrow aspiration and its related consequences. Inform details to get signature on the consent form. Allow the parent with the child during invasive procedure to gain cooperation, if they are available and willing to accompany the child and as per hospital policy.
- Preparation of child: Explain the procedure in age-appropriate simple language. Make the child clean and comfortable. Ensure patent IV access or perform IV cannulation for emergency medications. Hydrate the child with IV fluid, if needed. Ask the child to empty the bladder before going to the procedure room, if required. Discuss about use of anesthetic cream, medications for sedation and NPO status, as needed. Show the treatment room before procedure. Allow diversional strategies (music therapy, breathing techniques) to the child.

Performing the Steps of Procedure with Rationale/Point of Emphasis

1. Ensure local anesthetic cream applied to the site of bone marrow aspiration at least one hour before the procedure to decrease the pain sensation at aspiration site.
2. Verify legal signed consent form and verify the child's identity with two identifiers.
3. Confirm the NPO status, as directed by the physician.
4. Perform hand hygiene and wear protective gear as applicable.
5. Administer sedative drugs, as prescribed. Bone marrow aspiration is a painful procedure.
6. Collect and assemble all necessary supplies at the treatment room for organized approach.
7. Bring the child and parent/attendant into the treatment room. Place the infant or young child on the procedure table and allow attendant to ensure safety to prevent fall. Allow the older child to climb on the procedure table with precautions.
8. Assess the child's vital signs for baseline data and to ensure comfort level.
9. Position the child according to the aspiration site **(Figs. 3.14A to D)**. Place the child in supine position for aspiration from sternum and anterior iliac crest. Place the child in prone position with a small towel roll or pillow under the child's hips for aspiration from posterior iliac crest. For aspiration from the tibia, place the child in supine position with knee bent and supported by pillow or towel roll.

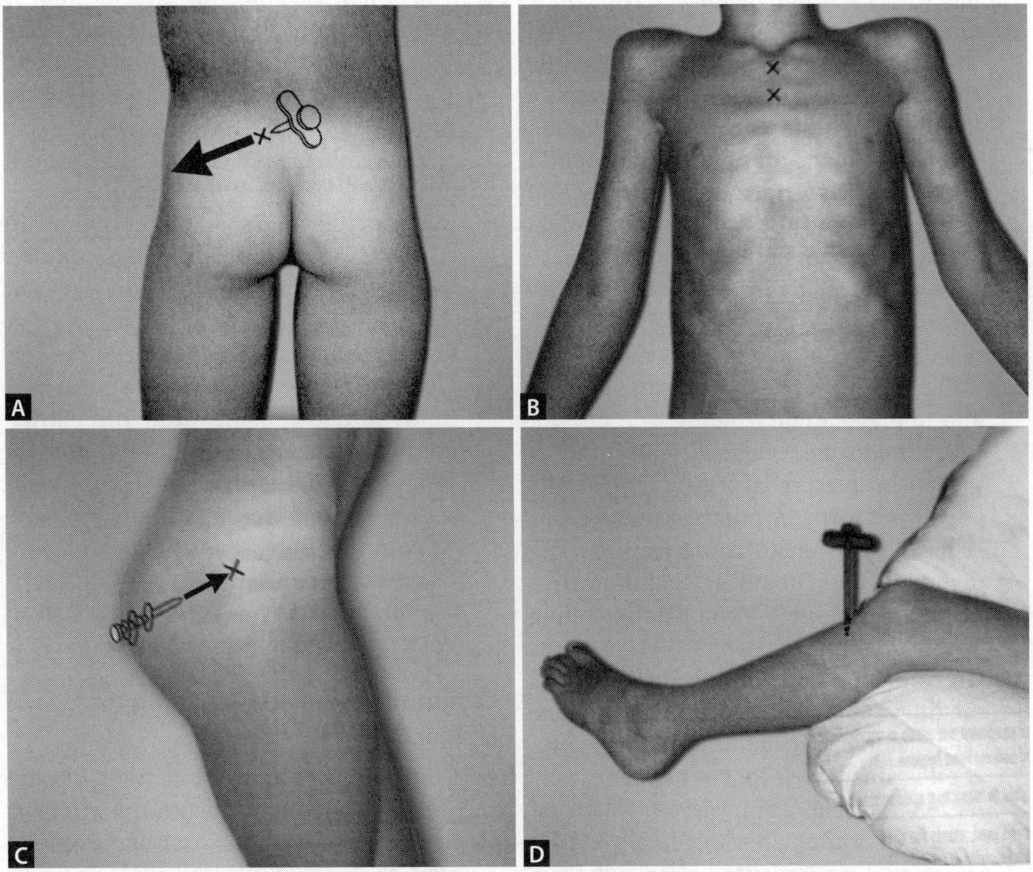

Figs. 3.14A to D: Sites for bone marrow aspiration: A. Posterior iliac crest. B. Sternum. C. Anterior iliac crest. D. Tibia.

10. Wipe the aspiration site with gauze pieces to remove the anesthetic cream.
11. Perform hand hygiene. Wear cap, mask, sterile gown and sterile gloves to assist during bone marrow aspiration. Ensure physician also don cap, mask, sterile gown and sterile gloves after surgical hand scrubbing, as standard precautions.
12. Assist the physician to prepare the aspiration site by cleansing with antiseptic solutions and to drape the selected site of aspiration with sterile towels or cut sheet. Ensure sterile technique is followed during the entire procedure of bone marrow aspiration.
13. Assist the physician to inject surface/local anesthetic drug (lidocaine) to ensure in pain relief during the aspiration procedure.
14. Assist the physician to introduce the bone marrow aspiration needle in the selected site with precautions. Help to collect the specimens in the containers and prepare the slides in sterile techniques. Aspiration may be difficult initially in some child (e.g., in case of leukemia), so several attempts may be necessary to collect required amount of specimens.
15. Observe the child during aspiration of the materials for any complications.
16. Ask the assistant to hold the child during procedure to decrease the movements and to prevent fall. Holding is important to maintain correct positioning and to prevent misplacement of aspiration needle and to complete the procedure with ease.
17. Allow the assistant to use age-appropriate diversion and breathing techniques to distract the child to enhance the coping skills.
18. On completion of the procedure, remove the drape and cleanse the area to reduce the risk for skin irritation. Make the child comfortable. Praise for cooperation.
19. Assess the aspiration site for signs of bleeding. Apply dressing using sterile gauze pad and secured with adhesive tape and bandage. Provide comfortable position to the child.
20. Label the specimens and send to the appropriate laboratory with filled up signed requisition form for examination.
21. Dispose all wastes and disposable items in appropriate containers as per BMW rules.
22. Remove gloves and perform hand hygiene to prevent cross contaminations.
23. Decontaminate, clean and sterilize the reusable items and reset for next use.
24. Assess the child's vital signs and signs of complications until he or she is fully awake. Check the dressing for bleeding. If dressing is saturated with blood, apply pressure using sterile gauze pad until bleeding ceases and inform the physician.
25. Assist the child to return to own bed/room and provide comfort.
26. Document the procedure of bone marrow aspiration, and about the specimens send for examination. Record all observational findings before, during and after the procedure.

Evaluation and Documentation

- Evaluate the child's vital signs and health status after the procedure and compare with baseline data. Evaluate for signs and symptoms of bleeding, infection and pain or any other complications
- Document the date, time and site of bone marrow aspiration and child's conditions before, during and after the procedure including vital signs, oxygen saturation and presence of any problems or complications. Keep record of bone marrow specimens send for laboratory examination and post-procedural instructions to the parents and child.

Communication and Teaching for Homecare

- Communicate with child and parents about the completion of procedure, child's health conditions, possible problems after the procedure and plan of future management based on findings of the bone marrow examination report

- Teach the parents about observation for bleeding from the aspiration site, fever, and unmanageable pain and discomfort. Instruct about hygienic care and cleanliness, use of pain relief medications (acetaminophen may be used, if needed, but not aspirin), restrictions of child's activity, dressing change time (as directed by physician), collection of bone marrow examination report, and routine care at hospital and at home after discharge. Discuss about plan of discharge, continued care at home with discharge advice and plan of follow-up visits.

PROCEDURE–30: LUMBAR PUNCTURE OF THE CHILDREN

Clinical Guidelines

- Lumbar puncture (LP) is an invasive procedure by insertion of hollow needle into the subarachnoid space of the meningeal sac below the end of spinal cord, in the intervertebral space of the lumbar region. The L3 - L4 interspace is the preferred site for lumbar puncture, but the L2 - L3 and L4 - L5 interspaces can also be used
- Lumbar puncture is performed under strict aseptic technique (a) to obtain cerebrospinal fluid (CSF) for analysis that helps in diagnosis of some conditions (such as severe headache, CNS infections or bleeding), (b) to administer medications to the brain and spinal cord (e.g., anesthetic drugs or chemotherapeutic agents), (c) to inject contrast dye for myelogram, and (d) to relieve from excess pressure of CSF or other fluids
- Informed written consent must be obtained before the procedure
- Lumbar puncture is done by the healthcare prescriber/physician with precautions
- Nursing personnel should present during the procedure to assist the physician to maintain sterile technique. Nurses are responsible to prepare the child before the procedure, to position and to support the child during the procedure of lumbar puncture. Nursing professionals are responsible to assess the child's vital signs and health status before, during and after the procedure.

Equipment Required

- Hand hygiene supplies and PPE to prevent transmission of microorganisms
- A sterile lumbar puncture tray containing all sterile items such as gloves, gown, cotton swabs, gauze pieces, dressing, small bowls, dressing forceps for skin preparation, sterile drapes/cut sheet, syringe (2 mL, 3 mL), needle (24 G, 25 G), lumbar puncture needle, three way stopcock, bandage, 3–5 CSF collection tubes, spinal fluid pressure manometer (optional)
- A clean tray containing lidocaine 1% injection vial/ampule, anesthetic cream, nonsterile gloves, caps, masks, apron/gown and items to manage any emergency conditions (syringe, needle, IV cannula, IV fluid, emergency medications), bottles of antiseptic solutions for skin preparation (alcohol, povidone-iodine), adhesive tape, scissors, stethoscope
- Lifting forceps or transfer forceps to handle the sterile items
- Articles for vital signs assessment, monitors and oxygen delivery supplies
- Extra pillow, blanket and sheets for positioning the child
- Laboratory specimen form and labeling items for the specimens
- Waste disposal containers as per BMW guidelines
- Consent form, child case sheet and documentation sheet for lumbar puncture.

Assessment and Preparation

- Assess child's pertinent history, vital signs and physical findings for signs of increased intracranial pressure. Assess child's age, developmental level, coping strategies, anxiety and level of understanding. Assess the parents for knowledge of reasons for the procedure, expected outcome and potential adverse reactions of lumbar puncture

- Self-preparation should be done with hand hygiene and use of protective items such as cap, mask, gown and clean gloves. Physician must perform surgical hand scrubbing and wear cap, mask, sterile gown and sterile gloves
- Environment should be clean, calm and well lighted. Lumbar puncture is usually performed in the treatment room. In emergency conditions, it can be done in the intensive care unit or in emergency room or at bedside
- All necessary articles should be collected and assemble near the procedure table in treatment room or at bedside. Aseptic technique must be followed using sterile supplies for the invasive procedure of lumbar puncture
- *Preparation of parents:* Explain the procedure according to parents' understanding level. Obtain informed written signed consent from the parent before the procedure. Discuss the role of parent to provide support to the child during the procedure and allow to participate to promote coping, if feasible
- Preparation of child: Explain the procedure to the child in age-appropriate simple language. Make the child clean and comfortable. Ask to empty the bladder before the procedure, if needed. Apply topical anesthetic cream to lumbar puncture site, as prescribed. Show the treatment room to the child and parent before procedure. Allow diversional measures to the child and involve parents. Prepare the child as per physician's instructions for diet, fluid and medications. Ask for cooperation from older child.

Performing the Steps of Procedure with Rationale/Point of Emphasis

1. Perform hand hygiene and set up all equipment and supplies using aseptic technique near the procedure table of treatment room for efficient time management.
2. Verify the child's identity and transfer the child to the treatment room.
3. Ensure consent form is signed and anesthetic cream is applied to the LP site, as directed.
4. Ensure physician is ready to perform the procedure and scrub hands, don cap, mask, sterile gown and sterile gloves for infection control measures:
5. Position the child on procedure table in one of the following methods **(Figs. 3.15A and B)**:
   i. *Knee-chest position:* It is best position for the infant to maximize separation of the vertebral bodies. Position the infant with back rounded and parallel to the side of the treatment table. Place the child on side-lying with lumbar area exposed. Hold the small infant in position by placing one hand over his

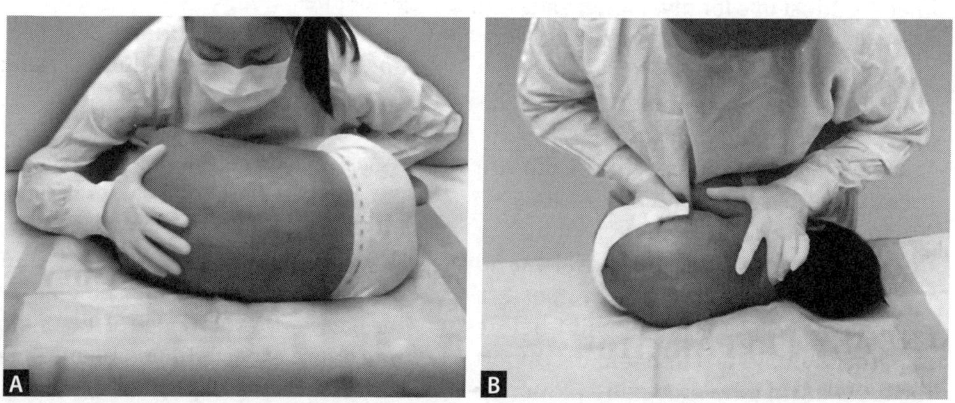

Figs. 3.15A and B: Positions for lumbar puncture: A. Knee - Chest position, B. Recumbent position.

or her neck and the other hand over the buttocks. Bend the child's back to the desired position.

ii. *Recumbent position:* It is best position for older infant or young child to maximize separation of vertebral bodies. Hold the older infant or young child in position by placing one hand behind child's neck or by placing one arm around the neck and grasping his or her hands. Place the other arm around the child's buttocks and grasp child's legs behind the knees. Give gentle pressure on neck and legs to bend the child's body as necessary.

iii. *Sitting position:* This is comfortable for the older child who is able to cooperate without restraint. An assistant should hold the child in the sitting position. Support the child in sitting position by having the child to sit at edge of the procedure table with shoulders and head bent forward. Place the child's elbows on the knees/thighs and the back arched.

iv. A small pillow or large stuffed animal can be placed in front of the chest of the older child and instruct the child to grasp it to make the desired position with ease.

6. Instruct the older child to stay as still as possible while the assistant continues to hold the child securely in position. The assistant or parent should present in the treatment room and should initiate distraction measures.
7. Assist the physician to identify the lumbar puncture site and for skin preparation using antiseptic solutions (such as alcohol-povidone iodine-alcohol) and sterile gauze/swabs in sterile aseptic technique. Skin should be cleaned around the puncture site with 10 cm diameter from inner to outer parts.
8. Assist to apply sterile drape or cut sheet over the back of the child, exposing the puncture area only, for preparation of sterile field of work.
9. Assist the physician to administer local anesthetic agent by intradermal injection of lidocaine around the area of puncture site to reduce the pain sensation.
10. Secure the child during insertion of lumbar puncture needle into the subarachnoid space by the physician and to prevent any complications.
11. Note the characteristics (flow, color and turbidity) of CSF. Normal CSF is clear. Red fluid indicates intracranial hemorrhage or a traumatic tap. Cloudy turbid fluid indicates infection. Yellow fluid indicates hyperbilirubinemia or hemolyzed RBCs.
12. Assess the child's respiration, heart rate, pain and any signs of complications during the procedure. Initiate emergency management, as needed.
13. Assess spinal pressure by using manometer and three-way stopcock, if required. It is done when the spinal needle is in position and free drip of CSF is established. Attach the spinal pressure manometer to the spinal needle using three-way stopcock. Normal CSF pressure in the relaxed child is 50–80 mm of H_2O.
14. Assist to collect CSF specimens in 3–5 sterile specimen tubes or as indicated.
15. Secure the child during removal of the LP needle. Assist the physician to wipe and clean the puncture site and to apply dressing and adhesive tape or bandage, as directed.
16. Observe the child for any complications after insertion of LP needle. Monitor throughout the procedure for tachycardia or bradycardia, decreased responsiveness, abnormal breathing, complaints of severe pain and sluggish or unequal pupil reaction.

    Brainstem herniation is a potential complication. Other complications include severe headache, back pain, nerve injury, breakage of needle in moving uncooperative child, etc.
17. Dispose the all wastes in the appropriate containers. Take care of reusable items.
18. Remove PPE. Perform hand hygiene. Document the procedure of LP.
19. Ensure that all specimens are correctly labeled and sent to the laboratory immediately with filled up laboratory form.

20. Transfer the child to his or her own bed. Make the child comfortable by lying flat in the bed. The child should remain lying flat for at least one hour after the procedure. Post-procedural headaches after lumbar puncture in children can be minimized by lying flat and providing good hydration.
21. Continue to monitor the child for post-procedural complications and for initiation of prompt management. Observe for changes in neurological status such as changes in level of consciousness, onset of high-pitched cry, restlessness, severe headache, bulging fontanel (in infants), numbness of legs, and for bleeding or leaking of CSF from the puncture site, redness at puncture site and fever.
22. Document the procedure of LP and all findings related to lumbar puncture.

Evaluation and Documentation

- Evaluate the child vital signs, response to the procedure and the presence of features for any complications related to the procedure of lumbar puncture
- Document the date and time of lumbar puncture, characteristics of CSF, date and time of CSF specimens sent for laboratory analysis, observational findings of vital signs and neurological status and name of the physician who preformed lumbar puncture.

Communication and Teaching for Homecare

- Communicate with the child and parents about the lumbar puncture procedure, possible outcome of the procedure, child's present health status and plan of further management
- Teach the parents about the need to have the child remain on bed rest following lumbar puncture and drinking of plenty of fluids. Discuss about the potential problems like severe headache, bleeding or leaking of fluid from the puncture site, redness and irritation at lumbar puncture site, fever, high-pitched cry and numbness of legs which require immediate attention. Instruct about hygienic care, diet, fluid intake, medications, future plan of treatment, discharge planning, continued care at home and follow-up care.

PROCEDURE–31: PRECAUTIONS DURING SEIZURES IN CHILDREN

Clinical Guidelines

- Seizures are common problems in children found as a symptom in various disease conditions. It occurs due to disturbances of the brain functions resulting from abnormal excessive electrical discharge from the brain. It is also termed as convulsions
- Common causes of seizures or convulsions in children are febrile seizures, epilepsy, CNS infections, metabolic disorders, intracranial hemorrhage, congenital CNS anomalies, traumatic injury, poisoning, brain tumor, postvaccination encephalopathy, etc.
- Seizure precautions are implemented for children with known seizure disorders, history of seizures in last 6 months or new onset of seizures and known risk factors for seizures from head trauma, severe electrolyte imbalance or drug overdose
- Seizure precautions must also be followed for first 24 hours postoperative or post-surgery on all children with a past history of seizures, if the current surgery requires the use of general anesthesia, narcotics or bowel-cleansing preparations
- Most breakthrough seizures occur as a result of missed seizure medications. Therefore, children whose diet status is NPO should have the order written as *"NPO, except for seizure medication"*. If the physician prefers nothing to be administered by mouth, then the IV route should be ordered for seizure medications.

Equipment Required

- Hand hygiene supplies for hand wash and hand rub to prevent cross infections
- Bed or crib with side rails and bed-pads to prevent injury

- Bedside oxygen delivery equipment including oxygen source, flowmeter, humidifier, nasal prong or oxygen hood and resuscitation bag-mask of age-appropriate size
- Suction apparatus, suction tube and suction catheter
- Pulse oximeter, multi-parameter monitor, cardiac monitor, apnea monitor, as available
- Vital signs measurement items–stethoscope, thermometer, sphygmomanometer with appropriate size cuff, bottle of 70% alcohol, cotton swabs in a covered container
- Blood glucose monitoring equipment: glucometer, test strip and other supplies
- Emergency Medication Tray with complete list of emergency drugs
- Medication administration articles including syringes, needles and other supplies
- Covered containers with mouth wipes, gauze pieces, cotton balls/swabs
- Seizure record, child treatment sheet and case sheet
- Waste disposal containers as per BMW rules.

Assessment and Preparation

- Assess child's seizure history including type of seizures, typical frequency of seizures, description of seizure events, typical length of seizure events, presence of aura, the child experience before seizures, birth history and perinatal illness/events and developmental milestones
  - Assess child's vital signs, present general health status and present body weight
  - Assess child's and family members' understanding level about seizures, precautions to be taken to prevent seizures and during seizures, need for medical assistance and use of anticonvulsive medications including purpose, side effects and importance of adherence to medication regimen
- Self-preparation should be done with practice of standard precautions of infection control
- Environment should be clean, calm, quite, well lighted and well ventilated
- Articles preparation should be done considering the need for prompt emergency management and organized approach. All required items must be ready in hand for time management and organized approach
- Preparation of parents: Explain the seizure precautions in simple language. Instruct the family members to report immediately if any abnormal signs are observed
- Preparation of child: Explain the seizure episode to the child with seizure disorders. Discuss about necessary precautions for seizures, in developmentally appropriate simple language, whenever possible.

Performing the Steps of Procedure with Rationale/Point of Emphasis

Preparation of Room/Area for Care of the Seizure Patient

1. Perform hand hygiene and collect all required equipment near the child
2. Follow basic safety measure and steps of preparation of child's bed/crib or room
3. Select age-appropriate bed or crib with side rails to prevent falls and injury
4. Apply pad on the side rails to prevent injury during seizure episodes
5. Set up suction apparatus at bedside with appropriate size suction catheter. Check the equipment for its working condition. Suctioning is required to prevent aspiration of secretions during postictal period of seizures
6. Ensure that the oxygen delivery system is ready for the child and working properly
7. Check the medication administration supplies including emergency medications are available within easy reach of the child for prompt initiation of treatment
8. Calculate weight-appropriate dosage for emergency seizure medications (e.g., Phenobarbital, phenytoin sodium, lorazepam) for the particular child and place a prepared document or chart at child's bedside for quick reference. Antiepileptic medications may be needed for prolonged seizures

9. Keep the child's bed in lowest position with side rails up and brakes locked
10. Keep ready or attach pulse oximeter and apnea/cardiac monitor to the child when unattended. This helps to identify changes in heart rate, oxygenation and respiratory status of the child which may indicate seizure activity
11. Ensure IV access is patent or place IV cannula for medications during or after seizures
12. Keep the seizure record ready at child's bedside to documentation of the event.

Nursing Care During Seizure Episode

1. Attend the child during a seizure episode promptly and manage skillfully. Ask for assistance from other nursing professionals and assistant/parent.
2. If the child is in standing position, place the child on floor or on bed or crib gently.
3. Place bedside curtains or close the room door, as appropriate, to protect other child and family members from having fearful and stressful experience of the seizure events.
4. Protect the child's head, as violent seizures may cause child's head to hit hard surfaces.
5. Place the child in side-lying position, if possible, to prevent aspiration of secretions. If the child has head or neck injury, then place in supine position only with precautions.
6. Loosen tight clothing, especially around the neck. It helps to maintain open airway.
7. Do not restraint the child during seizure episode. Restraint of movements could cause injury to the child and to the staff.
8. Do not force anything into child's mouth during seizures. Forcing tongue blades or other objects into child's mouth during seizure episodes may cause tooth loss or detachment, lacerations, vomiting or respiratory distress.
9. Remove objects from nearby area of the child, as those may cause injury.
10. Assess the child's airway, breathing and circulatory status and provide support, as needed. Most children with seizures require airway interventions (e.g., positioning to maintain patent airway and/or suctioning of secretions). But oxygen administration and/or bag-mask ventilation may be required for children with prolonged seizures.
11. Check the patency of child's IV access to administer medications. Seizures lasting for 5–10 minutes will likely require administration of anticonvulsive medications.
12. Obtain fingerstick blood glucose (capillary blood glucose) level from the child who presents with seizures and persistent altered level of consciousness to identify hypoglycemia and associated problems.
13. Stay with the child during seizure continuously and call for help whenever necessary. It helps in continuous monitoring of child's condition and to prevent complications.

Nursing Care after Seizure Episodes

1. Place the child in side-lying position to prevent aspiration in post-seizure phase.
2. Suction child's mouth and nose, if secretions present, to prevent aspiration.
3. Monitor child's vital signs and respiratory status including breath sounds, respiratory rate and depth, skin color, and pulse oximeter findings (SpO_2, heart rate) every few minutes until he or she regains consciousness. Measure child's BP and glucose level.
   i. Some children may have shallow ineffective breathing or may stop breathing in postictal phase. They require positioning to maintain patent airway, suctioning of secretions, oxygen administration or bag mask ventilation
   ii. Temperature readings will assist in identifying if the seizure is associated with fever (i.e., febrile seizures). Child with afebrile seizures often present with systemic hypertension and/or low blood sugar. Monitoring data will assist in investigations of origin of seizures
4. Ensure that the bed is in lowest position to prevent falls of disoriented child

5. Allow the child to take rest and sleep. Children are often tired or sleepy after seizures
6. Reassure and support the child and family members in simple language
7. Encourage questions and expression of feelings from child and family members regarding the seizure episode. Seizures are always frightening experience for both the child and those who witness the event
8. Dispose waste. Take care of reusable equipment and items
9. Perform hand hygiene and document the seizure episode in seizure record.

Evaluation and Documentation

- Evaluate child's health status after seizure episode and compare with baseline data. Evaluate child's and family member's understanding of seizure events and necessary precautions required to be followed for the event
- Document the seizure episodes on bedside seizure record, including date and time when seizure started, duration of seizures, description of seizure event (tonic or clonic or focal or multifocal or generalized) and presence of aura before seizure. Record the findings of vital signs assessment, color changes, presence of incontinence of urine and stool, postictal response, level of consciousness, presence of any injury, medications administered and nursing interventions provided for the child for seizures.

Communication and Teaching for Homecare

- Communicate with child and parents about the child's present health status, seizure episodes and plan of further management
- Teach the parents and the child in age appropriate language regarding precautions for seizures, use of medications, activity limitations, avoidance of swimming or alone in bathtub use, risk of injury during play, optimum rest and sleep, adequate diet and fluid intake, hygienic practices, routine care at hospital and at home after discharge, need for emergency medical help and plan of follow-up care.

PROCEDURE–32: CANCER CHEMOTHERAPY OF CHILDREN: ADMINISTRATION AND SAFE HANDLING

Clinical Guidelines

- Chemotherapeutic agents used to treat cancer patients are poisonous and pose risks to those who handle them, particularly pharmacist and nurses. The most important factor in reducing occupational exposure to antineoplastic agents is the use of appropriate protection during preparation and administration of these agent
- Antineoplastic agents kill cancer cells but also kill or injure normal cells that may consequently compromise patients comfort and safety due to related side effects or potential adverse effects. Bone marrow depression is common and potentially serious adverse effect leading to leukopenia and infections, thrombocytopenia, bleeding, and anemia. Other side effects include stomatitis, malnutrition, fluid electrolyte imbalance related to nausea, vomiting, hair loss, anxiety and depression, chemotherapy extravasation, drug allergy, etc.
- During chemotherapy to malignant children, nursing personnel are responsible for the prevention, early detection and prompt management of acute adverse reactions associated with cancer chemotherapy and to provide emotional support to the child and family
- Two chemotherapy-competent personnel should check the written directions and ensure that correct drug, dose, time, route, and patient are identified and relevant test results are noted. Ensure safe administration of correct type and dosage of antineoplastic agent
- All chemotherapy drugs doses are calculated independently by the physician, the pharmacist and the nurse. Counter

checking of calculations of drug doses must be done before administration. Verbal orders for chemotherapy administration are not acceptable

- Principles of pharmacological management must be followed for chemotherapy
- Strict sterile technique must be followed during preparation of chemotherapy medications
- IV access for chemotherapy administration should be completed with minimal trauma and repeated attempts must be avoided. An IV site for administration of chemotherapy should not be used if the site is more than 24 hours. If possible central line should be accessed and used for chemotherapy, especially for continuous infusion
- Optimal site for IV insertion for administration of chemotherapy include large healthy veins in the non-dominant arm (e.g., upper extremities, especially veins of the forearms). The dorsum of the hand, foot and antecubital fossa areas should not be used because of the increased risk for serious functional damage by infiltration of drugs
- IV insertion site should be visible, secured and stable at all times. Occlusive clear dressings are recommended for covering the site
- Venous integrity will be assessed before each administration of chemotherapy to validate blood return and adequate flow of medications. For chemotherapy by push-pull method, blood return will be assessed every 1–2 mL. For longer infusions, blood return should be assessed every hour
- Use of infusion pumps with high flow pressures are not recommended for peripheral IV line infusions
- "Chemotherapy Precautions" must be followed for the child who is receiving antineoplastic agents. Instructions must be given to the family members regarding these precautions those must also be practiced at home.

Equipment Required

- Hand hygiene supplies for prevention of transmission of microorganisms
- PPE (gloves, gown, face shield or goggles, face mask) for the nursing personnel both during chemotherapy preparation and administration
- Prescribed chemotherapy medications for the child
- IV access administration setup, connections, needles, syringes, IV filters
- Emergency medication tray with all necessary supplies and drugs
- Extra bed sheet, blanket and routine care supplies and equipment, as the child may not be able to move from the bed for long time
- Emesis basin, extra towel, mouth wash, mouth wipes, as required
- Waste disposal containers specific for chemotherapy as per BMW guidelines, including hard, plastic, puncture-resistant container that is disposable for any sharps, IV tubing, bags, bottles, needles, syringes that are contaminated
- Chemotherapy spill kit: Respirator mask, chemical splash goggles, non-permeable gown with cuffs and back closure, utility gloves, shoe cover, plastic scraper, disposable dustpan, disposable syringes, sharps container, plastic-backed absorbent towels, heavy-duty disposable bags, and hazardous label
- Chemotherapy documentation chart, child case sheet and treatment sheet.

Assessment and Preparation

- Assess child's vital signs, present health status, and signs of any chemotherapy complications. Assess the child's and family's level of understanding, anxiety, and readiness to learn and to accept the chemotherapy drugs. Determine the child's previous experience with chemotherapy, if any, and related side effects
- Self-preparation should be done with hand hygiene, use of PPE, and protective measures for prevention of hazards and occupational exposure of antineoplastic drugs, as per standard guidelines. Practice of strict sterile technique during preparation of chemotherapeutic agents and follow chemotherapy precautions

- Environment should be clean, calm, well-lighted and well-ventilated
- All necessary supplies and equipment should be arranged near the child at bedside or in treatment room, as per institutional policy
- Preparation of parent: Explain the effects of chemotherapy, its route, frequency, length of treatment, anticipated and possible adverse effects. Discuss about parent's role for prevention and management of adverse effects of chemotherapy. Obtain informed written consent from parent or legal guardian. Allow one parent with the child, as per unit policy
- Preparation of child: Explain the procedure of administration of chemotherapy in age-appropriate simple language. Make the child clean and comfortable. Administer antiemetic drug, as prescribed, before initiating chemotherapy. Play materials can be provided for distraction and to cope with stressful situation. Ask for cooperation.

Performing the Steps of Procedure with Rationale/Point of Emphasis

Administering Antineoplastic Chemotherapy to the Children

1. Verify the prescriber's/physician's direction for appropriateness of the antineoplastic drugs, its dose, diluent, route, frequency, and duration of treatment. This helps to ascertain that the child is receiving correct treatment course.
2. Calculate the amount of medications the child should receive. Recalculate the dose as prescribed by BSA or mg/kg and check against child's BSA or mg/kg. Verify that findings are consistent with the prescriber's directions, dosage limits and pharmacy preparation. Verify findings with second person (nurse, physician, or pharmacist) to ensure accuracy of medication administration.
3. Verify identification of the child before administration of chemotherapeutic agents.
4. Ensure informed written consent has been obtained from parents as legal approach.
5. Ensure that chemotherapy was prepared in biologically safe cabinet or hood in strict sterile technique. Healthcare provider should wear protective face shield/goggles, gown and gloves to prevent inhalation of drugs or direct skin contact or direct eye contact. This reduces the risk of inadvertent ingestion and contact with skin or eyes.
6. Ensure that the chemotherapy is in a sealed container or bag. This decreases risk of contamination to personnel or environment in case of accidental dropping.
7. Before administering the chemotherapy to the child, check the label of medication to become sure that correct solution is ready to administer. This decreases risk of error in administering wrong medication.
8. Perform hand hygiene and gather all necessary supplies for emergency and extravasation. This promotes efficient time management and provides organized approach.
9. Assess vital signs for baseline data, as chemotherapeutic agents may cause febrile or anaphylactic reactions. Child must be monitored for signs of adverse reactions throughout the period of administration of chemotherapy.
10. Perform hand hygiene and don all protective apparel including gloves. This reduces transmission of microorganisms and decreases risk for occupational exposure to cytotoxic agents.
11. Administer the medications using one of the following techniques:
    - ***Two-syringe method*** for IV bolus: Use one syringe to inject chemotherapeutic agent and other syringe to check for blood return and IV patency. Drug bolus should be completed in 3 minutes or less and blood return should be checked after every 1–2 mL of administered drug. Use the push-pull technique to administer a vesicant to the child. Push a very small amount, pull back on the plunger to obtain a

blood return and then push a small amount again. Continue until the total amount has been administered. Blood return is assessed every 1–2 mL. Slow IV push allows for continuous observation and immediate intervention, if required

- ***Side-Port boluses*** for peripheral IV sites: Prime the primary IV line with normal saline or with the same solution the chemotherapy has been mixed in. Prime the secondary line with antineoplastic agent, letting the vesicant run through the tubing and into gauze pad that is in a plastic bag. Dispose the gauze and the bag after the line is primed. Attach the secondary line into a side port of the primary line to allow free-flowing infusion of the chemotherapeutic agent. This method is used for medication that must be administered over a longer period of time than the medication that can be given via two syringe method
- ***Infusion pumps:*** Prime the primary IV line with normal saline or the same solution the chemotherapy has been mixed in. Prime the secondary line with the antineoplastic agent, letting the vesicant run through the tubing and into gauze pad that is in a plastic bag. Dispose the gauze and the bag after the line is primed. Attach the secondary line into a side port of the primary line and attach to a separate infusion pump, infusing at a rate consistent with the prescriber's direction. Access the central venous site as per institutional policy.
- Infusion pumps with high flow pressures can increase the risk of injury and are not recommended for peripheral line infusions. For pediatric patients, all chemotherapy should be given using a volumetric pump.

12. Administer chemotherapy agents through a central line, if possible, especially if it requires continuous infusion.
13. Assess the IV site. Gently drawback blood before starting to administer the drug through the tubing or a syringe. This helps to evaluate integrity of the IV line by validating presence of blood return and proper flow. Never test the line with the cytotoxic agent.
14. Administer chemotherapy by the prescribed route over the prescribed time frame. This helps to maintain safety and decreases risk for some side effects, especially anaphylaxis with some medications.
15. Monitor the child continuously for vital signs and for potential side effects during administration of chemotherapy. This ensures early identification of problems and for prompt initiation of management. Nurses are responsible for prevention, early detection and management of acute reactions of chemotherapy, such as hypersensitivity, anaphylaxis, hypotension, extravasation and nausea and vomiting.
16. Assess the effectiveness of measures used to control nausea and vomiting. Antiemetics should be administered before initiation of emetogenic chemotherapy and continued at regular intervals, as prescribed.
17. During chemotherapy administration, use measures to relax and comfort the child, such as minimizing stimuli from noises, light and bad odor.
18. On completion of administration of chemotherapy, flush the tubing, and IV line with normal saline or same solution that chemotherapy has been mixed in. This avoids substance incompatibility.
19. Remove and dispose IV tubing and medication solution bag, after the chemotherapy has been administered. Put contaminated items in a container that is puncture resistant and mark as "*Chemotherapy disposal only*". Seal the container and follow institution's policy for disposal of hazardous substances. The discarded items should include needles, syringes, IV tubing, discarded medicine bags, bottles, and gloves, and face shields/goggles. This reduces transmission of

microbial and antineoplastic agents and prevents cross contamination to others.

20. Dispose all materials those have come into contact with a cytotoxic drugs by placing the materials into a waste container designated for cytotoxic waste.
21. If any spills occur, follow institutional policy and guidelines for managing cytotoxic spills. A large spill is one in which more than 5 mL of a chemotherapy agent is released (e.g., breaking of glass bottle of chemotherapy drugs). Large spills must be cleaned up using chemotherapy spill kit. A small spillage is one in which less than 5 mL of chemotherapeutic agent is released due to disconnection or dislodgement of tubing. Small spills may be cleaned up using absorbent gauze by gloved hand. Remember, prevention of spills should be practiced with precautions, as it is easier than management of spills.
22. Remove gloves and perform hand hygiene to reduce transmission of microorganisms and contamination with antineoplastic agents. If there is any contact of skin with chemotherapeutic agent, then wash the area vigorously with soap and warm water to prevent skin reactions and irritation.
23. Place the child on chemotherapy precautions for 48 hours after the last dose of chemotherapy was administered. Any secretion from the child is considered contaminated with the chemotherapeutic agent. Universal precautions must be followed to decrease exposure by all caregivers to any secretions of the diseased child.
    It is assumed that anything that is soiled with bodily secretions of the child is contaminated with the chemotherapeutic agent. Thus taking precautions in decreasing exposure to the chemotherapeutic agent decreases the risk for contaminating others with the agent. Comply with confidentiality rules to implement strategy to alert other personnel that the child has received chemotherapy.
24. Evaluate child's present health condition, vital signs, and feature of complications
25. Document the procedure of administration of chemotherapy and assessment findings of child's health status.

Safe Handling of Chemotherapeutic Agents and Equipment

1. Use ***personal protective equipment (PPE).*** It is one of the best ways for nurses to prevent occupational exposure to chemotherapy agents.
   i. ***Gowns*** should be disposable, made of low-permeable fabric with closed front, long sleeves, and tight-fitting cuffs. Laboratory coats and cloths or patient gowns are not considered as PPE
   ii. ***Gloves*** should be disposable, powder-free, nonlatex, at least 0.007 inches thick with long cuffs. Some acceptable products are nitrile, polyurethane, or neoprene. Latex gloves should be used with caution because of latex sensitivities
   iii. ***Respirators and face masks*** must be worn for preparation and administration of antineoplastic drugs and when cleaning cytotoxic spills
   iv. ***Face shields or goggles*** should be used for protection from splashing or eye exposure. Splashing can occur when child vomits, spits, or struggles, when being given oral cytotoxic medication.
2. Ensure use of laminar airflow, eliminate exhaust with HEPA filter and have continuously running blower to decrease exposure to cytotoxic agents during preparation chemotherapy medications. Chemotherapy medication preparation and storage must be done with all precautions to prevent occupational exposure.
3. Prevent accidental ingestion of cytotoxic agents. It is prohibited to eat, drink, smoke, chew gum, apply cosmetics or store food in areas where chemotherapy is prepared or administered.
4. Use strict aseptic technique in preparation and administration of chemotherapy.

Chemotherapy Precautions

1. Wear gloves when handling diapers, urinals, emesis basin, soiled cloths, and bed linens.
2. Carry soiled items away from body or place them in a pillowcase or bag for transport.
3. Prelaunder contaminated linens before washing them with other cloths.
4. Label any linen that is soiled with the child's bodily secretions, as needing chemotherapy precautions when handled.
5. Label all specimens sent to laboratory, as being from a child undergoing chemotherapy.
6. Instruct the child to flush the toilet twice after each use, with the lid down.
7. Protect mattress and pillowcases using easily washable materials.
8. Wash reusable items such as emesis basin every day with soap and water. Wear gloves while completing this task. Always wash hand after removal of gloves.

Evaluation and Documentation

- Evaluate the child's response to chemotherapy, including presence of side effects. Evaluate child's and family understanding of chemotherapy regimen, medication side effects and effectiveness of measures to manage, and prevent side effects
- Document the date and time of chemotherapy, type of medication administered and its dose and diluent used. Record the site of administration of chemotherapy, precautions followed and appearance of IV access site, presence/absence of adverse effects, measures used to manage side effects, and child's tolerance of chemotherapy. Keep record of teaching completed with family and/or child and about family participation to provide comfort to the child during chemotherapy.

Communication and Teaching for Homecare

- Communicate with child and parents about child's present health status, possible side effects and further plan of treatment with discharge planning
- Teach the parents and child (as age-appropriate) about following:
  - To follow the discharge advice as prescribed by the physician/healthcare prescriber
  - Measures to prevent infections, e.g., good hand hygiene techniques, avoiding crowds, practicing general cleanliness and hygienic measures and oral hygiene
  - Clinical features of any infections (such as fever or chill, sore mouth, stomatitis)
  - Complications and side effects such as nausea, vomiting, loss of appetite, refusal to eat, diarrhea, and nose bleeds, excessive bruising, tarry stools, hair loss, etc.
  - To avoid use of aspirin or aspirin-containing products
  - Use of oral antifungal suspension to control fungal infections, as prescribed
  - To eat six small meals a day and to avoid hot and spicy food
  - To avoid extreme temperature, chemical treatments of hair, rectal suppositories and any kind of rectal manipulation
  - To minimize sun exposure and to use sunscreen
  - To consider that any secretions, blood, urine, emesis and stool of affected child are contaminated for 48 hours after last dose of chemotherapy that was administered
  - Safe handling of the chemotherapeutic agents must be done
  - To contact healthcare providers, if the child is having side effects and complications
  - Schedule date and time for next chemotherapy and follow-up visits
  - Keep contact with community health workers (ASHA, ANM, CHO), whenever needed.

PROCEDURE–33: TRANSITION MANAGEMENT: DISCHARGING AND TRANSFERRING THE CHILD

Clinical Guidelines

- Discharge planning should be initiated from the day of hospitalization of the child. Early discharge from healthcare facility is always expected after full course of treatment schedule without any complications
- Hospitalization is a stressful experience for both the child and parents. It disturbs family routines, relationship, and coping with financial constraints
- Before discharge from health care facility, ensure continuity of treatment of the child and supportive care at home along with follow-up visits
- Predischarge evaluation of home condition should be done to create continuity of therapeutic management between inpatient care and outpatient care. This will help to trouble-shoot problems in home environment those may interfere with child's continued care at home
- Child should always be discharged from hospital/health facility with parent or legal guardian with full signature including date and time and noting the relationship with child
- Transferring the child to another facility may required for better treatment facility depending upon the child's diagnosis and health condition, family preference and available resources. Standard guidelines should be followed to promote optimal outcome following transfer. Identification of indications of transfer must be done judiciously. Suitable transportation, preparation, and organization of transport, stabilization before transfer, communication, counseling, enroute care, and documentation are important aspects of referral or transferring the child to another facility
- Family members may want to take the child from the health care facility "Against Medical Advice (AMA)" or "Leave Against Medical Advice (LAMA)" before planned discharge for various reasons. Releasing the child against medical advice must be done with specific institutional guidelines to safeguard the child. Healthcare provider/prescriber should discuss the situation with the family with alternative solutions. Releasing the child in AMA may cause harm and even death of the child. It can be considered as medical neglect. Child protective social services may help the family to prevent the event to protect the child from harmful outcome. Parents or legal guardian can take the child home as "Discharge On Risk Bond (DORB)" according to the institutional/health care facility policy.

Equipment Required

- Child's case sheet with all documents of investigations and treatment
- Discharge certificate with medication prescriptions, as appropriate
- Written instructions for home care and follow-up visit appointments
- Carry bag for child's personal belongings
- Referral note and transport vehicle for transferring the child to another facility
- For transferring a critically ill child to another unit or healthcare facility the following additional equipment are needed – pulse oximeter, cardiac monitor, BP monitor, oxygen tank and tubing with delivery system, bag-valve mask device for ventilation support (whenever required and trained personnel are accompanying), emergency medications, and basic care supplies and equipment.

Assessment and Preparation for Planned Discharge of the Hospitalized Child

1. Begin discharge planning from the date of child's admission and continue the process throughout the period of hospitalization. This facilitates smooth transition of child to home and prepares the family members for continued care at home.

2. Collaborate with the healthcare prescriber/physician/surgeon and other multidisciplinary team members and parents in planning of discharge. This provides comprehensive approach to discharge needs, existing barriers and available resources.
3. Identify the child's primary caregivers in home setting. This helps to select appropriate individuals for teaching to continue care at home after discharge.
4. Assess the family's knowledge regarding the child's illness, possible complications, and treatment and care to be continued at home after discharge from hospital.
5. Assess the family's emotional preparedness for discharge to promote coping skills.
6. Monitor the parent's readiness and willingness to learn home care of the child. Provide ongoing teaching regularly and allow repeated opportunities to practice new skills. This reinforces parent's competence and decreases anxiety.
7. Assess child's self care ability and teach accordingly for continued care at home.
8. Review care and procedures that will need to be performed at home. Provide demonstrations and written instructions to parents and older child (age-appropriate) for those care and procedures. Evaluate parents and older child understanding and arrange for return demonstrations. If parents are unable to perform at safe level, then arrange for alternative caregivers (e.g., other family members). This ensures successful care of the diseased child at home with better outcome and recovery.
9. Provide information about available community healthcare resources (ASHA, ANM, CHO) and social support to help in continuity of care of the child.
10. Inform parents about anticipated date and time of discharge as soon as it is known. This allows the parent and family members to make necessary arrangements and helps to prevent last-minute delay.
11. Arrange for transportation, as per hospital policy, or instruct the parents to do it.
12. Teach parents about safety measures during transport and en-route care for the sick recovered child.

Performing the Steps of Procedure with Rationale/Point of Emphasis

Planned Discharge of a Child from Health Facility

1. Review healthcare prescriber's/physician's discharge certificate with order/advice for medications, treatment, and continued care at home. This helps as safeguard to double-check the accuracy of discharge orders/advices and to provide final discharge advice and necessary teaching with answering of questions.
2. Instruct the parents about prescribed medications, including the proper dose, route, time schedule and possible adverse reactions. This promotes proper drug administration.
3. Review the care and procedures that will need to be performed at home by the parents or the child, as appropriate. Provide demonstration and written instructions. Evaluate parent's understanding and ability to perform care of the child at home.
4. Discuss dietary or activity restrictions that are applicable for the child. Provide written instructions and answer to the questions as asked.
5. Ensure that the family will have all supplies what they need to provide ongoing care to the child at home. Confirm the arrangements for appropriate vendor or agency.
6. Instruct the parent regarding follow-up appointments and outpatients' procedures that are required. Provide written instructions with date, time, and place of follow-up visits. This promotes continuity of care after discharge.
7. Confirm transportation arrangements with the family. Inform about available social services, which can be utilized by the parent for transport to prevent unnecessary delay in discharge procedure.

8. Verify about the clearance from financial and official department. Instruct and refer the family members from getting clearance related to hospitalization.
9. Perform final physical assessment of the child before discharge. Notify any abnormal findings to the physician/healthcare prescriber. This may change in the discharge plan.
10. Gather child's all personal belongings which will be carried to home.
11. Collect hospital supplies and property separately. Make every effort to prevent hospital property from being removed with the child's belongings.
12. Allow the parent to dress up the child with separate personal clothing for transition to home during transport.
13. Obtain parent's signatures on the discharge instruction sheet and in hospital record. Instruct to bring the discharge certificate for next follow-up appointment of the child.
14. Answer to any final questions of the parents/child before leaving the hospital/healthcare facility. This ensures understanding of home care responsibilities for compliance with therapeutic regimen.
15. Follow facility policy for checking identification of the parents or legal guardian before releasing the child into their care. This is required as security safeguard.
16. Once the child and his or her family received discharge certificate, prescriptions, belongings and all discharge instructions, escort them to the lobby, either by walking or in a wheelchair. This ensures safety while exiting the hospital/healthcare facility.
17. Remind the parent about safety during transport and restraints system, if needed.
18. Complete discharge summary of the child in hospital record. Document child's physical conditions at discharge and care given to the child.
19. Once the child has left the patient care area, notify the housekeeping staff and arrange for the cleaning of the bed and room. This facilitates timely preparation of the bed and the room for the new patient.
20. Take care of all reusable items. Discard all waste. Reset the patient care area and bed for next patient. Perform hand hygiene.

Transferring a Child to Another Facility

1. Determine the need for transfer of the sick child to another facility with the attending healthcare prescriber/physician and the family, based on child's condition, availability of required treatment, resources at other facilities and the family's preference of the available options. This allows for most appropriate placement for treatment of the child
2. In collaboration with the receiving agency or facility to which the child will be transferred, determine the most appropriate mode of transport based on the child's physical condition. This ensures appropriate level of monitoring for the child to detect potential complications during transport
3. Select and arrange the mode of transport based on the urgency of the medical condition. A stable child may be transferred by car or van. A child requiring more intense physical monitoring must be transported in an ambulance. A long-distance emergency transfer may require air transport. Ensure that appropriate transportation is arranged in advance
4. Obtain transfer orders that identify the receiving facility and receiving healthcare prescriber. Identify healthcare provider who will be assuming legal responsibility for the child's care
5. Explain to the child (as appropriate) and the family about the purpose of transfer, risks, and benefits of transfer, name and location of receiving facility and how and when the transfer will take place. Provide the map, telephone number, and contact name of the new facility to the family members. This minimizes family's stress and anxiety. Family may arrange advance enquiry about the receiving facility

6. Obtain written informed consent from the parent or legal guardian for the transfer. If consent is not available, then both the indications for transfer and reason for not obtaining consent should be documented in the medical record
7. Obtain parent's or legal guardian's signature in the medical record and in transfer note
8. Prepare referral note or summary for the receiving facility with all necessary information to determine needed medications, therapies, nursing care and services. Standard referral note or summary format should be followed. This facilitates continuity of treatment and nursing care and assists in smooth transition care of the child in new facility.
   i. Some documents may need to be send before the child's departure to ensure new facility has full understanding of child's health status. Referral note is very useful document
   ii. The original medical records from transferring facility may not be allowed to send to the receiving facility, as institutional policy may not permit this
9. Perform physical assessment of the child prior to transfer and notify presence of any abnormal findings to the healthcare prescriber/physician. This may warrant a change in the transfer plan
10. Stabilize the severely ill child before transferring out to other facility, as the child's condition may deteriorate during transport
11. Explain enroute care of the child to the parents and accompanying person, as required. Ensure all facilities are available for enroute care during transfer in transport system
12. Ensure that all documentation in the child's medical record and case sheet is complete and accurate. This allows receiving facility to continue child's management accurately
13. Gather child's personal belonging and ensure that the child is transferred with all appropriate own belongings
14. Make every effort to prevent hospital property from being removed with the child's belongings to control hospital costs and financial loss
15. Have the parent assist the child to dress in personal clothing or street clothes for transfer
16. When transporter and vehicle arrives, check child's identification and obtain transporter's signature. This facilitates safe and legally appropriate transfer
17. When the child left the patient care area, notify housekeeping staff and arrange for cleaning of bed, surrounding area and room. This helps in timely preparation of bed and room for new patient
18. Check completion of all records related to transferring of the child to another facility
19. Take care of all reusable items. Discard all waste. Reset the patient care area and bed for next patient. Perform hand hygiene.

Releasing a Child against Medical Advice

1. If a parent expresses a desire to take the child from the hospital or healthcare facility before planned discharge, then notify the attending healthcare prescriber/physician immediately. Discuss the situation with the family to safeguard the child. Implement institution-specific guidelines.
   This gives an opportunity to explain the risks of leaving hospital against medical advice and advantages of continued hospitalization. Healthcare prescriber can give alternatives such as transfer to another facility or outpatient treatment.
2. If the parent persists in the decision to take the child from hospital against medical advice, then ask him or her to do signature in the presence of a witness on the AMA form. Preserve the signed AMA form in the medical record of the child. This provides legal verification of parent's informed choice to leave the facility with their child.
3. If the parent refuses to sign on AMA form, then note the parent's decision on the AMA form along with date, time,

and circumstances of refusal and name of person who refused to sign. Obtain the signature of a witness and file up the form in child's medical record with signature. It ensures legal documentation.

4. Perform documentation and send for review of quality management department.
5. Document a summary of the event in the child's chart/case sheet and preserve in child's permanent medical record.
6. Complete the AMA discharge procedure, as per hospital policy and as permitted by the parent to facilitate smooth transition of the child to home.
7. When the child left the patient care area, notify housekeeping staff and arrange for cleaning of bed, surrounding area and room. This helps in timely preparation of bed and room for new patient.
8. Take care of all reusable items. Discard all waste. Reset the patient care area and bed for next patient. Perform hand hygiene.

Evaluation and Documentation

- Evaluate the child's on-admission health condition with on-discharge or on-transfer health condition to identify the effectiveness of treatment and care provided to the child
- Document the followings in the child's record:
  - Date and time of discharge/transfer
  - With whom the child was discharged or transferred
  - Child's physical condition and assessment findings at discharge or transfer
  - Instructions/advice given regarding child's care at home or during transport
  - In case of transfer to another facility, document the reason for transfer, method of transport, and name of accompanying person.

Communication and Teaching for Homecare or Continued Care

- Communicate with child and parents about health status of the child on discharge or on transfer and regarding continued care required at home or during transport. Answer to the questions and concerns of the family members and child, as age-appropriate
- Teach the parents about child's illness, drug therapy, diet, activity level, other treatments, follow-up appointments, possible complications, conditions requiring immediate notification of healthcare prescriber/physician, health promotion behavior, and preventive measure of childhood diseases.

PROCEDURE–34: IMMUNIZATIONS IN CHILDREN

Clinical Guidelines

- Immunization is the protection of individuals or groups from specific diseases by vaccination or by injection of immunoglobulins
- National Immunization Schedule is usually followed for the children for maximum coverage in rural and urban areas. It includes most common vaccine preventable childhood diseases. The schedule has description of name of vaccine, when to administer the vaccine (i.e. age of the infants and children), maximum age of administration of the particular vaccine, dose, diluent, route, and site of injectable vaccine
- Vaccine recommendations are continuously reviewed and updated with research findings for evidence-based information and state health department consultations
- Reconstitution of vaccines before administration should be done as per standard guidelines of manufacturers to maintain its effectiveness of the vaccines
- For infants, BCG immunization is given in intradermal route at left upper arm, Hepatitis-B vaccine (HBV) is given intramuscular at anterolateral aspect of left mid thigh, Oral Polio Vaccine (OPV) is given by mouth, Pentavalent vaccine (i.e., combination of five vaccines - DPT, HBV, HIB) is given in intramuscular

route at anterolateral aspect of left mid-thigh, Rotavirus vaccine is given in oral route, Pneumococcal conjugate vaccine (PCV) is given in intramuscular route at anterolateral aspect of right mid-thigh, inactivated polio vaccine (IPV) is given in intradermal route in right upper arm, Measles vaccine is given in subcutaneous route at right upper arm, and Japanese encephalitis (JE) vaccine is given in subcutaneous route at left upper arm

- For children DPT booster dose-1 and dose-2 are given intramuscular at anterolateral aspect of left mid-thigh, MMR vaccine is given in subcutaneous route as measles vaccine, and Tetanus toxoid (TT) is given in intramuscular at mid-thigh or at upper arm. Other vaccines to the children such as Measles vaccine 2nd dose, OPV booster dose, JE 2nd dose are given in same route as administer in infants *(Refer: Appendix – XII: National Immunization Schedule)*
- For institutional delivery, neonates should receive BCG vaccine, Hepatitis B vaccine, "Birth dose" and OPV "Zero Dose" at birth as early as possible, or before discharge from healthcare facility. Hepatitis vaccine should be given within 24 hours of birth
- High body temperature and severe illness are reasons to delay immunizations until the child has recovered from acute stage of the illness. Minor illness, such as cold, otitis media, and mild diarrhea without fever, are not contraindications to immunizations
- Redness and tenderness at the site of injection, and low-grade fever are the most common side effects of vaccinations to the children
- Because of potential risk for anaphylaxis and allergic reactions with administration of vaccines, though rare, any child receiving a vaccine should be observed for several minutes for signs of immediate allergic and anaphylactic reactions, after the vaccine is administered to the child
- Immediate emergency interventions should be provided when the child experiences respiratory distress or decreased respiratory effort, change in responsiveness and hives as anaphylactic reactions or generalized urticaria
- If any adverse events following immunization (AEFI) occurs after use of any vaccine vial, do not use that vial for other child, mark the vial and preserve safely for AEFI investigation
- Cold chain must be maintained for all vaccines in recommended temperature to ensure the efficacy and potency of the vaccines for successful immunization program
- Refer and follow principles of pharmacologic management during immunizations
- Follow "Ten Rights" for administration of medications to the children.

Equipment Required

- Hand hygiene supplies for hand wash and hand rub to prevent cross infections
- Vaccines as per immunization schedule
- Cold-chain maintenance equipment, vaccine carrier, and ice packs
- Supplies for intradermal, intramuscular (IM), and subcutaneous (SC) injections with auto disable (AD) single use syringes of different sizes (0.1 mL and 0.5 mL) and 5 mL syringe for reconstitution of vaccines and diluents (as provided by manufacturer)
- AEFI management kit
- Sterile cotton swabs in covered container
- Marker to write the date and time of reconstitution on the vaccine vial
- Play material or personal toys of the infant/child for distraction during vaccination
- Waste disposal containers as per BMW guidelines
- Child's Immunization Record and Mother Child Protection (MCP) card.

Assessment and Preparation

- Assess the child for presence of signs and symptoms of any illness, known allergies, history of previous vaccines, history of complications with vaccination and immunocompromised status. Assess

the child for eligibility of immunization as per schedule and for possible contra-indications
  - Assess parent's readiness to learn and the barriers that affect child care especially cultural beliefs and practices of immunizations
- Self-preparation should be done with hand hygiene and other standard precautions
- Environment should be clean, calm, well-lighted, and free of overcrowding
- Articles preparation should be done as required for the vaccinations, in clinics or neonatal/pediatric/postnatal units or in immunization camps. Aseptic techniques must be followed for injectable vaccines. Ensure availability of all sterile items
- Preparation of parents: Explain the immunization procedure, purpose of the vaccination, route of administration, care of the child after administration and possible side effects. Giving instructions before administration of vaccines allows the parent to dedicate his or her attention to comfort the child after administration of vaccines. Allow the parent to hold the child during administration of immunization. Obtain informed consent from the parent or legal guardian for vaccinations
- Preparation of child: Infant should be hold by the parent in comfortable position. Explain the procedure to the older child in age-appropriate simple language. Ask for cooperation. Make the child clean and comfortable. Distract the child with play materials. Allow the child to remain on parent lap during vaccinations.

Performing the Steps of Procedure with Rationale/Point of Emphasis

1. Review the vaccination information with the parent and with immunization card. Answer questions regarding the immunizations to be given. This prepares the parents to assist during vaccine administration and to comfort the child.
2. Encourage the apparent to comfort and hold the child during and after administration of immunization. This ensures that parent is active and provide positive role to the child.
3. Provide distractions and pain relief measures as per standard guidelines.
4. Perform hand hygiene to reduce transmission of microorganisms.
5. Assemble and prepare all necessary supplies for vaccinations in the procedure room for time management and organized approach.
6. Obtain vaccines and read the label to verify the instructions. Check the expiration date, if the date expired, then it should not be administered. This helps to decrease the chance of vaccination error by ensuring "right vaccine".
7. Ensure proper maintenance of "cold chain" for the vaccine using "vaccine vial monitor" (VVM). Check for VVM on the cap of the vial. This VVM indicates whether the dry vaccine is usable or not. Once reconstitution of vaccine is done, VVM is not required, as the vaccines has to be used within 4 hours and it should be discarded after that period.
8. Prepare the injectable vaccine before the child enters into the room to reduce fear of needle and anxiety of the child and parent. Follow aseptic technique to prevent contaminations. Prepare vaccine for individual child.
9. Don gloves for preparation and administration of injectable vaccine in indicated dose, route and site to elicit immune response, as per standard guidelines.
10. Reconstitution of vaccines need to be done by mixing with diluents provided by manufacturer for the particular batch of vaccine. It is done immediately before use and should be marked with date and time of reconstitution. Put the reconstituted vaccine vial in the foam pad of vaccine carrier to maintain cold-chain. Use the reconstituted vials only for a single session, do not carry them from one session to another session.
11. Administer oral vaccines before giving injectable vaccines. Assist the parent to

hold the child in cuddle position on his or her lap with the head supported and tilted slightly back. Vaccinator should stand in one side. Open the infant's mouth with gentle pressure on the cheeks using your thumb and index finger. Don't give firm pressure to cause discomfort and noncooperation by the infant. Do not touch dropper to infant's mouth.

12. Position the child for injectable vaccines to keep the child still and in comfort. Positioning depends on the age of the child, route of injections, and number of vaccines to be given and ability of the caregiver/parent. Parent/family member/ assistant should hold the child steady to prevent injury and discomfort.
13. Ensure that the selected site of injectable vaccination is clean. Use of antiseptic agents at vaccination site is not recommended.
14. For intradermal (ID) administration of vaccines (BCG, IPV), gently stretch and support the skin with thumb and forefinger. Hold the syringe and needle almost flat along the infant's skin and gently insert the needle into the top layer of the skin.
15. For IM and SC administration of vaccines follow the same guidelines for giving IM and SC medications (*Refer the Procedure - 12 of this Unit - 3 - Intramuscular and Subcutaneous Injections)*.
16. If the child requires multiple injections, administer the injections in different extremities. If multiple injections are needed to be given in same extremity, leave at least one inch gap between the injection sites. Attempt to give injections that have the greatest chance of local irritation in an extremity of the child without other injection (e.g., PCV).
    This allows for optimal absorption of vaccine and decreases irritation at sites of injection and reduces overlapping local reactions.
17. Apply cotton swab or small adhesive bandages to immunization sites, as needed, to help in stopping bleeding and to provide comfort measures to the child.
18. Dispose used supplies, syringe and needle and other waste in appropriate containers after decontamination as standard precautions for infection control. Perform hand hygiene.
19. Instruct the parent about the due date and time of next schedule immunizations to improve compliance with immunization schedule and to reinforce the need of vaccinations of the child.
20. Document the vaccines administer to the child in child's personal immunization card/MCP card/medical record and in clinic/unit/camp records/registers.

Evaluation and Documentation

- Evaluate child's response to vaccine administration. Note immediate reactions, presence of local irritation at injection sites, and presence of any symptoms indicating anaphylaxis
- Document the following: (a) Name of vaccine, route, dose, site, date and time of administration, (b) Presence or absence of any adverse reactions, (c) Type of vaccine, vaccine manufacturer and lot number of vaccine, (d) Name and signature of healthcare provider who had administered the vaccines.

Communication and Teaching for Homecare

- Communicate with the parents about child's health status and care at home after immunization. Answer to questions in simple conversation when asked by the parents or family members
- Teaching should be given before administration of vaccinations and feedback should be taken after immunization to ensure the understanding of information
  - Instruct parent about care of the child after immunizations: (a) For discomfort at injection site, apply a cool clean washcloth to injection sites for 24 hours, followed by warm compresses,

if required, (b) Acetaminophen may be administered, as needed, in case of fever and pain. Aspirin should be avoided for the children, and (c) Not to apply anything on the injection site

- Instruct the parent to contact health-care provider or seek medical care if the child experiences – body temperature higher than 40.6°C or 105°F, seizures, change in level of consciousness, collapse, or shock-like state
- Discuss with the parents about recommended immunization schedule necessary for infants and children and the rationale for vaccination, routes of immunizations, possible adverse reactions of vaccinations and about the immunizations required for school entry
- Explain what vaccine is given to the child and what disease it prevents.
- Remind the parent when and where to come or visit for next vaccinations
- Provide both verbal and written information about the vaccines to be administered
- Instruct about the importance of preservation of immunization card/record of the children for future reference.

UNIT 4

Child Health Nursing Procedures for Surgical Conditions

INTRODUCTION

Surgical interventions in children are different than that of adults. It is always a potentially stressful experience for the children and family members. Potential threats for surgical operations for the children are physical harm, injury, fear of death, pain and discomfort, separation from parents and family, strange and unknown environment in the operating room (OR), fear of anesthesia and surgical interventions and postoperative problems.

Special attention must be given on emotional support, continuous monitoring for early detection of complications with preventive measures and standard precautions for infection control. Related teaching to the child and family members based on their level of understanding to prevent problems associated with the surgery should be emphasized.

Preparation of children for surgery and preoperative care should be based on child's age and developmental stage, personality level and past experience of surgery and hospitalization. It should be initiated from the planning of hospitalization for surgery. For the "day care surgery", preoperative care should be provided according to the type of surgery required for the child. In case of emergency surgical procedures, preoperative care should be modified according to the situation but the basic approach must be same as planned surgery.

Postoperative care must include physical care and psychological support along with related teaching to prevent complications. Immediate postoperative care can be arranged in the recovery room or in the post-anesthesia room or in the pediatric ward. Care after recovery from anesthesia usually organized in the pediatric surgical ward/unit for postsurgery care of the child including all routine care. Parents are allowed as per institutional policy. Teaching should be provided as incidental teaching and planned teaching for continuation of postoperative care at home after discharge from hospital or any health facility.

PROCEDURE–1: PREOPERATIVE CARE OF CHILDREN

Clinical Guidelines

- Extent of preoperative care depends upon type of surgery, i.e., planned elective surgery or emergency surgery or day care surgery. For elective and planned surgery all preoperative care can be performed systematically, but in emergency surgery priority interventions only can be performed depending upon the availability of time and facility
- Preoperative care must include complete preoperative assessment and presurgical checkup of the child. Preoperative fasting instructions and preoperative teaching to the child and parents according to their level of understanding are also very significant
- Preoperative preparation of the child should be done with psychological preparation, physical preparation and following protective measures for surgical interventions
- Informed surgical consent must be signed by the parent. Detailed explanation of the surgical procedure is very important for medicolegal aspect

- Family members of the children also need emotional support, explanation and teaching during preoperative phase of surgery to cope with situation and to obtain necessary cooperation from them. They usually help their children to adapt with the stressful condition and provide basic care according to their ability.

Equipment Required

- Hand hygiene supplies for hand washing and antiseptic hand rub
- Identification band for the child
- Surgical clothing for the child to dress up
- Stethoscope, thermometer, blood pressure monitor, pulse oximeter and other necessary articles and items to assess vital signs of the child
- Weighing scale to measure body weight before the surgical intervention
- Stadiometer or tape measure to measure the body height of the child
- Articles for administration of preoperative medications both intravenous (IV) and intramuscular (IM)
- Articles for IV cannulation and fluid therapy, as prescribed
- Child's case sheet with "Consent form" for legal guardian's signature
- "Preoperative Checklist" to counter check the preparation for surgery
- Documentation sheet and child case sheet
- Waste disposal containers as per bio-medical waste (BMW) rules.

Assessment and Preparation

- Assess child for present health condition, vital signs, body weight, developmental stage and level of cognitive function especially related to surgery
- Assess anxiety and level for understanding of child and parent to provide necessary support accordingly to promote coping in surgical interventions
- Assess ability of the child and parents for performance of postoperative self-care measures to plan for further management
- Self-preparation should be done with standard precautions, as needed
- Environment should be clean, calm, quite, well lighted and well ventilated
- All necessary items and supplies should be collected near the child
- Preparation of parents: Explain the purpose of surgery and possible post-operative complications. Allow parent to accompany the child to surgical waiting area. Encourage parents to ask questions and express their concern for the surgery
- Preparation of child: Prepare the child psychologically and physically, as required for the surgery. Explain the procedure to the child as per understanding level and age. Ask parent to interpret child's behavior and to assist the child to cope with the situation.

Performing the Steps of Procedure with Rationale/Point of Emphasis

1. Verify identification of the child with two identifiers. Check name, medical record number, sex, date of birth/age and parent's/legal guardian's name.
2. Confirm the type, site and laterality of the surgical procedure that to be done, with the parent and child, as appropriate.
3. Ensure the consent form is completed, signed and attached with child's case sheet.
4. Prepare the child and parent psychologically for the surgery, according to their level of understanding to promote cooperation and to reduce fear, anxiety, and negative reactions. Discuss about type of surgery, preoperative interventions, limitation of diet, OR environment, presence of surgical team members, type of anesthesia and possible postoperative interventions and problems.
5. Assess child's history of illness with special emphasis on previous OR experience and anesthesia, pain experience, allergic reactions and risk conditions.
6. Check the laboratory reports, identify abnormalities and inform to the surgery team.
7. Obtain baseline pertinent physical examination data. Check vital signs, current

body weight, height and elimination pattern (urine and stool). Identify any unusual trends or values beyond the normal range and inform to the surgery team immediately.

8. Provide preoperative teaching to the child and parents. Teach the child and parents about coughing and deep breathing mobility/exercises and other self-care measures, as possible. Instruct the child/parents regarding postoperative oxygen therapy, fluid therapy, tubes and drains. Describe about pain, discomfort, positioning, nausea, vomiting, temperature variations and any other anticipated problems related to the surgery.
9. Keep the child NPO as prescribed for preoperative fasting instructions.
10. Comply with facility standards for skin preparation by cleaning, bathing and shaving of operative area to reduce the risk of infections.
11. Dress the child for OR as per institutional policy.
12. Remove foreign objects (such as jewelry, hair pins) and prosthesis (such as eye glasses, lenses, orthodontic appliances and nail polish from fingers and toes) before sending the child and transporting to the OR
13. Examine child's mouth and search for potentially loose teeth. If identified, report to the OR nurse and anesthetist.
14. Encourage the child to void before transport to OR and before surgery, if possible.
15. Administer prescribed medications as per instructions before transport to the OR
16. Maintain fluid and nutrition balance with intravascular support, as prescribed
17. Accompany with the child to the OR and allow parents in OR waiting place.
18. Handover the child to the OR Nurse with detail information and records.
19. Keep record of preoperative preparation and care given to the child in child's case sheet and in hospital/facility record.
20. Report to the unit in-charge and surgical team about the preparation and care given the child along with any untoward events.

Evaluation and Documentation

- Evaluate child's and parent's understanding of surgical event, preoperative care, and postoperative care. Evaluate child's health status including vital signs, respiratory and neurologic status, mobility, and self-care ability. Compare with previous findings
- Document child's vital signs, body weight, height, NPO status and time of last food intake, allergy status, findings of history collection and physical examination, dental condition, removal of foreign objects, preoperative medications, fluid therapy, elimination patterns and operative site preparation.

Communication and Teaching for Homecare

- Communicate with child and family members about details of preoperative care, surgical procedure and postoperative care. Encourage to verbalize fears and anxiety
- Teach the child and parents about care of surgical site/wound, hygienic practices, hand washing, dietary limitations, medications and postoperative self-care measures. Instruct about continuation of postoperative care at home and time limit for restrictions of day to day activities. Inform about possible complications and danger signs which require medical attention and about importance of follow-up visits after discharge from the health facility.

PROCEDURE–2: POSTANESTHESIA AND POSTOPERATIVE CARE OF CHILDREN

Clinical Guidelines

- Postoperative care is provided as immediate care after surgical interventions or postanesthesia care and care after recovery from anesthesia. It may vary depending upon the type of surgery, i.e., major or minor surgery. Cardiac surgery, neurologic surgery and major abdominal surgery may require intensive care. Day care surgery can be even managed at home with appropriate instructions. Some surgical procedures may not need general anesthesia, so postoperative care for them may be planned in different ways. But overall purpose of postoperative care should be same for all surgery toward speedy recovery and prevention of complications

- Safety of the child during postanesthesia period is very important to prevent immediate complications. Use of sedation or restraints to restrict movement and to keep IV lines or tubes or drains in place should be emphasized. After recovery from anesthesia effects, child requires supportive and definitive care for recovery from consequences of surgical interventions and to restore normal activities and lifestyle
- Parents should be allowed in the postoperative period to provide support to the child and to reduce child's separation anxiety. They can provide basic care to the child as permitted by institutional policy, depending upon the child's health condition. Parents need necessary instructions and teaching to participate in postoperative care and thereafter. Both physical care and emotional care with necessary support should be ensured for the child with the help of the parents and family members
- Infection control measures must be followed along with standard precautions to prevent surgical site infections, postoperative respiratory infections, urinary tract infections and other infections to promote early discharge from hospital or health facility.

Equipment Required

- Hand hygiene supplies for hand washing, antiseptic hand rub and personal protective equipment (PPE) as needed
- Postoperative pediatric bed with all required articles and equipment
- Blanket, clothing and extra bedsheet to warm the child, if required
- Stethoscope, thermometer, blood pressure monitor, pulse oximeter, cardiopulmonary monitor and other necessary articles and items to assess vital signs of the child
- Articles for oxygen therapy and fluid therapy, as needed
- Articles for oral care and suction apparatus to remove secretions
- Emergency medications tray with syringes, needles, medications and other supplies
- Bedpan, urinal, cotton balls, diaper for young child
- Waste disposal containers as per BMW rules
- Postoperative monitoring record sheet and child case sheet.

Assessment and Preparation

- Assess the child's vital signs, effects of anesthesia and medications, blood loss, fluid and blood replacement in OR, procedural information and complications. Assess child for developmental stage and level of cognitive functioning. Explore parents' understanding and anxiety level for appropriate support
- Self-preparation should be done with maintenance of standard precautions
- Environment should be clean, calm, quite, well lighted and well ventilated
- All necessary articles and equipment should be arranged near postoperative bed
- Preparation of parents: Explain about the operative procedure and required postoperative care in simple local language. Answer to their questions on related issue
- Preparation of child: Receive the child from OR with all related information about the surgery, immediate postoperative attention and plan for further management.

Performing the Steps of Procedure with Rationale/Point of Emphasis

Immediate Care during Postanesthesia Recovery Period

1. Perform hand hygiene and ensure postoperative bed is ready to receive the child and other requirements are available

at bedside for easy access and prompt interventions.

2. Assess vital signs of the child quickly to evaluate the side effects of anesthesia and signs of impending shock or respiratory compromise. Connect all monitors and note the display. Compare all findings with preoperative baseline data
3. Assess airway clearance, cyanosis, pallor, level of consciousness, neurologic status, breath sounds, bowel sounds, bladder functioning or distention, status of IV lines, drains, tubes, skin integrity, pain status, positioning, presence of bleeding and condition of incision dressing. Frequency of these assessments should be done on the basis of child's surgical interventions and health condition. Compare all findings with baseline data.
4. Provide warming measures to the child to reduce postoperative shivering and hypothermia, whenever required.
5. Assess child and parents for fear, anxiety, level of knowledge and understanding with ability of postoperative self-care measures to provide necessary support and teaching.
6. Maintain adequate respiration function and provide support as required with clearance of airway by suctioning, oxygen therapy, coughing and deep breathing mobility (as indicated), chest physiotherapy, and incentive Spirometry, as required. Monitor breath sounds, oxygen saturation and blood gas, as applicable.
7. Maintain adequate intake, output and electrolyte balance by fluid therapy, as prescribed. Monitor IV infusion flow rate. Check nasogastric tube (if any) and follow the instructions for aspiration. Check the drainage tube (if present) and connect with bag for continuous drainage. Monitor signs and symptoms of fluid and electrolyte imbalance, all outputs (from tubes, drains, vomiting and other body fluids), and laboratory values of electrolytes assessment.
8. Keep the child NPO till complete awake or recover from anesthesia effect. Initiate diet from sips of clear fluids to full liquids to solid foods gradually, as indicated.
9. Restrain the child, whenever needed, to prevent dislodging of IV channel, drains, tubes and dressing. Monitor discomfort, restlessness and pain perception of the child.
10. Maintain neurologic status because medications, electrolyte and metabolic changes, pain and emotional factors can influence the level of consciousness. Monitor level of consciousness, color of extremities, skin temperature, capillary refill test (CRT), sensation, pain perception, restlessness and mobility. Change the child's position every 2 hours, as indicated and maintain patency and integrity of drainage systems.
11. Maintain urinary output because anesthetic agents may temporarily depress bladder tone and response. Accurate recording of intake and output helps to assess renal and circulatory functions. Monitor intake and output every 8 hours and notify if output is less than normal amount. Assess retention or incontinence of urine and catheterize as indicated. Provide perineal care and catheter care as per schedule.
12. Maintain normal bowel elimination as anesthetic agents may depress peristalsis and normal gastrointestinal (GI) function. Assess bowel sound, note signs and symptoms of abdominal distension, nausea, vomiting, abdominal pain, flatus and bowel movements. Compare with baseline pattern and inform the abnormalities.
13. Prevent infections of the surgical site and other systems. Maintain surgical site dressing integrity and patency of drainage systems, as required. Consult with surgeon regarding first dressing change and care of tubes and drains. Use sterile dressing technique in postoperative period. Maintain general cleanliness and hygienic practices including hand hygiene during

care. Assess clinical features of infections, redness, swelling, fever, increased pain and abnormal drainage or discharge.

14. Promote comfort and minimize pain sensation by non-pharmacological measures and medications, as prescribed. Change position and allow movements to relieve discomfort. Assess and reassess the pain perception of the child and modify interventions to control the pain and postoperative discomfort.
15. Administer all prescribed medications in due time and keep record.
16. Dispose all waste following BMW rules as standard precautions.
17. Maintain strict intake and output chart and document all findings.

Care during Ongoing Recovery Period before Discharge

1. Continue assessment to detect complications related to the surgical interventions.
2. Maintain adequate nutritional intake of the child. Alteration in nutritional, circulatory and metabolic state may predispose to infections and delayed healing. Do not force intake of solid food. Let the child eat what she or he feels like eating. Encourage intake of appropriate foods. Increase diet intake, as prescribed from clear liquids to full liquids to solid foods. Avoid greasy, spicy or rich foods in large amounts. Initiate dietary supplements or parenteral nutrition, as indicated.
3. Promote mobility and self-care activity. Encourage activity as tolerated by the child. Assist the child during mobilization, as feasible. Promote early ambulation. Plan about self-care activities with the child and involve the parent, whenever possible.
4. Provide sensory input to provide cognitive stimulation to the child. Orient the child to time, place, environment, and circumstances. Explain all procedures and instructions to the child using age-appropriate language.
5. Provide psychological support by involving parents in child's care and encouraging diversional and recreational activities to the child. Allow the child to verbalize her or his needs, concerns and questions.
6. Maintain adequate rest and sleep. Provide all hygienic care with special attention for oral care, skin care and care of bladder and bowel.
7. Ensure drains and tubes are removed in due time. Arrange for change of dressing of surgical site, if required. Provide wound care, as appropriate.
8. Administer medications and other supportive care, as prescribed.
9. Remove stitches or staples on the planned date before discharge.
10. Check discharge criteria, child's health condition and ability for perform continued home care before discharging the child from hospital
    Discharge criteria for same day surgery should be checked. These include: (a) child's vital signs are stable with no signs of respiratory distress, (b) child has no complications related to anesthesia, no excessive bleeding from wound, minimal nausea, vomiting and dizziness, (c) child's pain is well controlled and regained cognitive functioning, (d) Child ingests the recommended diet and retains fluid intake, (e) child has voided normally and (f) surgical site and wound healing is at optimum level and (g) child's parents understand continued postoperative care needs at home and features of complications.
11. Provide incidental and planned teaching in simple language to the child and parents. Explain discharge advice and take feedback about understanding of the information given.
12. Dispose all waste generated during care of ongoing postoperative recovery period .
13. Keep record of all observational findings and postoperative procedural activities in child's care sheet and facility record.

Evaluation and Documentation

- Evaluate child's health status and compare with baseline data. Evaluate child's and parents' understanding of surgical event and postoperative care

- Document child's vital signs, input and output, status of drains, tubes and dressings, findings of respiratory and neurological assessment and interventions, complications occurred, medications given, pain management and teaching provided.

Communication and Teaching for Homecare

- Communicate with child and parents about child's health conditions and plan of further management at hospital, continued care at home and schedule of follow-up care
- Teach the child and parents regarding continuation of care at home (about rest, dietary restrictions, medications, hygienic care, limitations of activities, incisional wound care, pain management, etc.), signs and symptoms of complications, emergency medical help and follow-up visits. Provide written instructions for home care with discharge certificate. Instruct to contact community health workers (ASHA, ANM, CHO), whenever required

PROCEDURE–3: REMOVAL OF SUTURES AND STAPLES IN CHILDREN

Clinical Guidelines

- In surgical interventions, sutures are used for stitching body tissues to make them united together with thread, wire or other materials. Surgical sutures can be classified into: absorbable or non-absorbable sutures. *Absorbable sutures* are sterile strand prepared with the collagen derived from healthy mammals or from a synthetic polymer. This type of suture does not require to be removed. *Non-absorbable sutures* are made from the material that are not absorbed by the body, such as silk, polymers, cotton or wire. These sutures are removed in due time or placed in the tissues deep to the skin where their presence will have minimal long-term consequences
- In surgical procedures, stapling is a means of fastening body tissues together by using special staples compatible with tissues. Staples are made of either titanium or an absorbable polymeric material. Stapling can usually be performed more rapidly than suturing and therefore may reduce total anesthetic or operative time
- The method of removal of sutures is determined by the suturing technique used in surgery. A running or continuous suture may need to be removed by gently pulling one end of the suture after the knot is cut. Interrupted sutures need to be removed by cutting sutures one after another. Reabsorbable sutures are meant to reabsorb over time. Ensure method of suturing technique before the planning for removal of them. Make the child and parents aware about the need of removal of sutures or about no need of removal
- Different parts of the body require suture or staple removal at different times. The general guidelines are as follows: Face - 3 to 4 days, Neck - 5 days, Scalp - 6 days, Chest and abdomen - 7 days, Arms and back of hands - 7 days, Legs and top of feet - 10 days, Back - 10 days, Palms and soles of feet - 14 days
- Suture and staple removal is performed using aseptic technique and all infection control measures to prevent surgical site infections.

Equipment Required

- Hand hygiene supplies for hand washing and antiseptic hand rub
- A sterile cover container/tray with all sterile articles namely dressing forceps, stitch cutter or suture scissors, dissecting forceps, staple remover, gloves, gauze pads and pieces, cotton swabs, drapes, small bowls
- A clean container/tray with normal saline, adhesive remover or solution (if needed), adhesive strips or bandages, cotton swabs, clean gloves, antiseptic solution, as prescribed
- Suture/Staple removal kit with all necessary items can be used, if available

- Waste disposal containers as per BMW rules
- Procedure documentation sheet and child case sheet.

Assessment and Preparation

- Assess the child and parents' knowledge and understanding level of the procedure to explain and to provide necessary support to them. Assess the need of the child for pain management and allergy to adhesive solution. Check vital signs and health status of the child with presence of any complications
- Self-preparation should be done with hand hygiene and practice of standard precautions
- Environment should be clean, calm, quite, well ventilated and well lighted
- All necessary items should be arranged in treatment/procedure room or at child's bedside, as indicated
- Preparation of parents: Explain the procedure of removal of sutures and staples in simple language. Encourage and allow them to remain with the child, whenever possible to gain cooperation from the child
- Preparation of child: Explain the child about the procedure as per level of understanding in age-appropriate language. Make the child clean and comfort. Provide distraction during the procedure. Manage pain by non-pharmacological measures, if required.

Performing the Steps of Procedure with Rationale/Point of Emphasis

1. Perform hand hygiene and arranged all necessary supplies for organized approach at procedure room or at the child's bedside.
2. Assist the child to be in comfortable position for the procedure. Be sure that the child's position does not create tension on the suture line.
3. Drape the child so that only suture area is exposed. Provide privacy and protect modesty.
4. Perform hand hygiene and don clean gloves to reduce transmission of microorganisms.
5. Remove old adhesive using adhesive remover, as needed.
6. Remove dressing that is placed over the suture line and discard in appropriate container.
7. Assess the site and suture line for redness, heat, swelling, foul smell and drainage. Note if the wound margins are well approximated. Inform and record all observational findings.
8. Remove gloves. Perform hand hygiene and wear sterile gloves.
9. Cleanse the incision site with saline soaked sterile gauze. Begin at the edges of the suture site and move around the skin, making increasingly larger circles until the area that was covered by the dressing is cleaned. Repeat if necessary with new gauze pad. Always wipe from the clean area to dirty area; innermost area to outermost area.
10. Remove the suture/staple in succession or skip every other one until reach the end and then return to the starting point and remove the rest. Dehiscence can be detected early, if removal of every second stitch is done and then every other suture/ staple can be left in place if needed.
11. For *Suture removal* perform the following steps (Refer **Fig. 4.1**):
    - Hold forceps in non-dominant hand and use them to grasp the suture near the knot. Gently lift the knot up off the skin while avoiding tension on the suture line
    - Place the curved edge of the scissors under the suture, either directly under or near the knot. When using a stitch cutter, place the curved edge of the cutter directly under or near the knot. Remember, exposed part of the suture may harbor pathogens that can trigger infection if pulled under the skin
    - Cut the suture. Pull out the suture in one piece with the forceps and discard the sutures onto a gauze pad. If using a stitch cutter, use an upward motion away from the child's body to "slice" the stitch. Adheres to the aseptic technique during removal of suture.

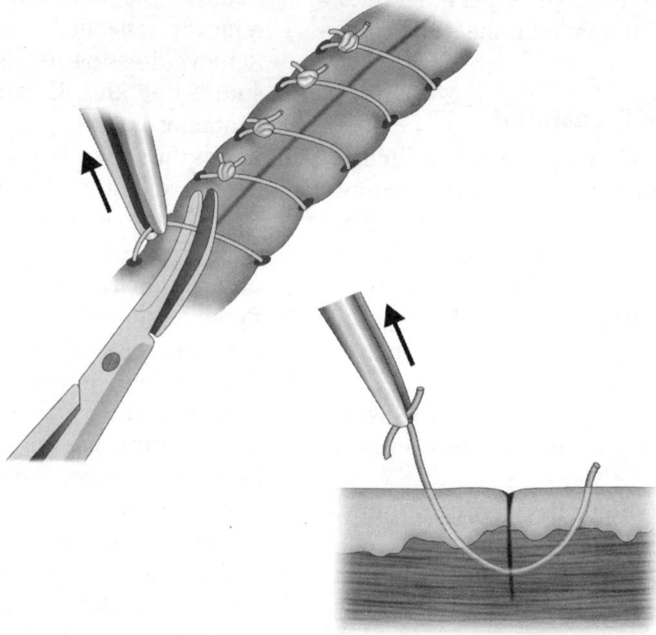

Fig. 4.1: Removal of surgical sutures.

12. For *staple removal* perform the following steps:
    - Place the bottom of the staple remover under the center of the first staple. If the staple is in at an angle, it should be straightened before attempting to remove to minimize damage to underlying tissue during the removal process
    - Keeping the lower jaw of the instrument against the skin, squeeze the handle of the staple remover together to close it. Lift the staple out of the skin in a swift smooth motion and discard the staple onto gauze pad. Adheres to the aseptic technique during removal of staple from the tissue.
13. Assess the suture site for approximation of margins, redness, heat, swelling, and drainage to identify any infection or incomplete healing. Inform and record the abnormalities.
14. Remove all sutures/staples when the wound is well healed.
15. Cleanse the incision site again with saline soaked sterile gauze, if needed (see Step 9).
16. Apply adhesive strips (i.e., Steri-Strips) to support the suture line to promote wound healing. Adhesive solution may be used to keep the adhesive strips in place.
17. Dispose the waste in appropriate containers following standard precautions.
18. Take care of instruments and reusable items by decontamination, cleaning and sterilization for next use.
19. Remove gloves. Perform hand hygiene. Document the procedure and all findings.

Evaluation and Documentation

- Evaluate the child's wound condition and features of surgical site infections. Evaluate the child's and parents' response to the procedure and level of understanding
- Document date and time of suture/staple removal, condition of the suture line, approximation of incision margins and presence of any abnormalities.

Communication and Teaching for Homecare

- Communicate with child in age appropriate language and with parents about

wound condition, presence of any complications and further plan of management and discharge
- Teach the parents about hygienic practices and overall cleanliness, diet, activity restrictions, wound care at home after discharge, signs of complications (fever, bad odor, pain, exudates, swelling), need for medical help and plan for follow up visits.

PROCEDURE–4: WOUND CARE OF CHILDREN

Clinical Guidelines

- Wound, a break in the continuity of body structures caused by surgery or trauma or violence, requires special care for appropriate healing. Wound care and wound management techniques may vary based on type of wound and the setting of the child care units (acute care, OPD based care or home based care)
- Strict aseptic technique must be followed to perform wound care in hospitalized children and in OPD settings to prevent further complications. Any wound that appears suspicious for infections should send for culture and sensitivity test
- Child having a wound should receive adequate systemic care to promote wound healing and to minimize the risk for complications. This includes adequate nutrition and fluids, systemic medications, aseptic technique of wound care and hygienic measures
- Pharmacological and non-pharmacological measures of pain management should be used before and during wound care to minimize child's discomfort.

Equipment Required

- Hand hygiene supplies and PPE for care providers to prevent cross infections
- Sterile cover container/tray with all sterile articles such as gloves, dressing forceps—two, dissecting forceps, sinus forceps, scissors, dressing towel/cut sheet, gauze pieces, cotton swabs, dressing pad, bandage and small bowls
- Clean container/tray with bottles of normal saline, alcohol 70%, povidone-iodine, medicated ointment, adhesive tape, scissors for wound dressing, unsterile cotton balls in a bowl and non-sterile gloves
- One extra sheet for privacy for the child
- Mackintosh/waterproof sheet and treatment towel to protect the child's bed/procedure table for contamination
- Transfer forceps in a sterile container to handle the sterile articles
- Color coded waste disposal containers and biohazard bags
- Large bowl with disinfectant solution (Hypochlorite solution – 0.5%) to decontaminate used instrument for wound care
- Documentation sheet for the wound care and child case sheet.

Assessment and Preparation

- Assess pertinent history focusing on primary reason of the wound. Assess child's vital signs, pain perception, and presence of any abnormal features. Assess level of anxiety and understanding level of the child and parents to provide necessary support and teaching related to wound care
- Self-preparation should be done with hand washing and practicing standard precautions
- Environment should be clean, well-lighted, and free from overcrowding. Usually wound care is given in the procedure room/treatment room
- All required items should be collected and arranged for easy access during procedure. Strict aseptic technique should be followed to prevent further infections of the wound
- Preparation of mother/parent: Explain the procedure to the parents and encourage for participation during the procedure, if they agreed
- Preparations of child: Explain the procedure to the child according to his

or her understanding level and ask for cooperation during wound care. Make the child clean and comfortable. Arrange for pain management, whenever needed.

Performing the Steps of Procedure with Rationale/Point of Emphasis

1. Perform hand hygiene and assemble all required supplies for easy access.
2. Position the child comfortably and conveniently to reach the wound site easily.
3. Maintain privacy by keeping other body parts well covered.
4. Protect the bed/table from soiling due to spillage and absorption of drainage.
5. Perform hand hygiene and wear nonsterile gloves.
6. Remove old dressing carefully. Untie the bandage. Remove adhesive tape slowly and carefully using water soaked cotton balls. Special precautions should be taken for neonates and young infants. Pull the tape on a horizontal plane, folding tape back onto itself while continuously wetting the adhesive-skin interface. Remove dressing gauze or gauze pad over the wound using one dressing forceps. It may be necessary to use normal saline/sterile water to loosen the dressing from the wound and thus to reduce pain during removal of old dressing.
7. Inspect the dressing for amount and color of drainage and odor. Dispose the old dressing in biohazard bag as per BMW rules. Serous and serosanguinous drainage are normal. Purulent drainage is abnormal.
8. Remove gloves, perform hand hygiene and wear sterile gloves. Take help from any assistant for handling sterile articles during wound care. Well practiced health professional can perform wound care with sterile technique using dressing forceps without taking help from other person and arranging all sterile items conveniently before wearing sterile gloves.
9. Cleanse the wound bed with normal saline or sterile water using cotton tipped applicator or gauze pieces using dressing forceps. Use antiseptic solutions (alcohol, povidone-iodine) on the wound with caution in weak dilutions. Cleanse the wound from clean area to dirty area.
10. Inspect the wound bed with attention to size, type of tissue in base, color, exudates, odor, any bleeding, non-viable slough, granulation tissue, condition of surrounding tissue and pain. Measure length, width, and depth of the wound using sinus forceps.
11. Remove all non-viable tissue gently by wound debridement as they hinder wound healing. Tough yellow tissue is non-viable slough and dark-brown black necrotic tissue of the wound is also non-viable.
12. Apply topical medications on the wound surface, as prescribed.
13. Apply primary dressing first then apply secondary dressing for absorption of drainage.
14. Secure the dressing with adhesive tape or with soft gauze bandage. Avoid adhesive tape when the dressing change frequency is more than once a day.
15. Dispose all waste in appropriate containers. Take care of reusable items and instruments.
16. Remove gloves. Perform hand hygiene.
17. Document the procedure of wound care and all related findings.

Evaluation and Documentation

- Evaluate the wound condition comparing with previous observations. Evaluate child's and parent's understanding of the importance of wound care and their ability to participate and perform the procedure, whenever required
- Document the location and appearance of wound site, contents of old dressing drainage, and condition of wound bed. Record date, time and type of dressing applied, child's tolerance of the procedure, use of pain medications/measures, involvement of the child and/or parent and teaching provided.

Communication and Teaching for Homecare

- Communicate with child and parents about condition of the wound and further plan of management. Answer to the questions as asked
- Teach the child/parents about hygienic practices, hand hygiene, cleanliness, and disposal of contaminated dressing, diet, fluid intake, medications and features of complications. Instruct the child/parent before discharge with written instructions about the wound care at home, if needed and plan for follow-up visits or medical help whenever necessary.

PROCEDURE–5: ASSESSMENT AND CARE OF CHILDREN WITH CAST

Clinical Guidelines

- Cast is a solid mold of a part, usually applied in situ for immobilization in case of fractures, dislocations, and surgical interventions and in any other severe injuries. It is usually made of POP, sodium silicate, starch or dextrin that is rubbed into crinoline then soaked in water, carefully applied to the immobilized part and allowed to harden
- Plaster cast is rigid dressing made of gauze impregnated with Plaster of Paris (POP), used to immobilize an injured part especially in bone fractures or surgery. Other synthetic casting materials such as fiberglass with polyurethane, are being used increasingly as preferred alternatives to plaster, especially for non-weight bearing parts of the body
- POP cast is easy to prepare, get desired shape when dried, do not shrink or cracked and act as very hard splint. It is a low cost material
- The purpose of POP cast is to maintain support and to improve bone alignment. It also helps to promote fracture healing and to correct deformity
- Management of the child in plaster cast and daily care is important for prevention of complications related to fracture and cast.

Equipment Required

- Hand hygiene supplies for hand washing and hand rub
- Waterproof apron to protect dress of doctor and assistant
- Clean unsterile gloves, as required
- Examination/treatment table for application of cast
- Cotton and bandage to protect the skin of the affected area
- POP or gypsum, bowl of water and long mackintosh
- Synthetic casting materials (such as fiberglass), if available
- Sponge holding forceps, cotton swabs and alcohol for skin preparation
- Articles for assessment of vital signs and physical examination
- Extra pillows or blanket roll to elevate the cast area
- Plastic wrap to protect the cast around genital area, if required
- Articles for administration of medications, as prescribed
- Wound care articles, if any wound is present
- X-ray view box and X-ray plates, as needed
- Routine child care articles including clothing and age appropriate diaper
- Marking pen or pencil to mark date of the cast
- Waste disposal contains as per BMW rules
- Procedure record sheet and child's case sheet.

Assessment and Preparation

- Assess the child's health status, vital signs, signs of infections and pain before and after application of cast. Review the indications of use of cast and the need for type of cast (Refer **Fig. 4.2**). Assess child and parents for anxiety and level of understanding for the importance of cast application to plan for necessary support, explanation and teaching
- Self-preparation should be done with the practices of standard precautions
- Environment should be clean, calm, well lighted and free from overcrowding

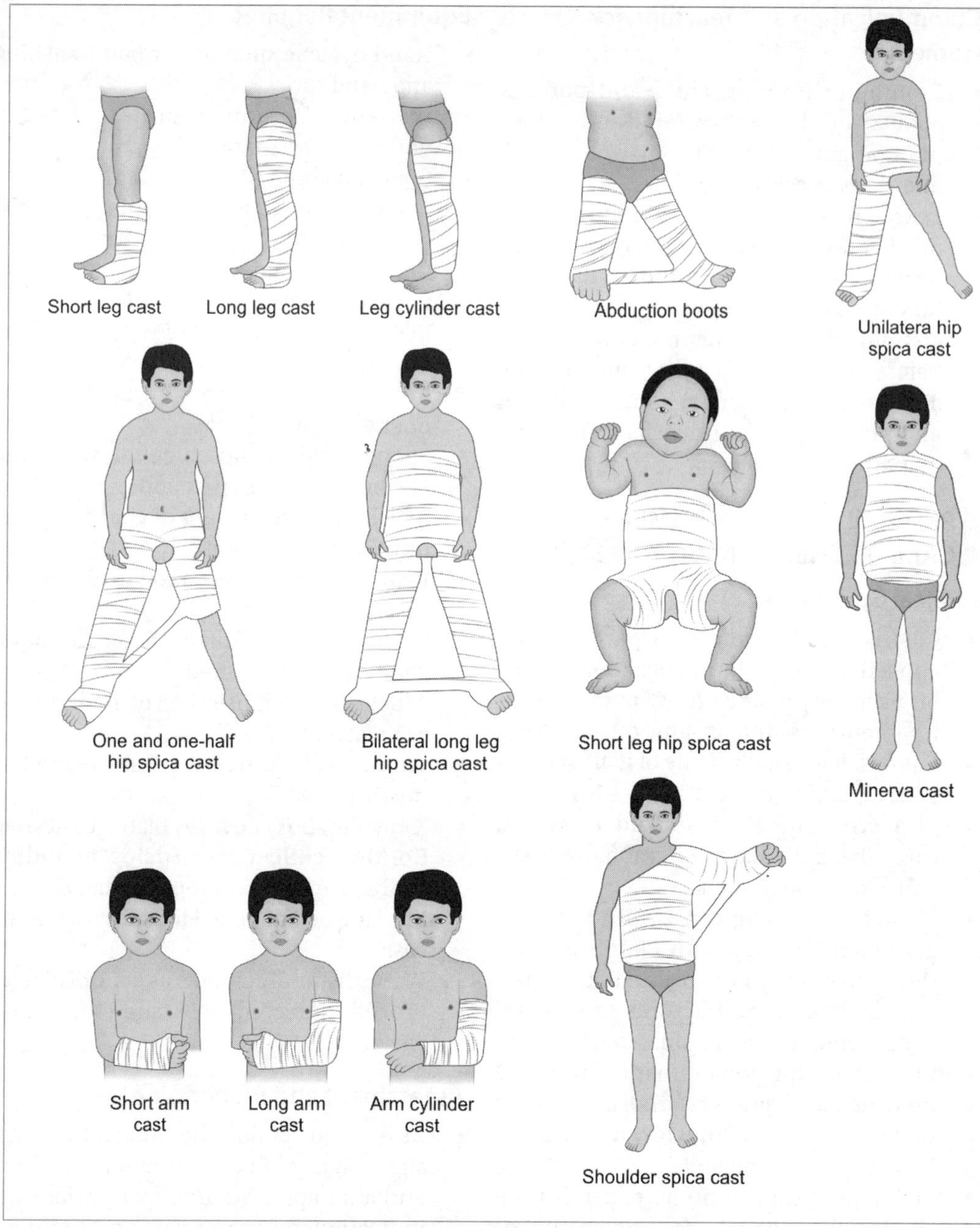

Fig. 4.2: Different types of casts in children.

- All required articles and equipment should be well arranged in the treatment room
- Preparation of parents: Explain the importance of the procedure of application of cast and plan of further management
- Preparation of child: Make the child clean, comfortable and explain as per level of understanding about application of cast and care of cast. Allow the parent during application of cast and thereafter, as feasible. Administer pain medication, if

prescribed. Use diversional activities and nonpharmacological measure to distract the child with cast.

Performing the Steps of Procedure with Rationale/Point of Emphasis

1. Perform hand hygiene. Don gloves, if appropriate. Wear protective plastic apron.
2. Assess the child for pain, using age-appropriate technique and use pharmacological and nonpharmacological measures for pain management. Assess for pain every 2–4 hours during acute phase and then along with vital signs assessment.
3. Assist the doctor during application of cast. Follow necessary precautions to prevent complications and promote healing.
4. Assess the child for the followings:
   - Vital signs to identify compromised circulation and tissue oxygenation
   - Pulse above and below the injured area for early detection and intervention of compromised circulation and compartment syndrome
   - CRT by pressing on fingers and toes (normal CRT 1-2 seconds), to find insufficient circulation to the distal extremity
   - Sensation of extremities by gently touching the fingers and toes for numbness, quality of response to stimuli, neurobehavioral response (such as rest, sleep, mood, level of consciousness, etc.). Assess neurovascular status every 4 hours for the first 48 hours after application of cast
   - Motor functions (presence of flexion, extension, abduction and adduction) of fingers and toes to identify the normal range of motion or impaired or absent motor functions
   - Skin integrity and presence of any skin disruptions. Assess skin around cast edges every 6–8 hours for irritation, rash or skin breakdown and skin over bony prominences for redness and tingling sensation. Check that the cast is not too tight anywhere
   - Compare the color and temperature of both limbs, above and below the injury site to diagnose compartment syndrome
   - Swelling of fingers or toes distal to fracture or surgical site to detect inadequate venous return. Swelling peaks within 24–48 hours. Delay in attending to swelling, even for as little as 4–6 hours, can lead to compartment syndrome and complete or partial paralysis.
5. Perform interventions to promote skin integrity, as indicated. (a) Protect edges of casts with cloth tape or cotton to decrease skin irritation; if the edges are rough; (b) Relieve the itching by blowing cool air into the cast or rubbing the skin around the cast edges or tap on the cast over the itchy areas. Never allow any stick or anything down the cast to scratch the itching area; (c) Provide daily bath (tub bath or sponge bath as feasible) to keep accessible skin areas clean to decrease skin irritation and itching. Wash fingers and toes near the cast with damp washcloth; (d) Provide perineal and perianal care for children with casts extending close to genital area to prevent contamination with urine and feces. Place diaper and plastic wrap to protect the skin from the wet cast.
6. Assess integrity of the cast because not intact cast impairs healing. Expose the wet cast to room air to dry and elevate the cast on pillows up to 4 inches above the level of heart. Handle the cast gently only with the palm of the hands. Plaster casts take 24–48 hours to dry. Synthetic casts dry within 30–60 minutes.
7. Inspect the cast for cracks, softening and excessive flaking or flattening. Flattened and flaking of the cast can cause skin irritation and undue pressure on bony prominences. Soft cracked cast will not provide support to maintain alignment of the fracture site.
8. Inspect the cast for signs of drainage or bad odor from the wound underneath the cast. Mark the circumference of the drainage on the cast as baseline parameter and to

detect whether there is more drainage or not.

9. Clean the surface of the cast, as needed. Plaster cast can be cleaned with toothpaste. Fiberglass casts can be cleaned with damp cloth.
10. Explain to the child in age-appropriate language and parents about the need for limited activity and required care with the cast.
11. Instruct the child and parents not to put any items down the cast and not to scratch under the cast with any object to prevent skin irritation and infections.
12. Assist the child to perform passive and active range of motion exercises of all extremities to prevent weakness and stiffness. This should be done 3–4 times a day to maintain functional ability of the extremities.
13. Assist the child to ambulate by the use of walker, crutches, cast shoes, or walking boot, or wheelchair, as indicated. For upper limbs sling can be used. Children in cast should be encouraged to be up and out of bed once the cast has dried and pain is well managed.
14. Collaborate with technician or physiotherapist to provide teaching regarding the use of ambulatory equipment such as crutch, walker, etc.
15. Provide diversional activities for the child on limited activity to adjust with the condition.
16. Provide comfort with suitable position of the extremities using extra pillows or sheet.
17. Prevent complications of immobility due to use of cast (such as constipation, pressure sore, pulmonary stasis, stress and anxiety, depression, etc.) and promote healing by ongoing nursing interventions and adequate nutrition.
18. Maintain cleanliness and hygienic care of the child. Involve parents, as feasible.
19. Take care of reusable articles and dispose the waste as per BMW rules.
20. Document and inform the procedure and all observational findings related to cast care.

Evaluation and Documentation

- Evaluate child's vital signs, neurovascular status, skin conditions at regular interval and compare with baseline data. Inform doctor about any abnormal findings. Evaluate child and parents for their anxiety and understanding to provide support, as needed. Evaluate parent's ability to perform the need based care to their child with the cast
- Document details of application of cast (date, time, type, indications, material used), all observational findings, medications administered, interventions done to prevent complications and to treat the problems, expected date of removal of cast and instruction given to the parents about care of child with cast.

Communication and Teaching for Homecare

- Communicate with parents and child, as appropriate regarding application of cast and care of the child with cast, plan of management at hospital, at home and removal of cast
- Teach the parents about cast care, medications, hygienic practices, skin care, toileting, positioning, neurovascular checks, mobility, precautions during transportation, comfort measures, appropriate clothing, diet and fluid intake, diversional activities, schooling and continuation of school activities, signs of complications, need for medical help, plan for removal of cast and follow-up care.

PROCEDURE–6: CARE OF CHILDREN WITH TRACTION

Clinical Guidelines

- Traction is the process of slowly or gently pulling or drawing the fractured or dislocated body parts to treat the underlying problems. It refers to the set of mechanisms for straightening broken bones or relieving pressure on the spine and skeletal system
- The purpose of traction is to guide the body parts back into place and hold it steady. It

may be used to stabilize and realign bone fractures and to reduce pain related to fracture. It is used to treat bone deformities (such as scoliosis) and to correct stiff constricted muscles, joints and tendons. It also helps to prevent muscle spasms and to relieve compression of nerves

- There are mainly two types of traction used for orthopedic patients: (1) skin traction and (2) skeletal traction. Different types of skin tractions (Refer **Fig. 4.3**) and skeletal tractions used with different indications, require special nursing considerations for optimum healing and recovery of the problems
- Skin traction refers to any traction apparatus where the pull force is applied to the affected body parts via the soft tissue. This traction is applied to the skin by using skin adherents, wraps, traction tapes or special foam boots
- Skeletal traction refers to any apparatus where the pull force is applied directly to the skeleton via of pins, wires, screws and/or tongs that are inserted into the appropriate area of bone. It is beneficial for unstable or fragmented fractures that are not amenable to surgical interventions. Skeletal traction would also be used if there is skin damage associated with the fracture. It is applied in strict aseptic technique
- Traction is applied by the technician or doctor with definite indications. Assist during application of traction following all precautions to prevent infections and other problems. Appropriate assessment and nursing interventions for the child with traction helps to prevent complications and promote healing with expected recovery

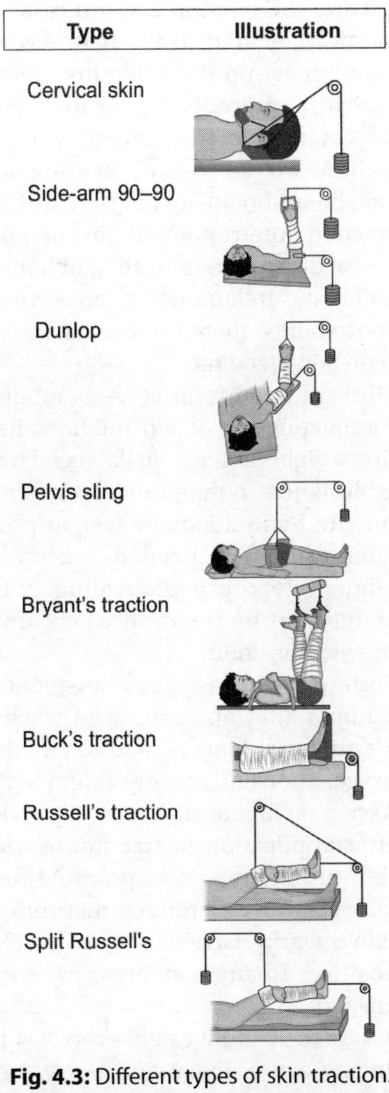

Fig. 4.3: Different types of skin traction.

Equipment Required

- Hand hygiene supplies for hand wash and hand rub and PPE
- Articles for physical assessment and assessment of vital signs
- Routine child care articles, clothing and age-appropriate diaper
- Skin care supplies, as required for the child with traction
- Extra pillows or blankets and sheets
- Waste disposal containers as per BMW rules
- Documentation sheet and child case sheet with traction.

Assessment and Preparation

- Assess child's vital signs, pain, muscle spasms, skin condition and presence of any abnormalities or features of complications
  - Review the diagnosis and type of fracture or surgery the child has sustained

- Check the type of traction used and its purpose. Observe amount of traction weights prescribed and used for the child
- Look for child's age, body weight, physical condition, and integrity of skeletal system
- Assess child and parents for level of anxiety and understanding regarding the use of traction and ability to participate during care of the child with traction

- Self-preparation should be done with standard precautions and hand hygiene
- Environment should be clean, well ventilated and free of overcrowding
- All care articles should be arranged at child's bedside for easy access
- Preparation of parents: Explain about the care to be provided to the child. Allow and encourage the parents to participate in routine care. Answer to their questions
- Preparation of child: Make the child clean and comfortable with the traction. Follow non-pharmacological measures to relieve pain and discomfort. Administer pain medication, if prescribed and indicated. Maintain adequate diet and fluid intake. Provide hygienic care to prevent infections. Assess and take care for normal elimination pattern. Allow age appropriate diversional and recreational activities. Listen child's concern, as expressed about the problems and discomfort related to traction.

Performing the Steps of Procedure with Rationale/Point of Emphasis

1. Perform hand hygiene and use PPE as appropriate.
2. Assess child's positioning in bed relative to traction. Proper alignment prevents pressure on the affected extremity, promotes healing and ensures good mechanical functioning of the traction equipment.
3. Maintain privacy and comfort of the child to get cooperation and relieve anxiety.
4. Reposition the child in supine position with alignment of shoulder, hip and legs in the midline position. Child's heel should not be digging into the mattress. The side-lying and semi-fowler position are contraindicated. Elevate head of the bed not more than 20 degrees to provide adequate counter-traction. If the force of pull of traction is greater than the counter-traction supplied by the body weight, then the child will slide toward the traction force. Child with lower extremity traction can be turned one-fourth to the uninvolved side for back care or to place bedpan, when needed.
5. Ensure the traction apparatus is appropriately secured to the bed. Assess the traction set-up including the amount of weight, as prescribed. Look for alignment of traction cords, integrity of rope, tightness of knots, and securing of tape. Bed linen should not interfere with line of traction. Interruption of "line of pull" can cause disruption of healing of bones and soft tissue. Inflammation can occur due to movements, therefore can cause spasm, pain and bleeding.
6. Observe weights for correct amount and for hanging free of bed and floor. Reposition weights as needed. Balanced traction is designed to maintain a constant pull on child and adequate weight provides counter-traction needed to keep bones aligned for optimal healing. Weights should not be removed when lifting or moving the child.
7. Perform neurovascular assessment every 4 hours after application of traction to identify problems related to circulation, oxygenation and sensory-motor activity.
8. Assess skin condition every 4 hours after application of traction to identify skin problems and to promote prompt interventions to reduce disruptions of skin integrity. Give back care and change position to prevent pressure sore, as needed.
9. Assess the child for pain every 2–4 hours during acute phase and every 4 hours

thereafter. Manage pain, as prescribed. Use diversional and recreational activities (such as toys, story book, music, video games, drawing, painting, etc.).

10. Assist child to perform passive and active range of motion exercises of all extremities at 6–8 hours interval. It helps to maintain muscle tone and prevent venous thrombosis.
11. Provide interventions to prevent complications of immobility due to application of traction (skin breakdown, pain, infections, etc.) and to promote healing.
12. Encourage intake of adequate fluid and appropriate foods to promote wound healing.
13. Notify all abnormal findings to healthcare prescriber/orthopedic surgeon immediately.
14. Perform specific interventions for skin traction: (a) Remove skin traction straps every 4 hours and boot every 8 hours to assess potential complications, as indicated and prescribed, (b) Check bony prominences for skin breakdown, abrasions and pressure area to assess compromised skin integrity, (c) Don gloves. Cleanse, dry and massage of the child's skin beneath the traction areas and dependent areas to promote circulation, (d) Replace the traction and remove the gloves, (e) Assess position of bandages, wraps or straps. Ensure wrapping material is not wrinkled on the skin to prevent skin breakdown; and (f) Assess for loosening or slipping of devices to prevent interruption of traction.
15. Provide specific interventions for skeletal traction: (a) Assess the pin site for signs of infections (redness, swelling or drainage) every shift. Children with skeletal pins are at higher risk of osteomyelitis, (b) Perform pin site care as needed and (c) Check that pins are secure and not slipping. Slippage or movement of the pins may interfere with the effectiveness of the traction. Loose pin site is at higher risk for infections.
16. Ensure child's comfort and pay attention to any concern.
17. Dispose all waste as per BMW rules.
18. Document all findings related to traction care in child case sheet and treatment sheet. Inform to appropriate authorities about abnormal findings.

Evaluation and Documentation

- Evaluate and compare health status, vital signs, neurovascular status, skin condition and pain of the child before and after application of traction. Evaluate the expected effectiveness of the traction applied to the child. Evaluate child's and parent's understanding of need to maintain proper body alignment and to report pain and any other abnormalities
- Document all activities, interventions, observational findings and teaching completed.

Communication and Teaching for Homecare

- Communicate with child and parents about child's health condition, traction integrity, plan of continuation of traction, possible complications and plan of further management and discharge from hospital
- Teach the parents about participation in routine care of the child with traction, maintenance of child's body alignment and reporting of problems related to tractions. Instruct about precautions during transportation after discharge from hospital to home, home care, signs of complications, need for emergency medical help and about follow-up appointments (date, time, place, documents needed, etc.)

PROCEDURE–7: SKELETAL PIN SITE CARE OF CHILDREN

Clinical Guidelines

- Skeletal traction is applied directly to the skeleton via of pins, wires, screws and/or tongs that are inserted into the appropriate area of bone. Skeletal pin site assessment for infections and appropriate treatment of complications are essential for expected healing and recovery

- The pin site should be assessed every 6–8 hours. First pin site redressing should be done within 24–72 hours after the insertion of skeletal pin, as per direction and presence of amount of drainage. After 48–72 hours, pin site care should be performed daily and then weekly for sites with mechanically stable bone-pin interfaces. Bath with medicated soap and drying the pin site with towel can be allowed 5–10 days after insertion of pin, if no such complications occurred.

Equipment Required

- Hand hygiene supplies including hand rub
- A sterile covered container/tray with sterile articles such as gloves, dressing forceps, absorbent nonstick dressing, gauze pieces, cotton swabs, applicators and small containers/bowls for sterile water and normal saline and antiseptic solution
- A clean tray with bottle of normal saline antiseptic solution, bandage
- Waste disposal containers
- Documentation sheet and child case sheet.

Assessment and Preparation

- Assess child for vital signs, integrity of skeletal traction, fever and pain, presence of features of infection or any other complications. Assess the extremity for neurovascular changes such as alteration of circulation, oxygenation, temperature and sensation.
  Assess the anxiety and level of understanding of the child and parents to plan for necessary support and teaching
- Self-preparation should be done with hand hygiene and following sterile technique
- Environment should be clean, calm, well lighted and well ventilated
- All required articles and supplies should be arranged at child's bedside. The procedure should be done with aseptic technique and standard precautions
- Preparation of parents: Explain the procedure and encourage for participation
- Preparation of child: Make the child comfortable and explain the procedure using age-appropriate language. Administer pain medication, as prescribed. Use diversional activities and relaxation techniques. These measures are more helpful to gain cooperation from the child, as pin site care is generally not painful

Performing the Steps of Procedure with Rationale/Point of Emphasis

1. Perform hand washing and arrange all necessary supplies for efficient time management.
2. Perform hand hygiene using hand rub or washing hand, as required. Don sterile gloves to reduce transmission of microorganisms. Sterile and aseptic technique must be followed during skeletal pin site care.
3. Remove the soiled pin site dressing using dressing forceps. Discard the dressing and the forceps (used to remove dressing) following BMW rules.
4. Inspect the wound of the pin site. Observe for redness, swelling, tenderness or purulent discharge to identify the presence of infections. Notify healthcare prescriber/orthopedic surgeon, if signs of infections and other problems are found.
5. Observe for loosening of the pin. Slippage or movement of the pin may interfere with the effectiveness of the traction. Excessive motion of the pin may result in increased drainage which can cause bacterial growth and infections.
6. Observe for skin adherence to pin. Adherence of skin may be painful and cause further tissue damage at the pin site.
7. Remove gloves and perform hand hygiene to reduce transmission of microorganisms.
8. Open sterile packs and container. Pour cleaning and antiseptic solution, as prescribed, into sterile containers in non-touch technique.
9. Don sterile gloves to maintain aseptic technique. Take help from assistant to maintain aseptic technique, whenever needed.

10. Cleanse the area starting at the pin insertion site and cleaning outward away from the pin site. Use sterile applicators or dressing forceps and gauze pads/pieces and antiseptic solution for cleaning the pin site. Use one applicator once. Remove exudates or dried crust or blood. Lightly massage the area..
    Chlorhexidine solution may be more effective in preventing pin site infections compared with other solutions. Removal of crust is recommended to allow exudates to escape from pin site, thereby preventing pin site contamination and abscess formation. Massaging of the area helps in preventing skin adherence to pin.
11. Allow the pin site to become dry after cleaning, as moisture encourages colonization of bacteria. Application of ointments is not recommended. Ointments applied to the site appear to block the normal drainage of exudates, thereby increasing the risk of infections.
12. Cleanse metal of pin using sterile water and sterile applicators or sterile gauze pads to remove bacteria and wound exudates.
13. Apply absorbent non-sticky dressing to the pin site. Apply wrapping bandage, if the site continues to have drainage. Dressing provides protective barrier against airborne infections and contamination by parent's or child's hands.
14. Dispose all waste in appropriate containers following BMW guidelines. Take care of reusable supplies by decontamination, cleaning and sterilization.
15. Remove gloves. Make the child comfortable. Perform hand hygiene.
16. Inform about any unusual findings to the appropriate authority for prompt interventions.
17. Document the procedure of pin site care and all observational findings.

Evaluation and Documentation

- Evaluate the child's health status and condition of the skeletal traction. Evaluate the pin site condition and compare with previous findings to identify the abnormalities. Evaluate child's and parent's understanding of procedure and ability to provide self-care
- Document the date and time of the procedure of pin site care with condition of pin site and surrounding skin including color, discharge, tenderness, swelling and skin adherence. Document child's health status, pain management done, presence of any unusual findings and teaching given to the child and parents.

Communication and Teaching for Homecare

- Communicate with the child and parents about child's health status, the importance of pin site care and discharge planning
- Teach the parents about hygienic practices, involvement in child care at hospital, pin site care and cleaning at home after discharge, precautions during transport, signs of complications, need for emergency medical help and plan of follow-up visits.

PROCEDURE–8: OSTOMY CARE OF THE CHILDREN

Clinical Guidelines

- Ostomy is an opening or stoma created by surgery from an area inside the body to the outside. It is commonly indicated in case of birth defect, cancer, abdominal or pelvic trauma and in many disease conditions
- Ostomy is a surgically formed fistula connecting a portion of the GI tract (such as gastrostomy, ileostomy, colostomy) or urinary tract (uretero-ileostomy, cystostomy) to the exterior of the body surface (usually through the abdominal wall) or in trachea (tracheostomy) to the neck
- Ostomy can be performed as temporary or permanent measures. Child and their family members should be assured that it is possible to carry normal activities with ostomy, only with minimum inconvenience
- Demonstration and return demonstration of ostomy care to the parents/family

members and to the child, as age appropriate, is essential and important part of this procedure
- The characteristics of the material excreted through the stoma will depend on the portion of the bowel to which it is attached. Excretions from the ileum will be fluid and quite irritating to skin and those from the upper right colon will be semi-fluid. The excretions from the upper left colon are partly solid and those from the sigmoid colon will tend to be solid. Understanding of these excretions is necessary to provide individualized site-specific ostomy care to the child
- Specific ostomy care involves stoma care and irrigation of bowel leading to the stoma, when indicated. Care of the stoma (ileostomy or colostomy) is directed toward maintaining the peristomal skin and mucosa of the stoma in healthy condition.
- All fecal stomas (ileostomy and colostomy) should be pouched. A protective barrier is necessary for these stomas. Pouch wear time for infants and children is generally 2–4 days. Successful stoma management can be measured by the maintenance of skin integrity and integrity of the stoma
- Older children and parents need to be taught ostomy care skills before discharge from hospital. Emptying and cleaning of ostomy pouch should also be taught for future practice to the older children, parents and care assistant
- Consultation and discussion with another children with ostomy and with their parents, who become competent in ostomy care will be very helpful.

Equipment Required

For Stoma Care in Immediate Postoperative Period

- Hand washing supplies and antiseptic hand rub
- Sterile or Clean gloves, as required and protective gown or apron
- Vaseline gauze or petroleum jelly and gauze pads/pieces
- Waste disposal containers as per BMW guidelines
- Documentation sheet and child case sheet.

For Application of Ostomy Pouch

- Hand hygiene supplies for hand wash and hand rub
- Basin of warm water, bottle of normal saline
- Clean gloves and protective gown or apron
- Washcloth, 4 × 4 size clean gauze, or soft paper towels
- Ostomy pouch and scissors
- Skin barrier paste and powder, as prescribed
- Waste disposal containers as per BMW rules
- Documentation sheet and child case sheet.

For Emptying and Cleaning Ostomy Pouch

- Hand hygiene supplies for hand wash and hand rub
- Clean gloves and protective gown or apron
- Basin or toilet facility
- Washcloths, diaper wipes, tissue papers or paper towels
- Waste disposal containers as per BMW guidelines
- Documentation sheet and child case sheet.

Assessment and Preparation

- Assess the child health status, ostomy-related problems and presence of any other problems. Assess child and parents to determine their current knowledge and ability to perform ostomy care to plan for necessary support and teaching sessions for them
- Self-preparation should be done with practice of standard precautions
- Environment should be clean, well-lighted and free from overcrowding
- All necessary articles and supplies should be arranged near the child
- Preparation of parents: Explain the procedure and encourage participating in

ostomy care. Describe the importance and precautions to be followed for ostomy care

- Preparation of child: Explain the procedure in age appropriate language. Make the child comfortable. Listen to her or his concerns and reply. Demonstrate the ostomy care procedure on a doll in presence of parents to relieve fear and anxiety. Encourage older child to assist during the procedure.

Performing the Steps of Procedure with Rationale/Point of Emphasis

Stoma Care without Appliance: Immediate Postoperative Period

1. Perform hand hygiene and arrange all necessary supplies near the child.
2. Perform hand hygiene and wear gloves to reduce transmission of microorganisms.
3. Cover the stoma site with Vaseline gauze or petroleum jelly and gauze pads/pieces, as directed until output begins from the stoma. This helps to keep the stoma moist and to protect from friction damage. Check the time of ostomy pouch application.
4. Follow any other directions for the child, as prescribed.
5. Observe the stoma condition for any abnormalities.
6. Remove and discard gloves. Perform hand hygiene. Document the procedure.

Routine Stoma Care

1. Perform hand hygiene and arrange all necessary supplies near the child.
2. Prepare pouch barrier for application (follow manufacturer instructions):
   - Measure the stoma with the "Measuring Guide" provided with the pouches. Pouch opening should be about 2 mm larger than the base of the stoma. Save the pattern to use as a guide in the future. In case of new ostomy, stoma size need to be checked each time the pouch is applied. The stoma will decrease in size after surgery, as the edema resolves
   - Trace the selected circle on the release paper on the back of the wafer or the pouch, if it is one piece system. It provides a guide to follow for cutting
   - Pull the front of pouch away from the wafer before cutting pouch opening or place fingers inside pouch to separate panels and to prevent puncturing the pouch using small rounded tip scissors. Cut the barrier on the marked circle
   - Smooth the cut edge by running a finger around the circle. Not all barriers can be smoothed. Some barriers may assist with the adhesion of the ostomy pouch to child's skin contours.
3. Position the infant and young child in supine position, restraining as necessary. Older child and adolescent may sit or stand, depending on which position is comfortable.
4. Make the child comfortable and maintain privacy. Keep the young infant warm. Allow the child and parent to participate actively, whenever possible.
5. Perform the procedure at bedside or in the washroom, based on accessibility.
6. Perform hand hygiene and wear gloves as standard precautions.
7. Remove old appliance or dressing and cleanse peristomal skin using warm water or normal saline. Cleaned skin allows better adhesion of pouch. Soap is not used, as it interferes with pouch adherence.
8. Dry the skin thoroughly. Apply skin preparations only if necessary and allow drying completely. Take special precautions for young infants for use of skin preparations.
9. Inspect the child's skin and stoma to detect any complications. Stoma should be pink to red in color and moist. Look stoma for color, tenderness to touch, swelling, peristomal hernia, prolapse, retraction and signs of infections around the stoma or incision.
10. Apply barrier powder on the skin, if it is reddened. Gently remove excess powder. Seal the powder with alcohol-free skin preparation. Allow drying completely. Powder can help with healing of peristomal

skin. Skin preparations help to seal around the stoma.

11. Apply a thin layer skin barrier on the pouch near the stoma-opening to paste and fill the gaps or to increase wear time and to protect the skin.
12. Remove paper backing and apply prepared pouch over the stoma. Press the pouch with fingertips, especially around base of the stoma. Hold with hands gently over the pouch for 1–2 minutes to improve adhesion of the pouch. This allows easy emptying of pouch.
13. Close bottom of the pouch with tail closure or clamp provided, to keep drainage in pouch. The tail closure on the infant and pediatric pouch needs to be rolled at least three times before folding ties in. When using a clamp to close the pouch, make sure that the end of the pouch is folded over just one time and clamp is closed.

    With infants and toddlers, it is easier to apply the tail closure before applying the pouch. Be careful not to pull on the pouch seal when applying tail closure. If clamp is not closed, pouch may come and leak from the weight of stool.
14. Dispose all waste in appropriate containers. Take care of reusable articles.
15. Remove gloves. Perform hand hygiene. Document the procedure and all findings.

Emptying and Cleaning the Pouch

1. Perform hand hygiene and arrange all necessary supplies near the child
2. Perform hand hygiene and wear gloves to reduce transmission of microorganisms
3. Position the infant or child supine or on side. Place the container under end of the pouch for easy emptying. Older children or teens may go into washroom and sit on toilet or can sit on the edge of their bed during the procedure
4. For younger children, unwind tail closure of the pouch and empty the contents into waste container or on the diaper. For older children, use clamp to open and turn bottom of pouch up to cuff
5. Empty contents of the pouch into waste container or toilet to remove feces
6. For infant and toddlers, cleanse bottom of pouch up to the tail closure both inside and out with paper towel tissue or diaper wipes. For older children and teens, cleanse bottom of pouch cuff with tissue paper or paper towel before uncuffing and closing the pouch. This helps to clean pouch bottom and decreases odor
7. Close the pouch with tail closure or clamp to allow the drainage inside the pouch
8. Inspect contents of the pouch for amount and for any abnormality. Discard the contents
9. Dispose all waste in appropriate containers. Clean the reusable articles
10. Remove gloves. Perform hand hygiene. Document the procedure and all findings.

Evaluation and Documentation

- Evaluate the child's health status after the procedure and identify problems. Evaluate the child's or parents' ability to perform self ostomy care
- Document date and time of the ostomy care, condition of stoma and skin around the stoma, type of output, application of specific pouch, parent's involvement and teaching of procedure to child and parents regarding ostomy care.

Communication and Teaching for Homecare

- Communicate with child and parents about child's health condition and condition of the ostomy. Discuss about plan of management and discharge from the hospital. Review the medical or surgical condition for which the ostomy was necessary
- Teach the child and parents for ostomy care at home after discharge from hospital and demonstrate the procedure. Instruct the parents about the signs of complications (any change in stoma or output such as skin breakdown, ribbon like stool, diarrhea, bleeding, no stool or no flatus, prolapse of the stoma), need for medical help, hygienic practices and

plan of follow-up visits. Inform about the vendor who can provide needed supplies for ostomy care at home.

PROCEDURE–9: CARE OF CHILDREN WITH GASTROSTOMY/JEJUNOSTOMY (SKIN CARE, TUBE CHANGE)

Clinical Guidelines

- Gastrostomy tubes (G-tubes) are placed either surgically, endoscopically or in some cases by interventional radiology. Gastrostomy tubes are placed directly into the stomach. Percutaneous endoscopic gastrostomy (PEG) tubes are placed endoscopically. After an established G-tube tract is formed (at about 6 weeks period), a skin-level G-tube device can be placed. The internal stabilizer for skin-level devices is either a balloon type or a mushroom type
- Jejunostomy tubes (J-tubes) can be placed through similar procedures. The distal tip rests in the jejunum but may originate through the stomach (G-J) or directly into the jejunum
- All long-term enteral indwelling feeding tubes (G-tube or PEG tube or J-tube) must have an internal stabilizer to keep the tube falling out. They must also have external stabilizer to keep the tube in the correct position and to prevent tube migration into the GI tract
- Children who are unable to take oral feeds and requiring enteral nutritional support for longer than 4–6 weeks should be considered as candidates for long-term enteral tube access. Common indications for these tubes are head or neck trauma or surgery, tumors of the esophagus, neurologic deficit, etc.
- Care of the indwelling enteral tube site should be performed every day preferably during bath or as needed to maintain skin integrity
- Indwelling enteral tubes are made of long-lasting material and should not require routine change unless they become accidentally dislodged or the integrity of the tube itself is breaking down. Follow manufacturer's instructions for routine time periods to replace enteral tubes in children receiving long-term enteral therapy.

Equipment Required

For Indwelling Enteral Tube Site Skin Care with Dressing Change

- Hand hygiene supplies for hand wash and hand rub
- Clean gloves to prevent cross infections
- Sterile covered container/tray containing all sterile items, such as gauze pieces, 2 × 2 split gauze in a sterile bowl, sterile water in a bowl, sterile normal saline in a bowl as cleansing solution, or as prescribed, two extra sterile small bowls, dressing forceps, three cotton-tipped applicators
- External anchor as needed according to hospital policy
- Skin barrier, liquid soap, antibiotic ointment (optional or as prescribed)
- Tape measure to measure the external part of the tube
- Waste disposal containers as per BMW guidelines
- Documentation sheet and child case sheet.

For Gastrostomy or Jejunostomy Tube Change or Replacement

- Hand hygiene supplies for hand wash and hand rub
- Clean gloves to prevent cross infections
- Sterile water in a covered bowl
- Water soluble lubricant
- Syringe – 5 mL size
- Catheter adapter (optional)
- Tape measure, Rubber band
- For external stabilizer: Gauze and tape or 1 inch foam tape
- Waste disposal containers following BMW rules
- Documentation sheet and child case sheet.

Assessment and Preparation

- Assess the followings:
  - Examine the child's health status, signs of poor wound healing, decreased muscle mass and poor dietary calorie

and protein intake to determine need for long-term enteral nutritional therapy

- Measure child's body weight daily during hospital stay and look for change of trends (e.g., increasing or decreasing) to identify nutritional adequacy
- Observe the skin and tube insertion site around the indwelling enteral tube for inflammation, tenderness, drainage or skin breakdown
- Check the patency of the indwelling enteral tube for clogging from formula or medications that have been administered through the tube
- Assess the cognitive level, readiness and ability to participate in the procedure
- Identify the stress and anxiety level of both the parents and child (as appropriate for age)
- Self-preparation should be done with maintenance of standard precautions
- Environment should be clean, calm, well lighted and free from overcrowding
- Articles and necessary supplies should be collected at child's bed side or at procedure room, as feasible
- Preparation of parents: Explain the purpose of the procedure, necessary precautions and possible complications. Allow the parent to participate and involve during the procedure. Reply to the questions as asked
- Preparation of child: Explain the procedure in age-appropriate language. Make the child comfortable. Take care of child's fear and anxiety. Use diversional measures.

Performing the Steps of Procedure with Rationale/Point of Emphasis

For Indwelling Enteral Tube Site Skin Care with Dressing Change

1. Perform hand hygiene and arrange all necessary supplies for skin site care and dressing change of long-term enteral indwelling tube. Dressing may be used as institutional preference or as prescribed.
2. Assist the child into a comfortable supine position to allow easy access to the tube insertion site and surrounding skin. This helps to gain cooperation during procedure.
3. Perform hand hygiene. Wear gloves for maintenance of standard precautions.
4. Remove old dressing, if used and discard in appropriate container.
5. Inspect the tube insertion site for any abnormalities and drainage.
6. Prepare cleansing solution. For newly placed tube (under 5 days), pour sterile normal saline or sterile water into a small bowl. Soap and water can be used for healed tube site.
7. For newly placed tube, cleanse the enteral tube insertion site gently in rolling motion using cotton-tipped applicator dipped in sterile normal saline or sterile water. Continue cleansing until all crusts and drainage has been removed
   - For established healed tube site, use soap and water for cleansing the tube site during bath. This cleansing prevents skin breakdown and infections of the tube site. Avoid excessive pulling on the enteral tube as it can cause pain and irritation/injury to the gastric mucosa.
8. Dry the insertion site with sterile gauze pieces to reduce moisture for preventing bacterial growth at the tube site.
9. For skin-level G-tube devices, rotate the device in full circle to prevent the device from adhering to gastric mucosal lining and skin (Refer the manufacturer's instructions). Rotating the J-tubes or G-J tubes is not indicated to avoid potential kinking of the tube.
10. Apply skin barrier and/or antibiotic ointment around the tube site, as prescribed. After the skin has healed, there should be very little or no discharge from the stoma, thus eliminating the need to apply ointment or dressing. Recommendations vary on use of

dressing, ointment or skin barriers on skin at tube site as a part of daily routine care.

11. When dressings are used, apply "pre-split 2 × 2 gauze" dressing, around the tube over skin and secure loosely with tape. Loose application promotes air circulation to the skin, thereby reducing moisture at the site and protects site from irritation.
    Do not apply "cut 2 × 2 make dressing" because threads adhere to stoma margins. Assess dressing frequently for the need to change the dressing. The tube site can be left open to air without any dressing, which may help in maintenance of skin integrity.
12. For newly placed PEG-tubes, secure a loop of tubing to abdomen. It helps to avoid tension, pulling and accidental dislodgement at site, which would impair healing process.
13. Make the child comfortable. Discard all waste. Take care of reusable articles.
14. Remove gloves. Perform hand hygiene. Document the procedure and all findings.

For Gastrostomy or Jejunostomy Tube Change or Replacement

1. Perform hand hygiene and arrange all necessary supplies for tube replacement.
2. Assist the child into a comfortable supine position to allow easy access to the tube insertion site and surrounding skin. It helps to improve tolerance to the procedure.
3. Perform hand hygiene. Wear gloves to reduce transmission of microorganisms.
4. Remove old dressing, if used and discard in appropriate container.
5. Inspect the tube insertion site for any abnormalities and drainage.
6. Assist the surgeon to perform the tube change and replacement procedure. Competent and skilled nurse also can perform this procedure. The new enteral tube with mushroom-type tip, PEG and jejunostomy tube should be removed and replaced by surgeon. Confident nursing professional can change and replace balloon-type G-tube, skin-level devices and/or Foley's catheter used as gastrostomy tube.
7. For enteral tube removal, deflate the balloon by connecting appropriate size syringe to the balloon port. Pull the tube out through the stoma and discard the tube.
8. Test the balloon of new balloon-type enteral tube by injecting designated amount of sterile water through balloon port lumen and then deflate. This helps to ensure the patency of new balloon-type tube (such as Foley's catheter).
9. When inserting balloon-type tubes, lubricate 3–5 cm of distal tip of the new tube liberally with water-soluble lubricant to reduce friction, prevent trauma and facilitate insertion. Then gently insert the enteral tube into stoma of the abdomen until stomach contents drain out of open end.
10. Auscultate for bowel sounds after replacement of the tube for early detection of any complications. Secure the tube in position with external anchor as appropriate, such as gauze bolster or by increasing the diameter of the tube by wrapping foam tape around the tube at skin level. Anchor stabilizes the tube, prevents excessive movements, and may reduce pressure and potential risk of dislodgement of tube.
11. Inflate the balloon of the inserted enteral tube with appropriate amount of sterile water through the balloon port. It prevents the tube from slipping out of place.
12. Gently pull backon the tube until slight resistance is met for balloon-type tubes. This allows to place the balloon snugly against abdominal wall to prevent leakage of fluid.
13. Measure external tube length for baseline measurement for an unmarked tube and Foley's catheter. G-tubes with balloon have centimeter marking on the tube that allow for baseline measurement.
14. Apply tube closure or insert catheter adapter and cap. It closes the feeding system and prevent leakage.

15. Clean and dress the tube insertion site to maintain skin integrity (as described in previous part of this procedure).
16. Make the child comfortable. Discard all waste. Take care of reusable articles.
17. Remove gloves. Perform hand hygiene. Document the procedure and all findings.

Evaluation and Documentation

- Evaluate the following:
  - Child's health status, presence of any problems and correct position of enteral tube
  - Child's bowel sound at least every shift to assess the motility and GI functions for tolerance of enteral feeding
  - Child's clinical features of infection such as drainage, pus, inflammation or tenderness at the enteral indwelling tube insertion site
  - Child's intake and output details and compare with recommended requirements
  - Child's and parents' level of understanding and anxiety regarding health condition
  - Ability to perform home base care of permanent G-tube/J-tube, as required
  - Document the date and time of enteral tube insertion, dressing change, skin care provided, tube replacement, and size of the tube, insertion site position (e.g., left upper quadrant of abdomen), enteral tube length measurement, medication administered, intake and output details, all observational findings and child's response to the procedure.

Communication and Teaching for Homecare

- Communicate with child and parents about the gastrostomy/jejunostomy care and its related issues. Discuss about their concerns and further plan of management
- Teach the child and parents about hygienic care, dietary intake, enteral tube feeding, continued stoma care and skin care at home, medications to be continued, possible complications related to stoma, need for necessary medical help and plan of follow-up visits. Explain about further treatment or surgery, if required for the child.

Demonstrate to the parents and check the ability to perform the required stoma care, skin care and tube feeding at home in simple ways as per level of understanding of the parents or family members.

If feasible, teach parents how to replace a dislodged tube. Provide the family with a set of Foley's catheter that are of same size and one size smaller than the inserted gastrostomy or jejunostomy tube to use as a short-term replacement, in case accidental dislodgement. Give emergency contact number of nearest health facility during discharge.

PROCEDURE–10: CARE OF CHILDREN WITH TRACHEOSTOMY

Clinical Guidelines

- Tracheostomy is a surgical opening of the trachea to provide and secure an open airway. It is performed in emergency situations (such as in case of upper airway obstruction) or electively to replace a temporary airway provided by endotracheal tube which is in place for more than several days or weeks
- Tracheostomy is indicated in case of respiratory muscle paralysis, child requiring long-term mechanical ventilation, spinal cord injury, upper airway obstruction, face and neck surgery or burns and carcinoma in neck or thyroid
- The purpose of tracheostomy care includes: (a) to keep the airway patent by suctioning, (b) to remove secretions, (c) to cleanse the tracheostomy area, and (d) to prevent infections and skin breakdown around the tracheostomy
- An assistant is always needed when tracheostomy care is performed. Sterile/aseptic technique must be followed during tracheostomy care
- Tracheostomy care include stoma care, cleaning of outer and inner cannula,

suctioning, tie change, and tracheostomy tube change, as required to provide safe effective management of the airway

- Vital signs of the child should be monitored frequently after the surgical intervention of tracheostomy. Warm humidified oxygen must be administered. Child is placed in semi-Fowler position to promote ease of breathing. Chest physiotherapy may be needed to promote aeration of lungs
- Meticulous oral hygiene must be maintained to a child with tracheostomy, along with other hygienic care, nutritious diet, adequate fluid intake and infection control measures
- After tracheostomy tube placement, stoma integrity and the area under the tracheostomy ties should be assessed every 2 hours for first 48 hours and then every 8 hours. Cleaning of fresh stoma should be completed every 8 hours or more frequently if indicated by the accumulation of secretions
- Frequency of tracheostomy tie changes varies from child to child based on type and condition of the tie used (soiled or wet or unraveling ends)
- Tracheostomy suctioning must be performed on the basis of clinical assessment and individual characteristics of the child (i.e., age, muscular and neurologic status, activity level, ability to generate an effective cough, viscosity and quantity of mucus and maturity of the stoma). Always perform suctioning if the child exhibits difficulty in breathing and if there is sound of mucus in the tracheostomy tube that cannot be removed by coughing by the child or when there is adventitious breath sounds

  In children with no evidence of secretions, perform a minimum of suctioning, at morning and at bedtime to check the patency of the tube. Sterile technique should also be followed during suctioning. At home, clean technique can be followed. Premarked suction catheters are recommended to ensure insertion of the catheter to the required depth. Routine instillation of normal saline in the tracheostomy tube would not be initiated to stimulate cough, to loosen or to make the secretions thin or to serve as vehicle to remove mucus
- Tracheostomy tube changes are performed to reduce the incidence of tube occlusion from increased secretions and to decrease the possibility of airway infections and airway granuloma. It is usually done about 5 days after the tracheostomy is performed and then weekly or as required. It should be done 2–3 hours after meals. Depth of suctioning should be reassessed and measured with any change in tracheostomy tube size.

  If accidental decannulation occurs, the tracheostomy tube is replaced with a tube of same size or one size smaller. If a tracheostomy tube cannot be placed, the child must be intubated. All tracheostomy tubes have 15 mm universal adapter to allow manual bag ventilation in an emergency
- All emergency equipment must be available at all times for suctioning, ventilatory breaths, for recannulation with extra tracheostomy tubes (one same size as being used by the child and one smaller size), tracheal dilator and tracheostomy obturator
- Tracheostomy tubes are available as metal, silicone and polyvinyl chloride (PVC) tubes. The tube has three parts, i.e., outer cannula, inner cannula and obturator. It can be cuffed and non-cuffed or plain. Type and size of tracheostomy tube is selected, based on child's age, indications of tracheostomy and other associated conditions
- If the child is discharged from hospital with permanent tracheostomy, then before discharge two adults family members who will be consistent caregivers at home must be trained in all aspects of child's care with tracheostomy
- Teach the parents and child about communication pattern. Question with simple yes and no answers, hand signals, simple sign language and board writing, as feasible

should be taught to the child for practice. Later, in permanent tracheostomy child is taught how to cover the tracheostomy with the cuff deflated to permit vocalization.

Equipment Required

For Tracheostomy Stoma Care and Cleaning of Cannula

- Hand hygiene supplies and PPE for health professionals involved in tracheostomy care
- A sterile covered tray containing sterile articles, such as gloves, gauze pieces, cotton swabs, towel, small container/bowl to soak inner cannula, sterile pipe cleaner, gauze pieces/gauze pads, small sponges, gauze or cotton swab applicators, small bowl/container with sterile water, washcloth, a small bowl with sterile normal saline, split gauze dressings, dressing forceps, tracheal dilator, extra tracheostomy tubes (one same size as being used by the child and one smaller size) and one extra obturator
- For changing tracheostomy ties: A sterile covered tray with sterile scissors, split gauze dressing and Twill tape or Velcro tape (as per hospital policy)
- Transfer forceps or lifter to handle sterile items
- A clean tray with shoulder roll or small rolled towel, bottle with hydrogen peroxide solution (1.5%), bottle of normal saline
- Stethoscope and manual ventilation bag
- Equipment for suctioning and oxygen therapy
- Waste disposal containers
- Documentation sheet for tracheostomy care and child case sheet.

For Suctioning in Tracheostomy

- Hand hygiene supplies and PPE for health professionals involved in tracheostomy suctioning and necessary care
- A sterile covered tray containing all sterile articles such as sterile gloves, suction catheters, suction tubing, gauze pieces, dressing, a small bowl with sterile normal saline, and a small bowl with sterile water
- Transfer forceps or lifter to handle sterile items
- Container for collection of secretions during suctioning
- Shoulder roll or small rolled towel
- Suction machine with all accessories and power connection
- Tracheostomy stoma care supplies, if necessary
- Articles for oxygen therapy and oxygen source
- Stethoscope and manual ventilation bag
- Waste disposal containers
- Documentation sheet for tracheostomy care and child case sheet.

For Tracheostomy Tube Change

- Hand hygiene supplies and PPE for health professionals involved in tracheostomy tube change and required stoma care
- A sterile covered tray with two sterile tracheostomy tubes of appropriate size with obturator in place, tracheal dilator, scissors, syringe, gloves
- Articles for tracheostomy tie change
- Tracheostomy stoma care supplies, if needed
- Transfer forceps or lifter to handle sterile items
- Water soluble lubricant, normal saline bottle
- Shoulder roll or small rolled towel
- Equipment for suctioning and oxygen therapy
- Stethoscope and manual ventilation bag
- Waste disposal containers as per BMW guidelines
- Documentation sheet for tracheostomy care and child case sheet

Assessment and Preparation

- Assess previous history of child's condition and indications of tracheostomy, current health status, care needs in relation to tracheostomy, condition of stoma and skin under the ties, need for suctioning the tube, range of motion of neck, breath sounds and work of breathing. Check the date of last tube change and presence of any problems.

Assess anxiety and level of understanding of both child and parents and their ability to perform this procedure of tracheostomy care
- Self-preparation should be done with hand hygiene and use of appropriate PPE. Ensure one assistant is ready to assist during the procedure of tracheostomy care
- Environment should be clean, calm, well lighted and free of overcrowding
- All necessary supplies should be arranged at the bedside of the child for stoma care, suctioning, tie change and replacement of tracheostomy tube with all emergency items
- Preparation of parents: Explain the purpose and precautions of tracheostomy care in details. Answer to their questions. Encourage the parent to participate during tracheostomy care. Teach the parents in simple language to perform the tracheostomy care at home after discharge in case of permanent tracheostomy. Allow the parents to stay with the child, as feasible
- Preparation of child: Make the child clean and comfortable. Explain the purpose of tracheostomy care in simple language as per understanding level. Use distraction measures to enhance cooperation. Perform suctioning of the tube before initiating tracheostomy care, as needed.

Performing the Steps of Procedure with Rationale/Point of Emphasis

Tracheostomy Stoma Care, Cleaning of Cannula and Tie Change

1. Perform hand hygiene and gather all necessary supplies near child's bed.
2. Open the sterile supplies pack carefully to prevent contamination. Take help of assistant to maintain asepsis and for easy completion of the procedure.
3. Place the child in supine position with neck slightly extended using shoulder roll. This straightens the airway and brings tracheostomy tube forward.
4. Perform hand hygiene. Don appropriate PPE and gloves. Face shield should be used if the child is infectious or has copious secretions.
5. Ensure one assistant is ready to assist during the procedure of tracheostomy care.
6. Cleanse the tracheostomy stoma and outer cannula as follows:
   - Cleanse the external end of the tracheostomy tube (outer cannula) with hydrogen peroxide-soaked gauze sponge to remove mucus and crusts. Make only one sweep with each gauze pad before discarding
   - Suction the tracheostomy tube before doing stoma care, if secretions presents, as needed
   - Clean the stoma area with hydrogen peroxide-soaked gauze sponges. It will assist in loosening dry crusts. Make only one sweep with each gauze pad before discarding
   - Use sterile cotton swab applicators to loosen and remove crusts from stoma site
   - Clean the stoma area with sterile water-soaked gauze sponges. Make only one sweep with each gauze pad before discarding. Ensure that all hydrogen peroxide is removed
   - Dry the stoma area with dry gauze sponges. Wetness will promote infections and skin irritation. Make only one sweep with each gauze pad before discarding
   - Use water-soaked gauze pads or wash-cloth to cleanse the neck under the ties. It maintains cleanliness of the skin and helps to prevent skin breakdown
   - Dry the neck area with dry towel or gauze pads. Moisture under the ties will increase bacterial growth and cause skin irritation.
7. Perform cleaning of the inner cannula as follows (Refer **Figs. 4.4A and B**):
   - Remove the inner cannula. Inner cannula designed for reuse can be removed for cleaning
   - If the inner cannula is reusable, clean that cannula by soaking it in a sterile bowl of half-strength hydrogen perox-

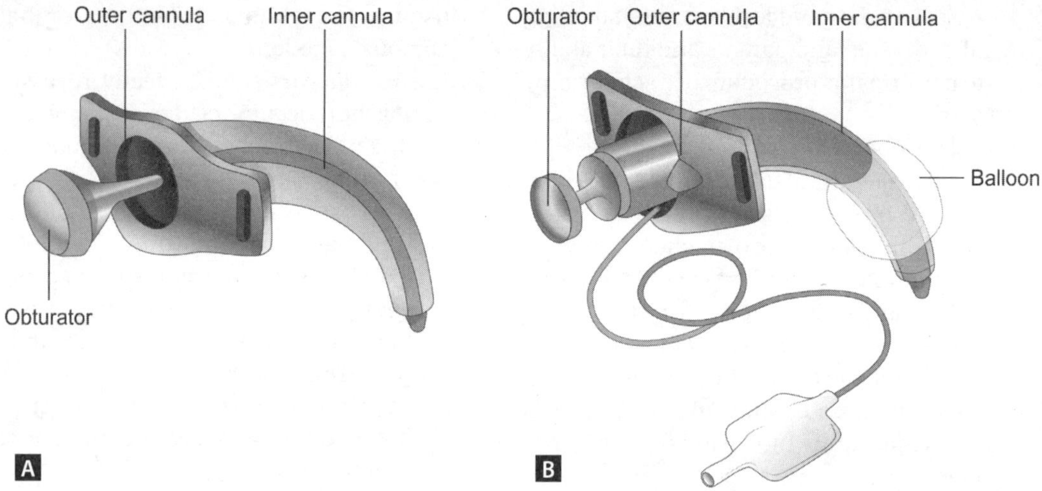

Figs. 4.4A and B: Parts of tracheostomy tube. A. Uncuffed. B. Cuffed.

ide solution and scrubbing. It helps to cleanse encrusted secretions from the lumen of the cannula. Use soft sterile brush for metal cannula or sterile pipe cleaners to remove all secretions from the inner cannula. Use of brush can damage plastic inner cannula

- Rinse the inner cannula in a bowl of sterile water. This helps to remove remaining debris and hydrogen peroxide solution from the cannula
- Reinsert the inner cannula. Turn the cannula 90 degrees from its usual orientation. Introduce the tip into the stoma and slowly advance the cannula while rotating it back 90 degrees to its final orientation. Lock the cannula into place by either pushing it in or twisting or squeezing the clips and clipping the cannula to the tracheostomy (Follow manufacturer instructions). Locking mechanism is used to prevent accidental removal of the tracheostomy tube.

8. Changing Tracheostomy ties:
   - Cut the old ties while holding tracheostomy tube securely in place. A second person must assist by holding the tracheostomy tube. This will decrease the chance of accidental dislodging of tracheostomy tube and minimizes irritation and coughing due to tube manipulation
   - Remove the old ties carefully and replace the tracheostomy ties to keep the neck area clean and dry. Follow manufacturer instructions for Velcro ties. For Twill ties, grasp slit end of sterile/clean tape and thread one end through the opening on the side of the tracheostomy tube. Pull other end of tape securely through the slit end of the tape. Repeat on other side. Securely tie the tapes with square knot on the side or back of the neck. Tying the tie too tightly may lead the vascular obstruction and skin breakdown. Tying too loosely may lead to decannulation
   - If split gauze dressing is prescribed as dressing under outer cannula, then secure the dressing in place. Use prepackaged split gauze to prevent threads to pull away and lodged in the trachea. Dressing is recommended if the child has increased secretions. But there is chance of stoma infections due to dressing moisture
9. Dispose all waste in appropriate containers. Take care of reusable items.
10. Remove gloves and used PPE. Perform hand hygiene.
11. Make the child comfortable. Remove the shoulder roll and elevate the head at 30

degrees to facilitate easy breathing. Assess for presence of any problems.

12. Document the procedure and all related findings.

Suctioning of Tracheostomy Tube

1. Perform hand hygiene. Gather the necessary supplies near the child.
2. Verify that the suction machine manometer is set between 80 and 100 mm Hg.
3. Ensure all necessary articles for suctioning are well functioning. Suction catheter should be one half of the internal diameter of tracheostomy tube. Correct size suction catheter minimizes the chance of creating negative pressure that could lead to atelectasis.
4. Place the child in supine position with neck slightly extended. Older children can raise his or her head into "sniffing position". Extension of neck enables the suction catheter to more easily follow the natural curve of the trachea.
5. Open the sterile tray containing necessary articles for suctioning tracheostomy tube. Pour small amount of sterile normal saline into small sterile bowl/disposable container. Normal saline is used to lubricate the tip of the suction catheter and to cleanse the catheter during suctioning.
6. Perform hand hygiene. Wear protective gear/PPE, and don sterile gloves.
7. Ensure one assistant is ready to assist during the procedure of tracheostomy suctioning.
8. Determine the length of catheter to be inserted in the tracheostomy tube during suctioning. Shallow suctioning can be done by inserting the catheter just into the hub of the tracheostomy tube to remove secretions that the child has coughed up to the opening of the tube. Premeasured technique involves inserting the catheter to a premeasured depth to the tip of the tracheostomy tube. Deep suctioning involves inserting the catheter until resistance is met, but it can cause epithelial damage.
9. Pick up the sterile suction catheter and attach to the suction tubing. Do not touch the part of suction catheter which will be inserted into the tracheostomy tube.
10. Ensure suction tubing is attached and suction machine is turn on with functioning.
11. Lubricate the suction catheter with normal saline for easy passage into the tube.
12. If the child has a mask applied over the tracheostomy tube to deliver oxygen and humidification, move the mask aside during suctioning to access entrance into the tube.
13. Insert the suction catheter gently by twirling or rotating the catheter between the fingers and thumb. This reduces friction and helps in easy insertion of catheter.
14. Use premeasured technique to insert catheter to the exact depth into tracheostomy tube.
15. Do not apply suction while the catheter is being inserted.
16. Apply intermittent suction during withdrawing the suction catheter. Gently rotate or twirl the catheter between thumb and forefinger and withdraw the catheter.
17. Complete suctioning in 5 seconds or less using premeasured technique. Prolong suctioning results in hypoxia and can lead to atelectasis. In deep suctioning, complete suctioning in 15 seconds or less.
18. Do not introduce saline into the tracheostomy tube in an attempt to loosen the mucus.
19. Rinse the suction catheter tip in a container of sterile water. It helps in unclogging the catheter and the tracheostomy tube with mucus.
20. Assess respiratory status (respiratory rate, breath sounds, oxygen saturation) and determine the need for post-suctioning hyperventilation or hyperoxygenation breaths (using bag ventilation).
21. Repeat the suctioning procedure until breath sounds are relatively clear. Too many suction attempts can irritate the mucosal lining of the trachea.
22. Cleanse the suction catheter and tubing (as required) by placing the tip of catheter in the container of sterile water and applying suction. It helps to prevent contamination.

23. Detach the suction catheter from suction tubing and dispose. Turn off the suction machine. Dispose all wastes and disposable items. Take care of reusable articles.
24. Discard gloves and protective gear. Perform hand hygiene.
25. Remove the child's shoulder roll and place the child in comfortable position with head elevated on 30 degrees to facilitate easy breathing.
26. Document the procedure of tracheostomy suctioning and all associated findings.

Tracheostomy Tube Change

1. Perform hand hygiene and assemble all necessary supplies near the child's bed
2. Select appropriate size tracheostomy tube. The tube must fit into the airway and fulfill the functional need of the child. Tracheostomy tube size and type is determined based on child's tracheal size and shape, indications for the tracheostomy, lung mechanics, upper airway resistance and the needs of the child for speech, ventilation and airway clearance. During second replacement of tube at bedside, select next smaller size from that of present use, because the stoma may become slightly smaller over time
3. Place the child in supine position with neck slightly extended using shoulder roll
4. Inspect tracheostomy tube for stiffness, cracks, splits and damage. Damaged tubes must be discarded and replaced with new tube
5. Perform hand hygiene and wear appropriate protective gear and sterile gloves
6. Ensure one assistant is ready to assist during the procedure of tracheostomy tube change
7. Attach tie to the opening on one end of new tracheostomy tube (see previous part of this procedure). Ensure that the obturator is inserted in the new tube
8. Lubricate the end of the new tracheostomy tube with water-based lubricant or as per prescription to prevent trauma to tracheal tissue during insertion. Place back of the new tracheostomy tube in open pack and prevent contamination
9. Remove old ties with precaution to prevent skin injury. Assistant should hold the tracheostomy tube in place
10. Remove old tracheostomy tube. Insert new tube gently and quickly, pushing back and down in an acting motion to follow the natural curve of the trachea
11. Stabilize the flanges of the outer cannula with the fingers of one hand
12. Immediately remove the obturator with other hand, to keep the tracheostomy patent
13. Assess the patency of the new inserted tracheostomy tube using stethoscope to auscult the air entry/air movement and breath sounds. If there is no air movement, the procedure will need to be repeated. Tracheal dilator can be used to keep the trachea open. A tracheostomy tube whose distal position is not collinear with the trachea may cause complications, such as esophageal obstruction, partial occlusion of the tracheostomy tube tip by the tracheal wall, tracheoesophageal fistula, and tracheal wall erosion
14. Hold the outer cannula of the tracheostomy tube in place and secure the tracheostomy ties. Assistant should help to hold the tube in place or to secure the ties
15. If a cuffed tracheostomy tube is used, inflate the cuff to the proper volume using a syringe. Cuff pressure should be kept as low as possible to protect the airway
16. Provide ventilation/oxygenation breaths as needed using manual ventilation bag based on child's respiratory status or presence of respiratory distress during the procedure
17. Dispose all wastes and disposable items. Take care of reusable supplies
18. Discard gloves and protective gear. Perform hand hygiene
19. Place the child in comfortable position. Remove shoulder roll. Allow the child's head to keep elevated on 30 degrees to facilitate easy breathing

20. Document the procedure of tracheostomy tube replacement and all related findings.

Evaluation and Documentation

- Evaluate child's tolerance for the procedure and present health status. Compare with previous findings. Report to appropriate authority for necessary interventions
- Document and report the followings:
  - Date and time of the procedure performed for tracheostomy care
  - Child's tolerance and any difficulties encountered while performing the care
  - Use of oxygenation during the procedure
  - Quality of breath sounds and respiratory status before and after procedure
  - Appearance of stoma and skin under ties (irritation, redness, edema, subcutaneous air)
  - Characteristics of secretions (color, consistency, odor)
  - Depth used to insert premeasured catheter during tracheostomy suctioning
  - Size and type of the tracheostomy tube in place or replaced
  - Type of tracheostomy tie used and presence of dressing around stoma site
  - Teaching completed for the parents/family members and their response regarding involvement and participation in tracheostomy care of the child

Communication and Teaching for Homecare

- Communicate with the child and parents/family members about child's present health status, condition of tracheostomy, procedure performed, important findings, further plan of management and discharge planning from health facility/hospital
- Teach the child/parents/family members about the followings for the care at home:
  - Explain the basic anatomy of trachea and indications of tracheostomy for the child
  - Discuss about identification of respiratory problems (change in respiratory rate, cyanosis, difficulty in breathing) and other signs of illness (fever, change in amount, color, odor and consistency of secretions, presence of any bleeding from tracheostomy stoma, etc.) which required immediate medical attention
  - Demonstrate tracheostomy tube cleaning (with soap, warm water), drying and disinfection using commercial disinfectant or by boiling, if suitable
  - Explain about the actions to be taken at home in the event of tube obstruction, accidental decannulation, respiratory distress, bleeding and other problems
  - Demonstrate use of gloves, method of suctioning, stoma care, and portable oxygen therapy, use of manual resuscitation bag and replacement of tracheostomy tube, if feasible. Consider the ability of the parents or any other family members to teach these techniques depending upon their understanding level
  - Discuss about recommended diet, fluid intake, permitted activities, hygienic care, cleanliness, infection control practices (hand washing, use of hand rub, disposal of waste) and safety measures (avoid all dust, smoke, powder, pet hairs, sprays, water sports)
  - Inform about the vendor to arrange necessary supplies of tracheostomy care at home and to keep all emergency supplies related to tracheostomy care with the child in hand
  - Instruct about plan for follow-up care (date, time, place, documents)
  - Inform about further treatment plan for definitive management of the underlying condition which necessitate tracheostomy of the child
  - Give emergency contact number of nearest health facility during discharge

APPENDICES

Appendix – I: WHO Growth Chart for Boys

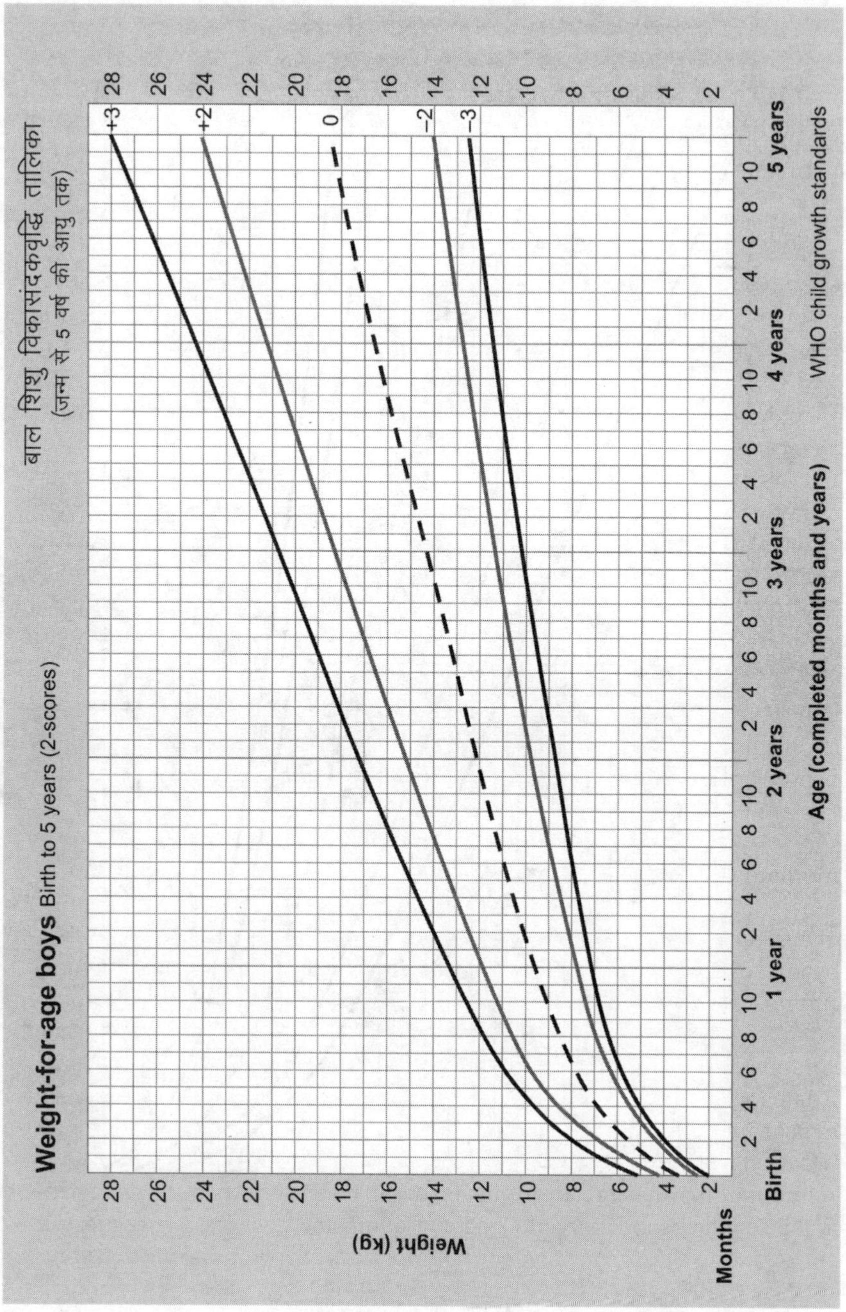

(For color version, see Plate 2)

Appendix – II: WHO Growth Chart for Girls

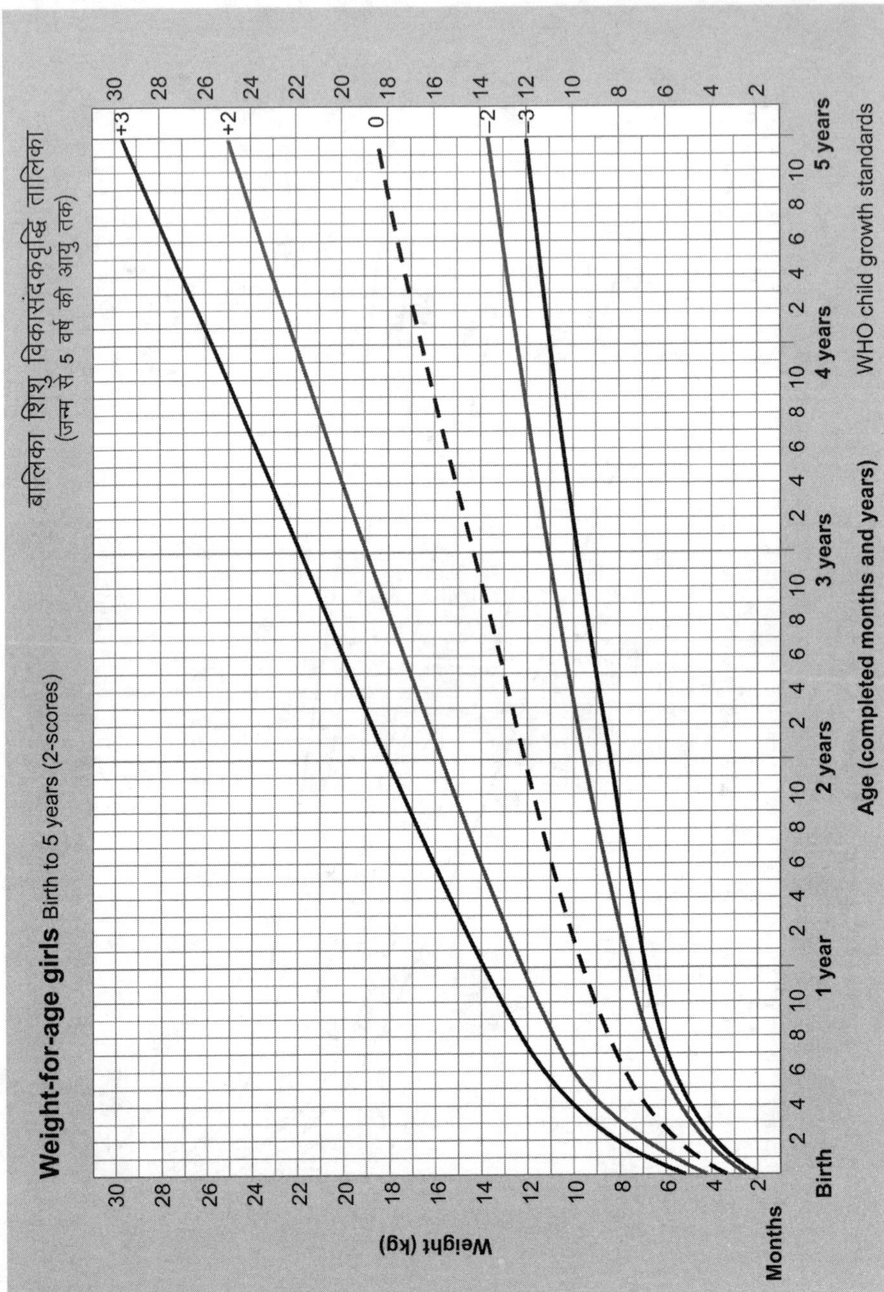

(For color version, see Plate 3)

Appendix – III: Average Height and Weight of Indian Boys and Girls

	Height in centimeters		*Weight in kilograms*	
Age in years	*Boys*	*Girls*	*Boys*	*Girls*
1	72.5	72.5	8.5	7.5
2	87.5	86.6	12.6	12.3
3	96.2	95.7	14.6	14.4
4	103.4	103.2	16.5	16.4
5	108.7	108.1	18.5	18.4
6	118.9	117.3	22.1	21.4
7	123.9	122.7	24.5	24.8
8	127.9	126.8	26.4	26.1
9	133.6	132.3	30.0	29.7
10	138.5	138.5	32.4	33.5
11	143.4	144.1	35.3	36.5
12	148.9	150.3	38.8	42.6
13	154.9	153.0	42.9	44.4
14	161.7	155.1	48.3	46.7
15	165.3	155.3	52.2	47.2
16	168.4	155.4	55.5	49.8
17	169.9	156.4	59.0	49.9
18	169.9	156.8	61.1	50.1

Source: ICMR—Growth and development of Indian infants and children

Appendix – IV: Five Moments of Hand Hygiene

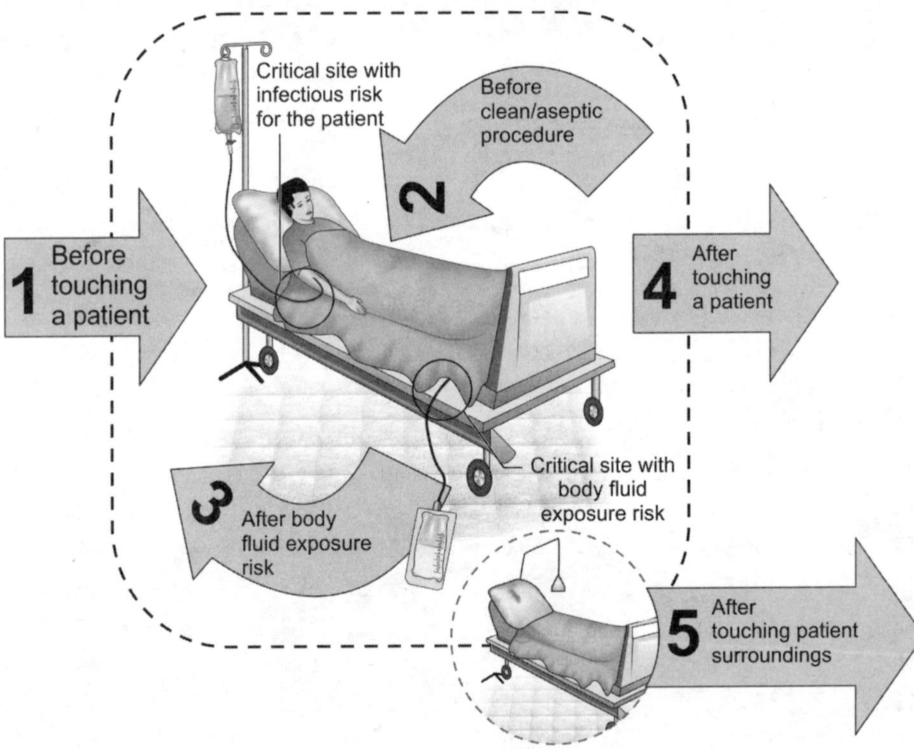

Appendix – V: WHO Steps of Hand Wash

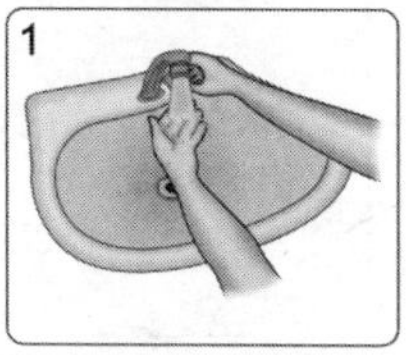

Wet hands with water

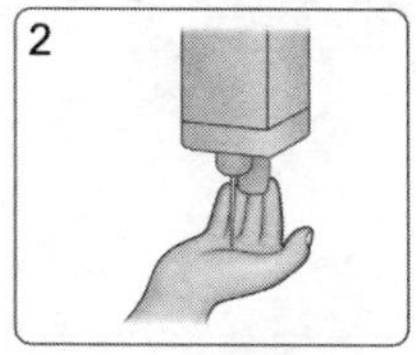

Apply enough soap to cover all hand surface

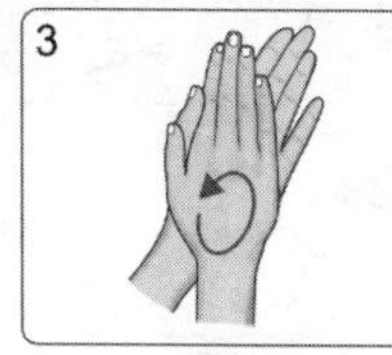

Rub hands palm to palm

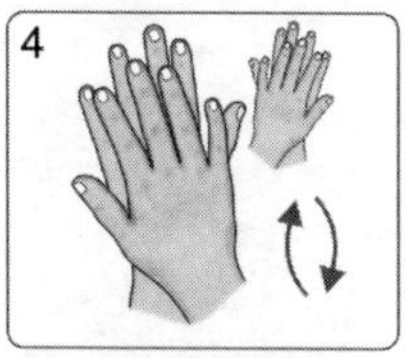

Right palm over left dorsum with interlaced fingers and vice versa

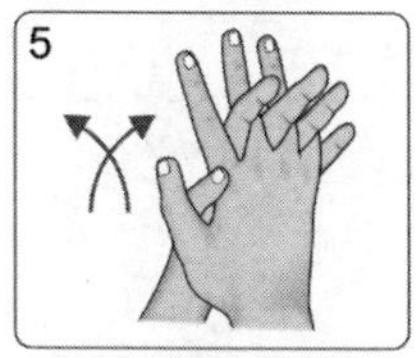

Palm to palm with fingers interlaced

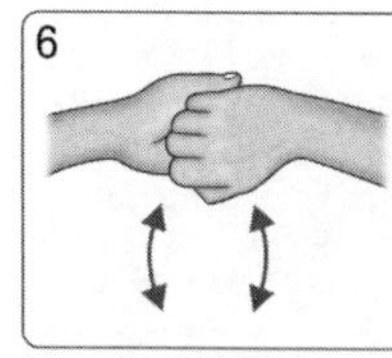

Backs of fingers to opposing palms with fingers interlocked

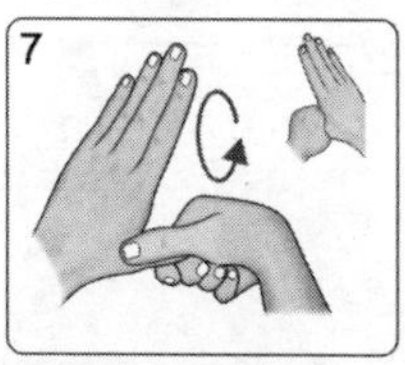

Rotational rubbing of left thumb clasped in right palm and vice versa

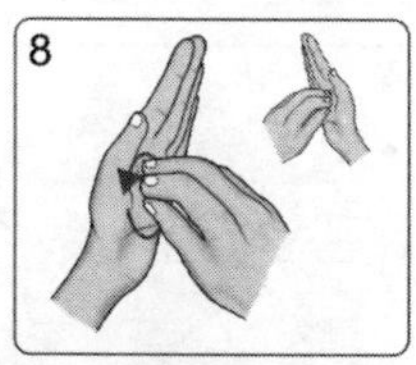

Rotational rubbing, backwards and forwards with clasped fingers of right hand in left palm and vice versa

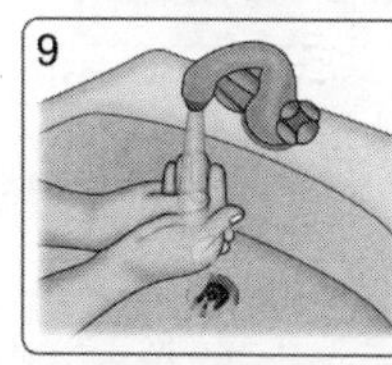

Rinse hands with water

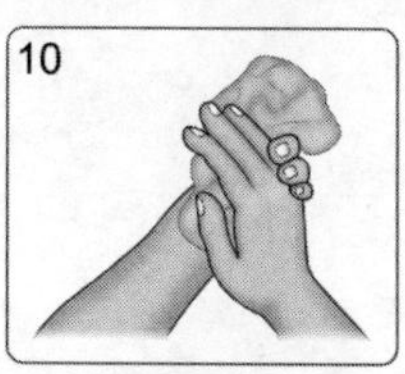

Dry thoroughly with a single use towel

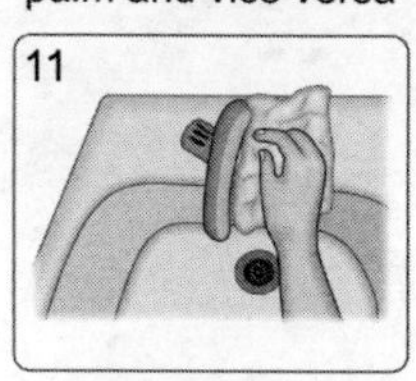

Use towel to turn off faucet

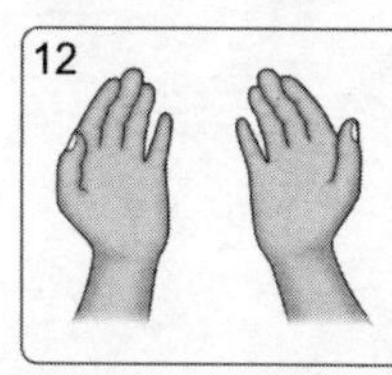

...and your hands are safe

Appendix – VI: WHO Steps of Hand Rub

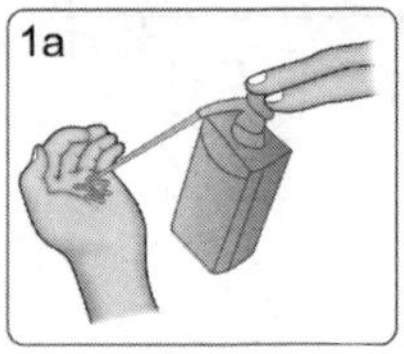

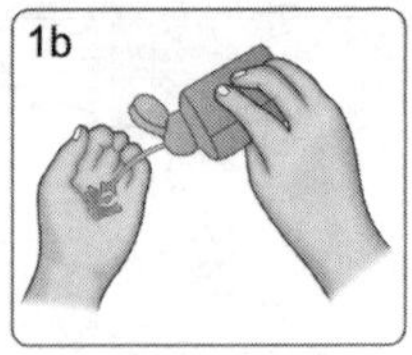

Apply a palmful of the product in a cupped hand, covering all surfaces

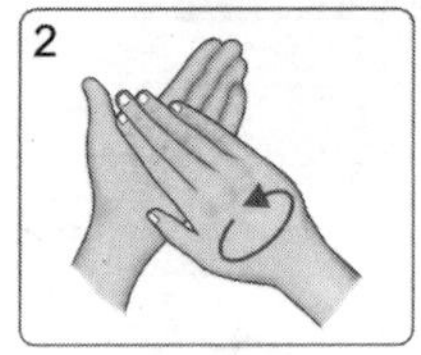

Rub hands palm to palm

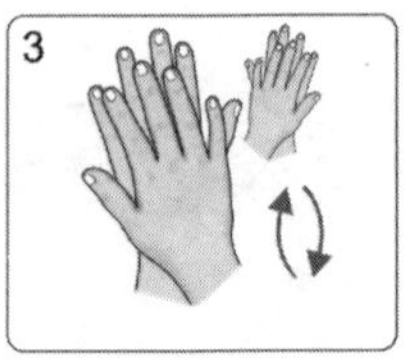

Right palm over left dorsum with interlaced fingers and vice versa

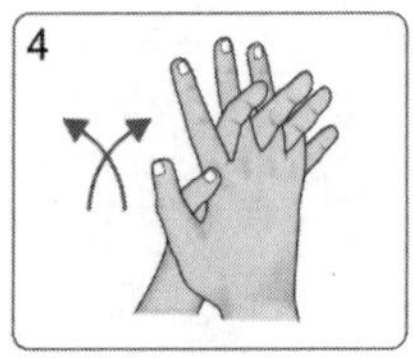

Palm to palm with fingers interlaced

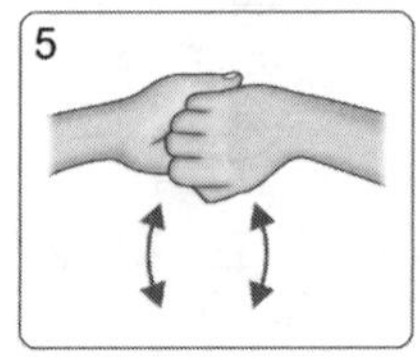

Backs of fingers to opposing palms with fingers interlocked

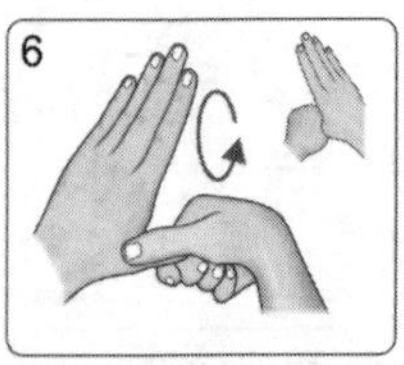

Rotational rubbing of left thumb clasped in right palm and vice versa

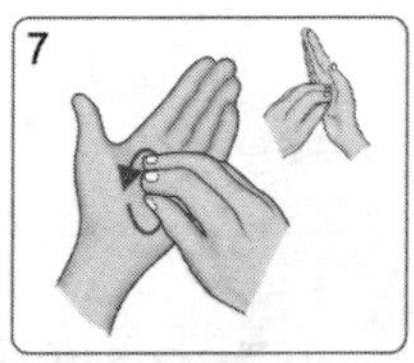

Rotational rubbing, backwards and forwards with clasped fingers of right hand in left palm and vice versa

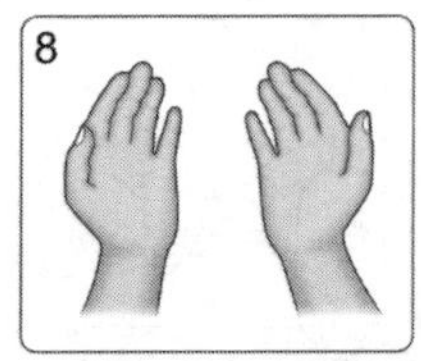

Once dry, your hands are safe

Appendix – VII: WHO's The Glove Pyramid

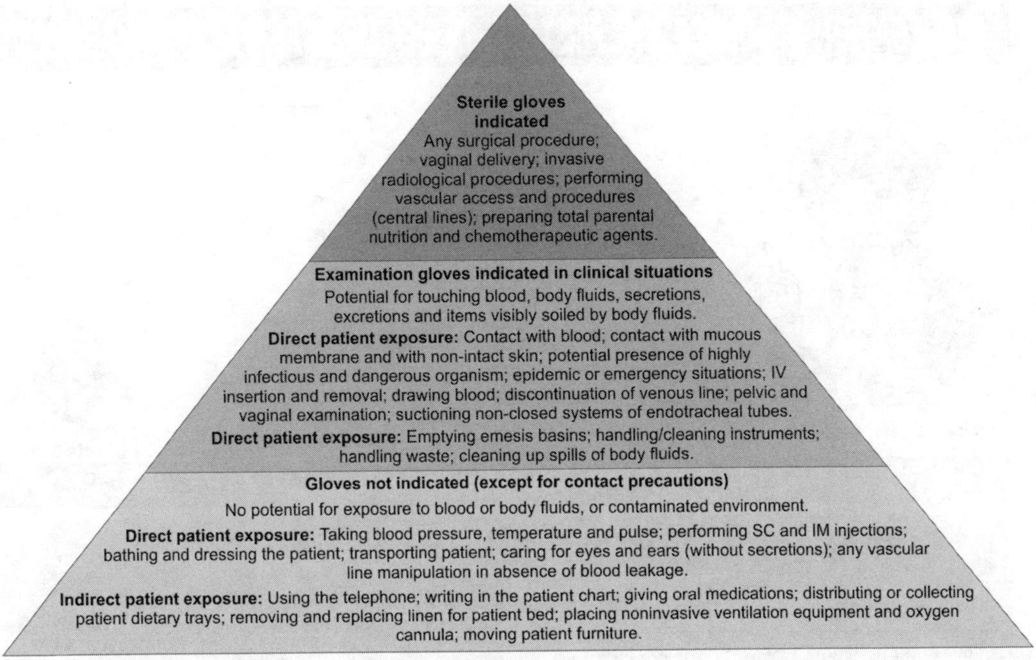

Appendix – VIII: Segregation of Bio-Medical Waste (BMW)

SEGREGATION AT SOURCE - THE FIRST STEP IN BIO - MEDICAL WASTE MANAGEMENT

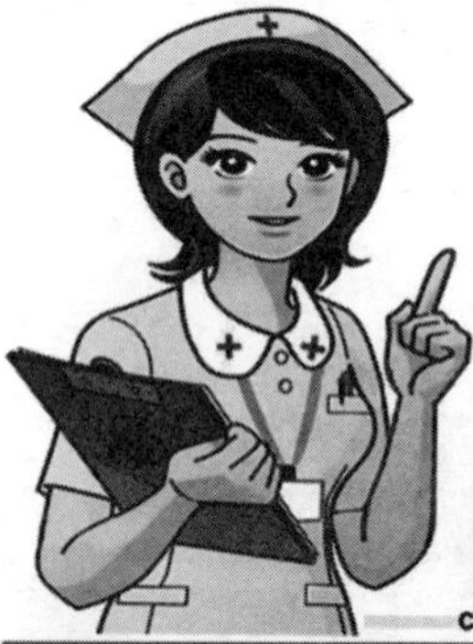

CYTOTOXIC HAZARD

BIO-HAZARD

THINK BEFORE YOU THROW

SEGREGATION OF BIO-MEDICAL WASTE

Yellow waste	White (PPC)	Red waste	Blue waste
• Human body parts • Placenta • Human tissues • Cotton waste • Bandages • Specimens • Non-chlorinated blood bags • Discarded-lenen, beddings, infected mattresses and clothings • Solid plaster, casts • Expired medicines and cytotoxic drugs • Any surgical wastes	• Needles after burning • Blades • Lancets • Scalpels • Any discarded and contaminated metal sharps	• Disposable syringe without needle • Saline bottles • Urine bag • I.V tubes • Catheters • Stents • Gloves • Aprons • Any other tubings	• Broken/discarded glass • Vials and ampules • Glass bottles excluding Cytotoxic wastes • Broken slides • Metallic body implants • Any other glassware

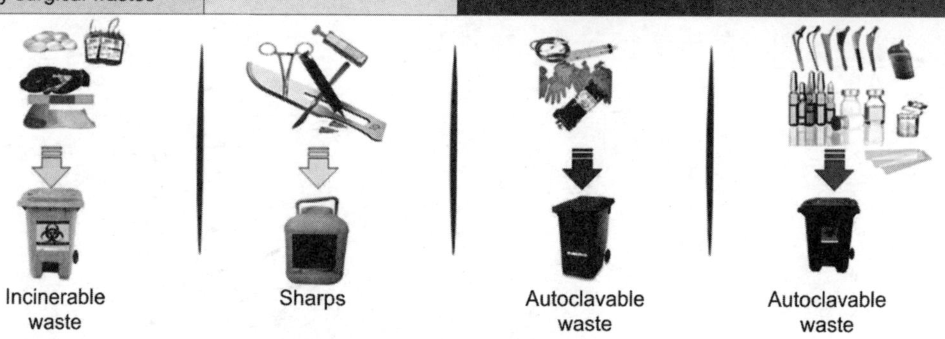

(For color version, see Plate 4)

Appendix – IX: Neonatal Resuscitation Algorithm

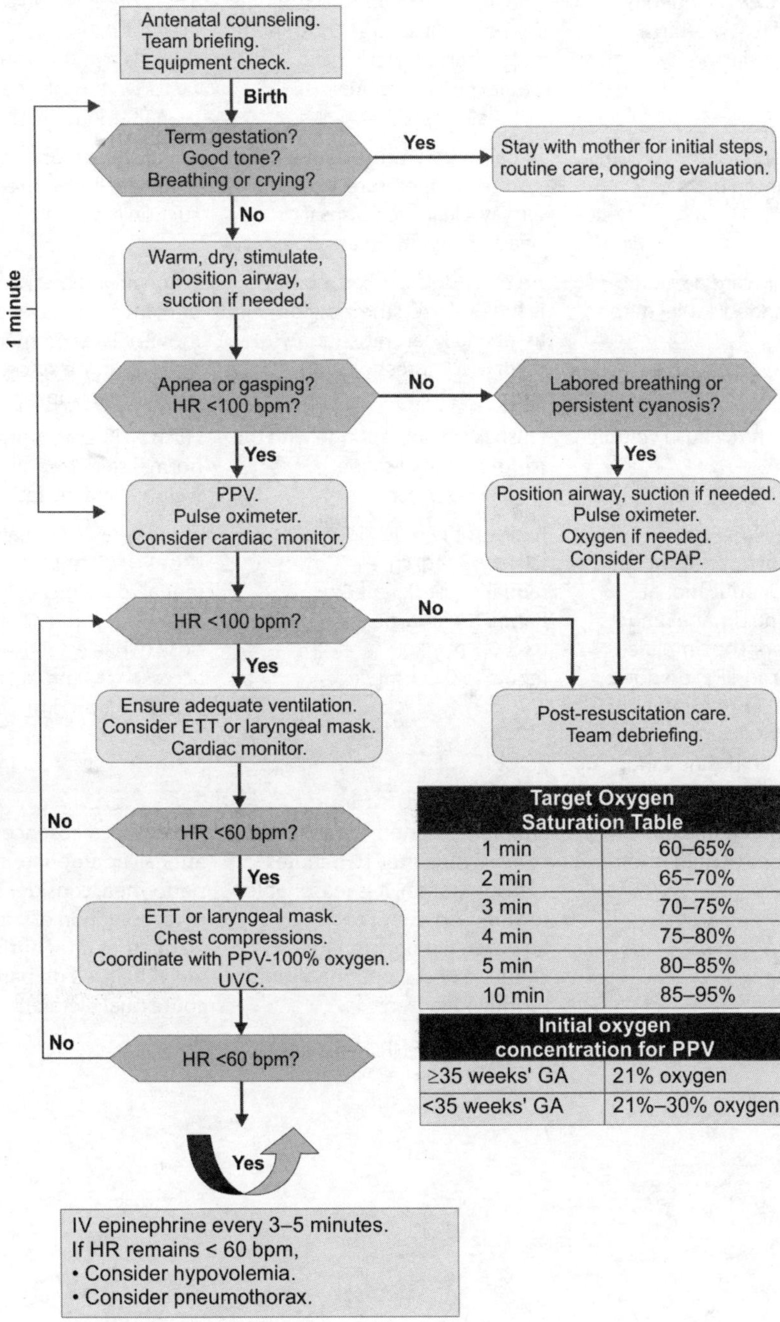

Target Oxygen Saturation Table	
1 min	60–65%
2 min	65–70%
3 min	70–75%
4 min	75–80%
5 min	80–85%
10 min	85–95%

Initial oxygen concentration for PPV	
≥35 weeks' GA	21% oxygen
<35 weeks' GA	21%–30% oxygen

Overview of significant NRP 8th Edition practice changes		
Change	*NRP 7th Edition*	*NRP 8th Edition*
Umbilical cord management plan added to 4 pre-birth questions, replacing "How many babies?"	The 4 pre-birth questions: (1) Gestational age? (2) Amniotic fluid clear? (3) How many babies? (4) Additional risk factors?	The 4 pre-birth questions: (1) Gestational age? (2) Amniotic fluid clear? (3) Additional risk factors? (4) Umbilical cord management plan?
Initial steps reordered to better reflect common practice.	Initial steps: Warm and maintain normal temperature, position airway, clear secretions if needed, dry, stimulate.	Initial steps: Warm, dry, stimulate, position airway, suction if needed.
An electronic cardiac monitor is recommended earlier in the algorithm	An electronic cardiac monitor is the preferred method for assessing heart rate during cardiac compressions.	When an alternative airway becomes necessary, a cardiac monitor is recommended for the most accurate assessment of the baby's heart rate.
Epinephrine IV/IO flush volume increased	Flush IV/IO epinephrine with 0.5 to 1 mL normal saline.	Flush IV/IO epinephrine with 3 mL normal saline (applies to all weights and gestational ages).
Epinephrine IV/IO and endotracheal doses have been simplified for educational efficiency. The dosage range is unchanged. The simplified doses (IV/IO and ET) do not represent an endorsement of any particular dose within the recommended dosing range. Additional research is needed.	Range for IV or IO dose = 0.01-0.03 mg/kg (equal to 0.1-0.3 mL/kg) Range for endotracheal dose = 0.05-0.1 mg/kg (equal to 0.5-1 mL/kg).	The suggested initial IV or IO dose = 0.02 mg/kg (equal to 0.2 mL/kg) The suggested endotracheal dose (while establishing vascular access) = 0.1 mg/kg (equal to 1 mL/kg).
Expanded timeframe for cessation of resuscitative efforts	If there is a confirmed absence of heart rate after 10 minutes of resuscitation, it is reasonable to stop resuscitative efforts; however, the decision to continue or discontinue should be individualized.	If confirmed absence of HR after all appropriate steps performed, consider cessation of resuscitation efforts around 20 minutes after birth (decision individualized on patient and contextual factors).

(IV: intravenous; IO: intraosseous; ET: endotracheal; HR: heart rate)

Appendix – X: New Ballard Score

MATURATIONAL ASSESSMENT OF GESTATIONAL AGE (New Ballard Score)

NAME ____________ SEX ____________
HOSPITAL NO. ____________ BIRTH WEIGHT ____________
RACE ____________ LENGTH ____________
DATE/TIME OF BIRTH ____________ HEAD CIRCUMFERENCE ____________
DATE/TIME OF EXAM ____________ EXAMINER ____________
AGE WHEN EXAMINED ____________
APGAR SCORE: 1 MINUTE ________ 5 MINUTES ________ 10 MINUTES ________

NEUROMUSCULAR MATURITY

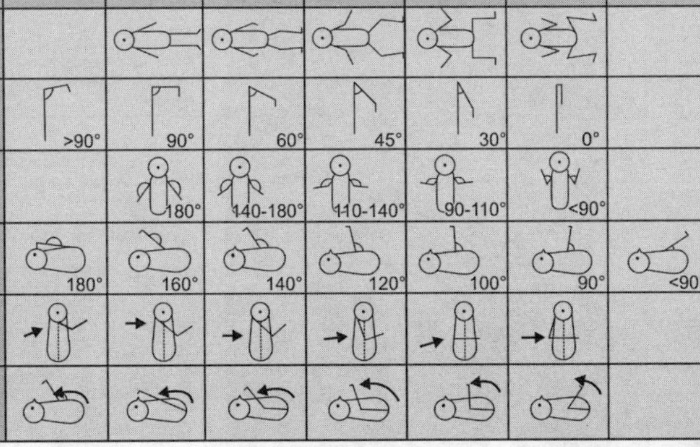

Neuromuscular maturity sign	SCORE –1	0	1	2	3	4	5	Record score here
Posture								
Square window (Wrist)	>90°	90°	60°	45°	30°	0°		
Arm recoil		180°	140-180°	110-140°	90-110°	<90°		
Popliteal angle	180°	160°	140°	120°	100°	90°	<90°	
Scarf sign								
Heel to ear								
							Total neuromuscular maturity score	

PHYSICAL MATURITY

Physical maturity sign	Score –1	0	1	2	3	4	5	Record score here
Skin	Sticky friable transparent	Gelatinous red translucent	Smooth pink visible veins	Superficial peeling and/or rash few veins	Cracking pale areas rare veins	Parchment deep cracking no vessels	Leathery cracked wrinkled	
Lanugo	None	Sparse	Abundant	Thinbing	Bald areas	Mostly bald		
Plantar surface	Heel-toe 40-50 mm:-1 <40:-2	>50 mm no crease	Faint red marks	Anterior transverse crease only	Creases ant. 2/3	Creases over entire sole		
Breast	Imperceptible	Barely perceptible	Flat areola no nud	Stippled areola 1–2 mm bud	Raised areola 3–4 mm bud	Full areola 5–10 mm bud		
Eye/Ear	Lids fused loosely:- 1 tightly:- 2	Lids open pinna flat stays folded	Sl. curved pinna; soft; slow recoil	Well-curved pinna; soft but ready recoil	Formed and firm instant recoil	Thick cartilage ear stiff		
Genitals (Male)	Scrotum flat, smooth	Scrotum empty faint rugae	Testes in upper canal rare rugae	Testes descending few rugae	Testes down good rugae	Testes pendulous deep rugae		
Genitals (Female)	Clitoris prominent and labia flat	Prominent clitoris and small labia minora	Prominent clitoris and enlarging minora	Majora and minora equally prominent	Majora large minors small	Majora cover clitoris and minora		
							Total physical maturity score	

SCORE

Neuromuscular ________
Physical ________
Total ________

MATURITY RATING

Score	Weeks
–10	20
–5	22
0	24
5	26
10	28
15	30
20	32
25	34
30	36
35	38
40	40
45	42
50	44

Gestational age (weeks)

By dates ________
By ultrasound ________
By exam ________

Reference
Ballard JL, khoury JC, Wedig K, et al. New Ballard score, expanded to include extremely premature infants. *J Pediatr* 1991; 119; 119:417-423. Reprinted by permission of Dr Ballard and Mosby-Year Book, Inc.

Appendix – XI: Routine Examination of Newborn Infants

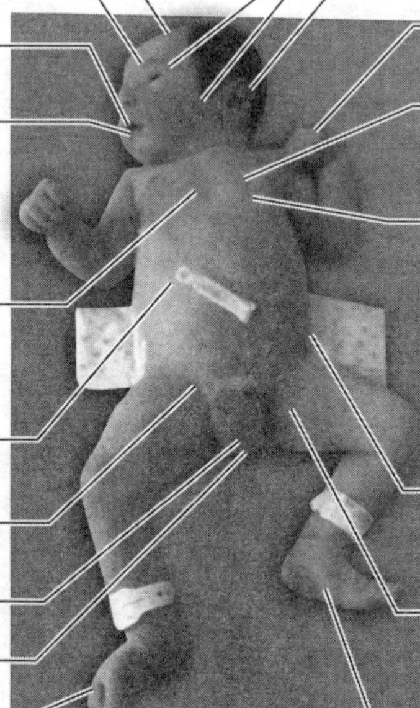

Measurements (at 40 weeks):

	50th centile	10th–90th (centile)	Comments
Birth weight	3.5 kg	(2.8–4.5 kg)	Maximal occipitofrontal diameter
Head circumference	35 cm	(33.5–37 cm)	Routinely measured in USA, not in UK
Length	51 cm	(48–53.5 cm)	Inaccurate unless hips and knees are straightened

Appendix – XII: National Immunization Schedule

Vaccine	*Due age*	*Max age*	*Dose*	*Diluent*	*Route*	*Site*
			For Infants			
BCG	At birth	till one year of age	(0.05 mL until 1 month) 0.1 mL Beyond age 1 month	Yes Manufacturer supplied diluent (Sodium chloride)	Intradermal	Upper Arm-LEFT
Hepatitis B-Birth dose	At birth	within 24 hours	0.5 mL	NO	Intramuscular	Anterolateral side of mid-thigh-LEFT
OPV-O	At birth	within the first 15 days	2 drops	-	Oral	Oral
OPV 1, 2 & 3	At 6 weeks, 10 weeks and 14 weeks	till 5 years of age	2 drops	-	Oral	Oral
Pentavalent 1, 2 and 3** (Diphtheria + Pertussis + Tetanus + Hepatitis B + Hib)	At 6 weeks, 10 weeks and 14 weeks**	1 year of age	0.5 mL	NO	Intramuscular	Anterolateral side of mid-thigh-LEFT
Fractional IPV (Inactivated Polio Vaccine)	At 6 and 14 weeks	1 year of age	0.1 mL	NO	Intradermal	Upper Arm - RIGHT
Rotavirus‡ (Where applicable)	At 6 weeks, 10 weeks and 14 weeks	1 year of age	5 drops	NO	Oral	Oral
Pneumococcal Conjugate Vaccine (PCV) (where applicable)	At 6 weeks and 14 weeks At 9 completed months - booster	1 year of age	0.5 mL	NO	Intramuscular	Anterolateral side of mid-thigh-RIGHT
Measles/Rubella 1st dose##	At 9 completed months-12 months	5 years of age	0.5 mL	YES Manufacturer supplied diluent (Sterile water)	Subcutaneous	Upper Arm-RIGHT
Japanese Encephalitis-1 @ (where applicable)	At 9 months-12 months @	15 years of age	0.5 mL	YES-Manufacturer supplied diluent (Phosphate Buffer Solution)	Subcutaneous	Upper Arm-LEFT
Vatimin A (1st dose)	At 9 months	5 years of age (1 lakh IU)	1 mL	-	Oral	Oral

Contd...

Contd...

Vaccine	*When to give*	*Max age*	*Dose*	*Diluent*	*Route*	*Site*
For Children						
DPT Booster-1	16-24 months	7 years of age	0.5 mL	NO	Intramuscular	Anterolateral side of mid-thigh-LEFT
Measles/Rubella 2nd dose ##	16-24 months	5 years of age	0.5 mL	YES Manufacturer supplied diluent (Sterile water)	Subcutaneous	Upper Arm-RIGHT
OPV Booster	16-24 months	5 years	2 drops	NO	Oral	Oral
Japanese Encephalitis-2 @ (where applicable)	16-24 months @	till 15 years of age	0.5 mL	YES Manufacturer supplied diluent (Phosphate Buffer Solution)	Subcutaneous	Upper Arm-LEFT
Vitamin A $ (2nd to 9th dose)	At 16 months. Then, one dose every 6 months	up to the age of 5 years	2 mL (2 lakh IU)	-	Oral	Oral
DPT Booster-2	5-6 years	7 years of age	0.5 mL	NO	Intramuscular	Upper Arm
Td	10 years and 16 years	16 years	0.5 mL	NO	Intramuscular	Upper Arm

* Give Td-2 or Booster doses before 36 weeks of pregnancy, However give these even if more than 36 weeks have passed. Give Td to a woman in labour, if she has not previously received Td.

** Pentavalent vaccine is introduced in place of DPT and HepB 1, 2 and 3.

‡ Rotavirus vaccine is being introduced in phases.

MR vaccine introduced in phases replacing measles vaccine in the UP schedule. It first dose delayed beyond 12 months ensure minimum 1 month gap between 2 MR doses.

@ JE vaccine has been introduced in select endemic districts. If first dose delayed beyond 12 months ensure minimum 3 months gap between 2 JE doses.

$ The 2nd to 9th doses of vitamin A can be administered to children 1-5 years old during biannual rounds, in collaboration with ICDS.

➢ Human Papilloma Virus (HPV) Vaccine-presently not in schedule.

➢ Td-Tetanus diphtheria to replace TT-to be added in schedule.

Appendix – XIII: Basic Life Support –CPR for Children

Maneuver	*Infant*	*Child (1–8 years)*	*Child and adult (Above 8 years)*
➢ Airway	➢ Head tilt-chin lift ➢ If trauma is present, use ➢ Jaw-thrust	➢ Same as infant	➢ Head tilt-chin lift or jaw thrust in trauma
➢ Breathing			
– Initial – Subsequent	➢ Two breaths at 1–1½ sec. per breath ➢ 20 breaths/min	➢ Same as infant ➢ 20 breaths/min	➢ Two breaths at 1.5–2 sec. per breath ➢ 10–12 breaths per minute
➢ Circulation			
– Pulse check – Compression area – Compression width – Compression depth – Rate	➢ Brachial/Femoral ➢ Lower half of sternum ➢ 2 or 3 fingers together ➢ 0.5″ – 1″ Approximately ⅓ – ½ the depth of the chest ➢ At least 100/min	➢ Carotid ➢ Lower half of sternum ➢ Heel of one hand ➢ 1″ – 1.5″ Approximately ⅓ – ½ the depth of the chest ➢ 100 per min	➢ Carotid ➢ Lower half sternum ➢ Two hand stacked ➢ 1.5″ – 2″ ➢ 80–100/min
➢ Compression – Ventilation ratio	➢ 5 : 1 (Pause for ventilation)	➢ 5 : 1 (Pause for ventilation)	➢ 15 : 2 (one rescuer) ➢ 5 : 1 (two rescuer)
➢ Foreign body airway obstruction	➢ Back blows or chest thrusts	➢ Heimlich maneuver	➢ Heimlich maneuver

Adapted from M Singh. Medical Emergencies in Children, 3rd edition. Sagar Publications, New Delhi, 2000.

Appendix – XIV: Balanced Diet for Children and Adolescents

	Toddlers		Preschooler		School age children				Adolescents					
									Boys		Boys		Girls	
	1–3 years		4–6 years		7–9 years		10–12 years		13–15 years		16–18 years		13–18 years	
	Veg (g)	Non-veg (g)	Veg (g)	Non-veg (g)	Veg (g)	Non-veg (g)	Veg (g)	Non-veg (g)	Veg (g)	Non-veg (g)	Veg (g)	Non-veg (g)	Veg (g)	Non-veg (g)
Cereals	150	150	200	200	250	250	320	320	430	430	450	450	350	350
Pulses	50	40	60	50	70	60	70	60	70	50	70	50	70	50
Green leafy vegetables	50	50	75	75	75	75	100	100	100	100	100	100	150	150
Other vegetables, roots and tubers	30	30	50	50	50	50	75	75	150	150	175	175	150	150
Fruits	50	50	50	50	50	50	50	50	30	30	30	30	30	30
Milk	300	200	250	200	250	200	250	200	250	150	250	150	250	150
Fats and oils	20	20	25	25	30	30	35	35	35	40	45	50	35	40
Meat, fish and eggs	–	30	–	30	–	30	–	30	–	30	–	30	–	30
Sugar and jaggery	30	30	40	40	50	50	50	50	30	30	40	40	30	30
Roasted peanut	–	–	–	–	–	–	–	–	–	–	50	50	–	–

Suggested Reading

1. American Academy of Pediatrics, Neonatal Resuscitation Guidelines, 8th Edition, 2021.
2. Bowden VR, Greenberg CS. Pediatric Nursing Procedures, 4th edition, 2015, Wolters Kluwer Lippincott Williams and Wilkins, Philadelphia.
3. Cloherty and Stark's Manual of Neonatal Care, 8th Edition, 2017, Wolters Kluwer, South Asian Edition.
4. Datta P. Pediatric Nursing, 4th Edition, 2018, Jaypee Brothers Medical Publishers, New Delhi.
5. Deorari AK, Paul VK. Neonatal Equipments, 5th Edition, 2020, CBS Publishers, New Delhi.
6. Deorari AK, Paul VK, Neonatal Nursing Procedures, 5th Edition, 2018, Noble Publications, New Delhi.
7. Disque K. Pediatric Advanced Life Support (PALS) Provider Handbook, 2016, https://t.me/Anesthesia_Books. Save a Life Initiative, Satori Continuum Publishing, Las Vegas, USA.
8. Dorland's Illustrated Medical Dictionary, 33th Edition, 2019, Elsevier.
9. Government of India, Ministry of Health and Family Welfare, Training Module for Facility Based Newborn Care, 2014.
10. Government of India, Ministry of Health and Family Welfare, Facility Based Newborn Care Training Module for Neonatal Resuscitation, 2014.
11. Government of India, Ministry of Health and Family Welfare, Guidelines for Implementation of KAYAKALP Initiative.
12. Gomella T. Neonatology, 8th Edition, 2020, McGraw Hill Companies, New York.
13. Gupta P. Essential Pediatric Nursing, 5th Edition, 2022, Jaypee Brothers Medical Publishers, New Delhi.
14. Gupte S. The Short Textbook of Pediatrics, 13th Edition, 2020, Jaypee Brothers Medical Publishers Pvt. Ltd, New Delhi.
15. Kliegman RM, et al. Nelson's Textbook of Pediatrics, Elsevier, 1st South Asia Edition, 2015.
16. Marlow DR, et al. Textbook of Pediatric Nursing, 1st South Asia Edition, 2013, Elsevier.
17. Nettina SM. Lippincott Manual of Nursing Practice, 11th Edition, 2012, Lippincott Williams & Wilkins. Philadelphia.
18. Paul VK, Bagga A. Ghai Essential Pediatrics, 9th Edition, 2019, CBS Publishers and Distributors Pvt. Ltd, New Delhi.
19. Singh M. Care of the Newborn, 9th Edition, 2021, CBS Publishers and Distributors Pvt. Ltd, New Delhi.
20. Singh M. Pediatric Clinical Methods, 6th Edition, 2020, CBS Publishers and Distributors Pvt. Ltd, New Delhi.
21. Singh M. Essential Pediatrics for Nurses, 3rd Edition, 2014, CBS Publishers and Distributors Pvt. Ltd, New Delhi.
22. Taber's Cyclopedic Medical Dictionary, Volume-I and Volume-II, 21st Edition, 2009, Jaypee Brothers Medical Publishers, New Delhi.
23. West Bengal Nursing Council. Nursing Theories and Practices, Volume - I and Volume - II, 2019, Kolkata.
24. WHO Collaborating Centre for Training and Research in Newborn Care, AIIMS, New Delhi, Facility-Based Care of Preterm Infant, Part - I and Part - II, 2018 - 2019.
25. WHO Collaborating Centre for Training and Research in Newborn Care, AIIMS, New Delhi, Newborn Nursing for Facility-Based Care Level II units, 2014–2015.
26. WHO Guidelines on Hand Hygiene in Health Care.
27. WHO Department of Communicable Disease Surveillance and Response - Prevention of Hospital-Acquired Infections.
28. Wong DL, et al. Wong's Essential of Pediatric Nursing, 1st South Asia Edition, 2018, Elsevier.
29. Wong DL et al. Wong's Nursing Care of Infants and Children, 11th Edition, 2012, Elsevier.
30. Wong DL. Clinical Manual of Pediatric Nursing, 8th Edition, 2011, Mosby.

INTERNET REFERENCES

1. www.ncbi.nlm.nih.gov
2. www.newbornwhocc.org
3. www.who.int
4. www.nhm.gov.in>index1
5. www.researchgate.net>....>Newborn
6. www.journals.elsevier.com>paediatric
7. www.nnfi.org>cpg-guidelines
8. www.indianpediatrics.net
9. www.thelancet.com>article>
10. www.sciencedirect.com>article>
11. www.pediatricnursing.org
12. www.sciencedirect.com>journal>
13. www.scimagojr.com>journalsearch
14. www.indianjournals.com
15. www.ipinnovative.com>journals
16. www.unicef.org>reports

Index

Page numbers followed by *f* refer to figure and *t* refer to table.

C

I

N

O

T

U

V

W

Z